The Complete Collection of Barbara O'Neill

Lost Cures for Ultimate Vitality

1,200+ Herbal Remedies and Holistic Secrets based on Dr. Barbara's Natural Healing Research

Jacqueline Bridge

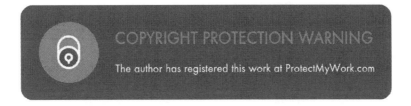

Table of Contents

FOREWORD

Dear Reader,

Welcome. I want to begin by thanking you, wholeheartedly, for picking up this extraordinary collection of study materials. In your hands, you now hold a key—a key to unlocking a treasure trove of knowledge that has the potential to transform not only your health but your entire approach to well-being.

You may have found your way here out of curiosity or perhaps out of a deep need for answers to questions about health and vitality that conventional wisdom has failed to address. Maybe you are searching for natural solutions for a specific ailment, or perhaps you seek a holistic approach to enrich your lifestyle. Whatever brought you to this moment, I want you to know that you are in the right place. This book was created with you in mind.

This book is unlike any other resource. Inside, you will discover 50 mini-books, each meticulously crafted and dedicated to exploring specific health topics, disorders, or broader areas of wellness. These books are not just theoretical or academic; they are rooted in the real-world experience and natural healing principles that Barbara O'Neill has spent her life researching, applying, and teaching. Her methods have helped countless people reclaim their health, and now this knowledge is being passed on to you.

What makes this collection so special is its focus on holistic healing. It views the body, mind, and spirit as interconnected parts of a whole, which means healing one aspect of yourself will inevitably benefit all aspects. This is not about quick fixes or masking symptoms. It's about getting to the root cause of illness, understanding your body's natural rhythms, and supporting it with time-honored, nature-based remedies. In these 50 books, you will find over 1,200 herbal remedies, offering natural solutions for a wide array of health concerns. From boosting your immune system to enhancing your mental clarity, from improving digestive health to finding relief from chronic pain—there is something here for everyone.

I understand that embarking on a collection of this magnitude can feel overwhelming at first, but let me reassure you—this book has been carefully organized to guide you through each topic in a clear, approachable manner. The 50 books are divided into sections, with each one focusing on a specific area of health. This structure allows you to dip into the chapters that are most relevant to your needs, while also providing a coherent, overarching narrative that ties everything together. Not only are the topics covered extensively, but the sheer variety of remedies means that you have options—

there is no one-size-fits-all solution, and Barbara O'Neill has ensured that this collection reflects that diversity.

One of the most powerful aspects of Barbara O'Neill's work is that it offers hope. It offers hope to those who feel stuck in cycles of illness, to those who have tried everything and are still searching for answers, and to those who simply want to live their lives in a way that feels vibrant and full of energy. I want you to know that this book holds the potential to change lives—not just in the way you manage your health, but in how you see yourself as an active participant in your own well-being.

By engaging with this material, you are taking a step toward reclaiming your health and vitality. The knowledge contained within these pages is a gift, one that has been carefully curated to help you on your path to healing. But the real power lies in you—in your willingness to learn, to try new things, and to trust in the process of natural healing. As you explore these remedies and practices, you may find that you are not only healing physically, but that you are also nurturing a deeper sense of connection to yourself, to the earth, and to the life force that flows through all living things.

Before you dive into the wealth of information ahead, I want to express once again how grateful I am that you are here. By choosing this book, you are choosing to invest in yourself, in your health, and in your future. This is no small decision, and I want to honor the commitment you are making.

As you move forward, remember to be patient with yourself. Healing is a journey, not a destination, and the path you are on is one of growth and discovery. There may be moments of challenge, but there will also be moments of profound insight and transformation. Trust in the process, and trust in the wisdom that Barbara O'Neill has so generously shared.

Thank you for being here. Thank you for your openness, your curiosity, and your courage. May this collection inspire you, nourish you, and guide you on your journey to ultimate vitality.

With deep appreciation,

Jacqueline Bridge

Section I: Foundations of Natural Healing

Book 1: The Basics of Herbal Medicine

Introduction to Herbalism

Herbalism, or herbal medicine, is a practice that stretches back to humanity's earliest interactions with nature. For thousands of years, cultures around the world have turned to herbs as the primary source of healing and health maintenance. From the rich botanical traditions of ancient Egypt, Greece, and Rome, to the time-honored practices of Ayurveda in India and Traditional Chinese Medicine (TCM), herbs have been valued for their potent medicinal properties. These plants are more than just therapeutic agents—they are a bridge connecting humans to nature's profound healing power. Herbalism's philosophy revolves around supporting the body's intrinsic ability to heal itself. It is a holistic practice, integrating physical, emotional, and spiritual well-being into the healing process. Unlike many modern pharmaceutical approaches that focus on symptom suppression, herbal medicine seeks to address the root cause of ailments and restore the natural balance of the body.

Herbal medicine has always been intertwined with cultural identity and tradition, and its application varies widely depending on geographical and cultural contexts. In Traditional Chinese Medicine, for example, herbs are used as part of a comprehensive system that includes acupuncture, dietary therapy, and qi cultivation practices. The aim is to harmonize the body's yin and yang energies, using herbs to nourish deficiencies, clear heat, and restore vitality. In contrast, Ayurvedic herbalism, which has its origins in India over 5,000 years ago, categorizes herbs based on their effects on the body's doshas—Vata, Pitta, and Kapha. Each herb is selected to balance these doshas and support the body's innate ability to self-heal through practices that include both physical and spiritual purification.

In Europe, the Greco-Roman tradition laid the groundwork for what would later evolve into modern Western herbalism. Influential physicians such as Hippocrates and Dioscorides documented the medicinal uses of hundreds of plants. This knowledge was preserved and expanded upon during the Renaissance and eventually formed the foundation for the herbal practices of the early settlers in North America. Indigenous peoples of the Americas also developed their own complex herbal systems, often blending their practices with the European methods introduced by settlers.

Today, herbalism has experienced a resurgence in popularity, as people seek more natural and holistic approaches to health. Modern herbalism draws on this diverse heritage, integrating scientific research with traditional knowledge to validate the effectiveness of various herbs. As a result, herbal medicine is once again being recognized not only as an alternative to conventional treatments but as a complementary system that can work alongside modern healthcare.

Key Herbs and Their Properties

The world of herbal medicine encompasses thousands of plants, each with unique properties and therapeutic uses. Some herbs, however, have stood out for their wide-ranging benefits and versatility, earning a place in every herbalist's toolkit. One such herb is **Chamomile (Matricaria chamomilla)**, known for its calming effects on the nervous system. Chamomile has been traditionally used to ease anxiety, promote restful sleep, and soothe digestive upsets. Its anti-inflammatory properties make it useful for topical applications as well, helping to heal minor skin irritations and wounds.

Another foundational herb is **Echinacea (Echinacea purpurea)**, prized for its immune-boosting properties. Echinacea is commonly used to reduce the severity and duration of colds and other respiratory infections. It stimulates the body's defense mechanisms, enhancing the activity of white blood cells. In contrast, **Ginger (Zingiber officinale)** is a warming herb with a long history in both Ayurvedic and TCM traditions. Known for its ability to alleviate nausea, improve circulation, and reduce inflammation, ginger is often used in digestive tonics and remedies for joint pain.

Turmeric (Curcuma longa), with its vibrant yellow color, is celebrated for its potent anti-inflammatory and antioxidant properties. Curcumin, the active compound in turmeric, has been extensively studied for its role in reducing chronic inflammation, a common underlying factor in many diseases, including arthritis and cardiovascular conditions. Meanwhile, **Garlic (Allium sativum)** is a powerful antimicrobial herb that has been used for centuries to fight infections and support cardiovascular health. Its ability to lower blood pressure and cholesterol, combined with its immune-boosting properties, make garlic a staple in herbal protocols for overall health.

Each of these herbs exemplifies the range of actions that plants can have on the body. Some herbs are gentle and can be used daily to promote wellness, while others are more potent and suited for addressing specific health concerns. Understanding these properties and selecting the right herbs for individual needs is a core skill in herbal medicine.

Methods of Preparation and Use

The preparation and use of herbs are as important as the selection of the herbs themselves. Depending on the type of herb and the condition being treated, there are various methods to unlock the therapeutic properties of plants. One of the simplest and most widely used preparations is **herbal tea**, or **infusion**. Infusions are typically made from the leaves and flowers of plants, where boiling water is poured over the herbs and allowed to steep for a period of time. This method is ideal for extracting the delicate volatile oils and nutrients that might be destroyed by prolonged heat exposure.

For denser plant materials such as roots, barks, and seeds, a **decoction** is often recommended. Unlike infusions, decoctions require simmering the herbs in water for a longer duration to release their medicinal compounds. This method is commonly used for herbs like ginger or burdock root, where a stronger extraction is necessary to access the beneficial properties.

Another popular preparation is the **tincture**, an alcohol-based extraction that captures both water- and fat-soluble constituents of an herb. Tinctures are highly concentrated and can be taken in small doses, making them convenient for herbs that might not be palatable in tea form, such as valerian or goldenseal. The alcohol acts as a preservative, allowing tinctures to have a long shelf life.

For topical use, herbs can be incorporated into **salves**, **balms**, and **oils**. These preparations are made by infusing herbs into carrier oils and then combining them with beeswax or other natural thickeners to create a semi-solid product. Such preparations are ideal for healing skin conditions, reducing inflammation, and providing localized pain relief.

In some cases, herbs are dried and encapsulated for easy consumption, particularly when the taste of the herb is unpleasant, or the dosage needs to be precisely controlled. **Capsules** are commonly used for bitter herbs like gentian or strong adaptogens like ginseng, allowing for accurate and convenient dosing.

Each preparation method serves a specific purpose, and choosing the right one depends on the desired therapeutic outcome. By understanding these methods, herbalists can tailor their remedies to maximize the healing potential of each herb. This foundational knowledge of preparation techniques is key to harnessing the full power of herbal medicine.

Book 2: Detoxification and Cleansing

Importance of Detoxifying the Body

In today's world, our bodies are constantly exposed to a barrage of toxins from the environment, food, water, and even personal care products. The importance of detoxifying the body cannot be overstated, as it plays a critical role in maintaining overall health and well-being. The human body has a natural detoxification system that involves the liver, kidneys, lungs, digestive system, skin, and lymphatic system. These organs work synergistically to process and eliminate toxins, protecting the body from their harmful effects. However, when the body's natural detox pathways become overloaded or impaired, toxins can accumulate and contribute to a range of health problems, including chronic fatigue, digestive issues, skin problems, hormonal imbalances, and a weakened immune system.

The liver is the body's primary detox organ, responsible for filtering toxins from the blood and converting them into less harmful substances that can be excreted. It is supported by the kidneys, which filter waste from the blood to be eliminated through urine. The skin, often referred to as the "third kidney," also plays a vital role in expelling toxins through sweat. The lungs filter out environmental pollutants we breathe in, while the digestive system removes waste from food and absorbs essential nutrients. The lymphatic system, meanwhile, transports toxins away from cells and tissues, acting as a crucial drainage system that needs regular maintenance.

When the natural detox pathways are functioning optimally, they efficiently eliminate toxins and support overall health. However, modern lifestyles, high-stress levels, and poor dietary habits can place an immense burden on these systems. The accumulation of toxins may manifest as unexplained symptoms like brain fog, joint pain, or even autoimmune conditions. Therefore, incorporating regular detoxification practices, supported by herbal remedies, is essential for sustaining a healthy body and preventing toxin buildup. Detoxification is not about extreme cleanses or quick fixes; it is about supporting the body's natural processes to ensure that it operates at its best. A well-balanced detox program should be gentle yet effective, targeting key organs and pathways to rejuvenate and restore balance.

Natural Detox Methods

Detoxification can be approached through various natural methods, each targeting different systems and organs within the body. Among these methods, herbal detox protocols, fasting, and juicing are widely used for their ability to cleanse the body deeply while nourishing it with essential nutrients.

Herbal Detox Protocols involve using specific herbs known for their ability to enhance the body's natural detox pathways. These protocols may include liver cleanses using herbs like milk thistle and dandelion root, kidney cleanses using nettle and parsley, and lymphatic cleanses utilizing red clover or cleavers. Herbal detox protocols are designed to be gentle, allowing the body to gradually release toxins without causing a sudden overload to the system. The herbs chosen are tailored to support particular organs, thereby maximizing the detoxification process.

Fasting is another time-honored method of detoxification. Intermittent fasting, in particular, has gained popularity for its benefits in promoting autophagy—a natural process in which the body breaks down and recycles damaged cells and toxins. During fasting, the digestive system gets a rest, allowing the body to divert energy toward repair and detoxification. Water fasting, in which only water is consumed for a set period, is more intense and should be done with caution, ideally under the guidance of a healthcare professional. Fasting not only supports detoxification but also helps to reset eating habits and improve insulin sensitivity.

Juicing is a popular detox method that involves consuming fresh vegetable and fruit juices to flood the body with vitamins, minerals, and antioxidants while reducing the digestive load. Juice cleanses are typically done for 1 to 7 days and can help to detoxify the liver, kidneys, and digestive system. They are often used as a bridge to more sustainable dietary changes. Ingredients like beets, carrots, leafy greens, and apples are common in detox juices due to their liver-supporting and alkalizing properties. The key to an effective juice cleanse is to balance the natural sugars from fruits with plenty of green vegetables to keep blood sugar levels stable.

Herbal Cleanses specifically target organs like the liver, kidneys, and colon. For example, a liver cleanse might involve taking a combination of milk thistle, dandelion root, and turmeric to stimulate bile flow and repair liver cells. A kidney cleanse may include uva ursi, marshmallow root, and juniper berries to support urinary tract health. Colon cleansing, which can be done using psyllium husk, flaxseeds, and ginger, helps to clear the digestive tract of waste and improves nutrient absorption.

Each of these detox methods can be adapted to individual needs, making it easy to design a personalized detox plan that aligns with one's health goals and lifestyle. The best results come from combining different approaches, such as integrating herbal teas into a fasting regimen or using detox baths alongside juicing to support the skin's elimination pathways.

Herbal Cleanses and Supplements

The key to a successful detox is choosing the right herbs and supplements that can assist each of the body's detoxification pathways. Certain herbs have specific actions that make them particularly effective for cleansing, while supplements provide essential nutrients and compounds that support detoxification on a cellular level.

For **liver detoxification**, herbs like **milk thistle**, **dandelion root**, and **burdock root** are highly recommended. Milk thistle contains silymarin, a compound that protects liver cells and promotes regeneration. Dandelion root stimulates bile production, which helps to break down and eliminate fats and toxins. Burdock root is a blood purifier that aids in clearing toxins from the bloodstream.

To support **kidney function**, **nettle leaf**, **parsley**, and **uva ursi** are frequently used. Nettle leaf acts as a diuretic, increasing urine flow and helping to flush out toxins. Parsley is rich in antioxidants and promotes kidney health, while uva ursi is known for its antibacterial properties, making it useful for urinary tract support.

For **digestive health**, herbs such as **ginger**, **fennel**, and **peppermint** can be very effective. Ginger warms the digestive tract and enhances circulation, while fennel relieves bloating and gas. Peppermint is soothing and helps to relax the muscles of the gastrointestinal tract, reducing symptoms of digestive distress.

Lymphatic cleansing can be supported by using herbs like **cleavers**, **red clover**, and **echinacea**. Cleavers stimulate the lymphatic system, encouraging the drainage of toxins and waste. Red clover acts as a gentle purifier, aiding in the elimination of metabolic waste, while echinacea enhances immune function, making it a valuable addition to any lymphatic cleanse.

For **skin health**, herbs like **calendula**, **neem**, and **Oregon grape root** are excellent choices. Calendula is known for its anti-inflammatory and wound-healing properties, neem is a powerful antibacterial herb that helps with skin infections and detoxification, and Oregon grape root is effective against a range of skin conditions due to its antimicrobial and anti-inflammatory actions.

In addition to herbs, supplements such as **chlorella**, **spirulina**, and **activated charcoal** can further enhance the detoxification process. Chlorella and spirulina are nutrient-dense algae that bind to heavy metals and other toxins, facilitating their removal from the body. Activated charcoal, on the other hand, is highly absorbent and can trap toxins in the digestive tract, preventing their reabsorption.

By strategically combining these herbs and supplements, a comprehensive detox program can be created that targets multiple detox pathways, ensuring a thorough and effective cleanse. The next section will delve into specific recipes and formulations to guide you through the process of creating your own detox remedies.

Remedies for Detoxification

1. Liver Cleansing Tea Blend

Ingredients: 1 tablespoon dandelion root, 1 tablespoon burdock root, 1 teaspoon milk thistle seeds, 1 teaspoon licorice root, 1 teaspoon ginger root.

Preparation: Combine all herbs in 4 cups of water. Bring the mixture to a boil, then reduce the heat and let it simmer for 15 minutes. Strain and store the tea in a glass jar.

Suggested Usage: Drink 1 cup twice daily for 7 days to stimulate liver function and support detoxification.

Benefits: This blend helps cleanse the liver, promotes bile production, and enhances liver cell regeneration.

2. Kidney Flush Juice

Ingredients: 1 cup fresh parsley, 2 stalks of celery, 1 cucumber, juice of 1 lemon, 1 cup water.

Preparation: Blend all ingredients until smooth. Strain if desired for a clearer texture.

Suggested Usage: Drink first thing in the morning on an empty stomach for 3-5 days.

Benefits: Supports kidney function, enhances urinary flow, and helps flush out toxins from the urinary tract.

3. Colon Cleanse Smoothie

Ingredients: 1 tablespoon ground flaxseed, 1 tablespoon chia seeds, 1 apple (cored), 1 handful of spinach, 1 banana, 1 cup water.

Preparation: Blend all ingredients until smooth and serve fresh.

Suggested Usage: Consume once daily for 5-7 days to promote colon health and regularity.

Benefits: Provides high fiber content to aid in digestion, supports gut health, and gently eliminates waste from the digestive tract.

4. Detoxifying Herbal Bath Soak

Ingredients: 1 cup Epsom salt, ½ cup baking soda, 10 drops lavender essential oil, 2 tablespoons dried rosemary.

Preparation: Mix all ingredients thoroughly and store in an airtight container. Add 1 cup of the mixture to warm bathwater.

Suggested Usage: Soak in the bath for 20 minutes to encourage toxin release through the skin.

Benefits: Relaxes muscles, draws out impurities, and supports skin detoxification.

5. Lymphatic Drainage Tea

Ingredients: 1 teaspoon cleavers, 1 teaspoon red clover, 1 teaspoon calendula.

Preparation: Steep all herbs in 2 cups of boiling water for 10 minutes. Strain before drinking.

Suggested Usage: Drink twice daily for 14 days to promote lymphatic health and drainage.

Benefits: Stimulates lymphatic system activity, promotes detoxification, and helps reduce inflammation.

6. Gentle Detox Green Smoothie

Ingredients: 1 cup kale, 1 cucumber, 1 green apple, ½ cup cilantro, juice of 1 lemon, 1 cup coconut water.

Preparation: Blend all ingredients until smooth. Adjust with additional coconut water for desired consistency.

Suggested Usage: Drink in the morning as a light breakfast for 5-7 days to support general detoxification.

Benefits: Provides essential vitamins and minerals, alkalizes the body, and supports gentle detoxification through the liver and kidneys.

7. Digestive Reset Tea

Ingredients: 1 teaspoon ginger root, 1 teaspoon fennel seeds, 1 teaspoon peppermint leaves.

Preparation: Steep all ingredients in 2 cups of hot water for 10 minutes. Strain before drinking.

Suggested Usage: Drink 1 cup after meals for 5 days to promote digestive health and ease bloating.

Benefits: Eases digestive discomfort, reduces gas and bloating, and supports overall digestive function.

8. Heavy Metal Detox Smoothie

Ingredients: 1 cup spinach, 1 cup blueberries, 1 tablespoon chlorella powder, 1 tablespoon ground flaxseed, 1 banana, 1 cup almond milk.

Preparation: Blend all ingredients until smooth. Serve immediately.

Suggested Usage: Consume once daily for 7-10 days to aid in removing heavy metals and toxins from the body.

Benefits: Helps bind and eliminate heavy metals, provides antioxidants, and supports cellular health.

9. Blood Purifying Herbal Infusion

Ingredients: 1 teaspoon burdock root, 1 teaspoon red clover, 1 teaspoon nettle leaf.

Preparation: Combine herbs in 3 cups of boiling water and steep for 15 minutes. Strain before drinking.

Suggested Usage: Drink 1 cup three times daily for 10-14 days to support blood purification and overall health.

Benefits: Cleanses the blood, supports liver and kidney function, and promotes healthy circulation.

10. Skin-Clarifying Detox Bath

Ingredients: 1 cup bentonite clay, ½ cup sea salt, 10 drops tea tree oil, 1 tablespoon dried chamomile flowers.

Preparation: Mix all ingredients and add to a warm bath. Stir well to dissolve.

Suggested Usage: Soak for 20 minutes to draw out toxins and soothe the skin.

Benefits: Purifies the skin, reduces inflammation, and promotes a healthy complexion.

11. Liver Repair Elixir

Ingredients: 1 tablespoon turmeric powder, 1 teaspoon ginger root powder, 1 tablespoon apple cider vinegar, 1 teaspoon raw honey, 1 cup warm water.

Preparation: Mix all ingredients in a glass and stir until well blended.

Suggested Usage: Drink once daily for 14 days to support liver repair and reduce inflammation.

Benefits: Promotes liver cell regeneration, reduces oxidative stress, and supports bile production.

12. Kidney Detox Herbal Decoction

Ingredients: 1 teaspoon uva ursi leaves, 1 teaspoon marshmallow root, 1 teaspoon corn silk, 1 teaspoon dandelion leaf.

Preparation: Simmer all herbs in 3 cups of water for 20 minutes. Strain and serve.

Suggested Usage: Drink 1 cup twice daily for 7 days to promote kidney cleansing and urinary health.

Benefits: Supports kidney function, enhances urinary flow, and helps eliminate waste products.

13. Anti-Inflammatory Detox Tonic

Ingredients: 1 cup pineapple juice, 1 teaspoon turmeric powder, 1 teaspoon ginger juice, 1 pinch cayenne pepper, juice of 1 lime.

Preparation: Combine all ingredients and mix well. Serve immediately.

Suggested Usage: Drink once daily for 10 days to reduce inflammation and support detoxification.

Benefits: Reduces systemic inflammation, supports liver health, and promotes healthy digestion.

14. Herbal Detox Lemonade

Ingredients: Juice of 2 lemons, 1 tablespoon raw honey, 1 teaspoon cayenne pepper, 2 cups filtered water, 1 teaspoon grated ginger.

Preparation: Combine all ingredients and stir until well mixed. Serve chilled.

Suggested Usage: Drink throughout the day for 3 days as part of a short detox regimen.

Benefits: Stimulates digestion, supports liver detoxification, and boosts immunity.

15. Gut-Healing Detox Broth

Ingredients: 4 cups bone broth, 1 cup chopped cabbage, 1 cup chopped carrots, 1 tablespoon minced garlic, 1 tablespoon fresh ginger, 1 teaspoon turmeric, 1 cup kale, 1 teaspoon apple cider vinegar.

Preparation: Combine all ingredients in a pot and simmer for 30 minutes. Serve warm.

Suggested Usage: Consume 1-2 cups daily for 5 days to soothe the gut and promote healing.

Benefits: Supports gut health, reduces inflammation, and provides nutrients that aid in digestive repair.

16. Herbal Liver Support Capsules

Ingredients: 1 tablespoon dried milk thistle seed powder, 1 tablespoon dried dandelion root powder, 1 tablespoon turmeric powder, empty vegetable capsules.
Preparation: Mix all powdered herbs in a bowl. Using a capsule machine, fill each capsule with the herbal blend. Store in a glass jar away from direct sunlight.
Suggested Usage: Take 2 capsules twice daily for 14 days to support liver detoxification and health.
Benefits: Supports liver cell regeneration, enhances bile flow, and protects the liver from oxidative damage.

17. Deep Cleanse Detox Soup

Ingredients: 4 cups vegetable broth, 1 cup chopped celery, 1 cup chopped carrots, 1 cup chopped cabbage, 1 cup broccoli florets, 1 tablespoon minced garlic, 1 tablespoon grated ginger, 1 teaspoon turmeric powder, 1 teaspoon cayenne pepper, juice of 1 lemon.
Preparation: Combine all ingredients in a large pot. Bring to a boil, then reduce heat and simmer for 25 minutes until vegetables are tender. Serve warm.
Suggested Usage: Eat 1-2 bowls daily for 5-7 days as part of a deep detox program.
Benefits: Promotes detoxification through the digestive system, supports immune health, and provides anti-inflammatory nutrients.

18. Bloating Relief Tea

Ingredients: 1 teaspoon fennel seeds, 1 teaspoon peppermint leaves, 1 teaspoon chamomile flowers, 1 teaspoon lemon balm leaves.
Preparation: Steep all ingredients in 2 cups of boiling water for 10 minutes. Strain before serving.
Suggested Usage: Drink 1 cup after meals as needed to alleviate bloating and digestive discomfort.
Benefits: Reduces bloating, soothes the digestive tract, and relieves gas and cramping.

19. Full-Body Cleanse Juice Shot

Ingredients: 1 tablespoon fresh ginger juice, 1 tablespoon fresh lemon juice, 1 tablespoon apple cider vinegar, 1

tablespoon fresh turmeric juice, pinch of cayenne pepper.
Preparation: Mix all ingredients thoroughly in a small glass. Drink immediately.
Suggested Usage: Consume once daily in the morning for 7-10 days to kickstart the body's detox processes.
Benefits: Stimulates digestion, boosts metabolism, and helps the body eliminate toxins more effectively.

20. Anti-Parasitic Herbal Infusion

Ingredients: 1 teaspoon wormwood, 1 teaspoon black walnut hull, 1 teaspoon clove buds, 1 teaspoon thyme.
Preparation: Combine all herbs in 2 cups of hot water. Steep for 15 minutes, then strain.
Suggested Usage: Drink 1 cup twice daily for 5-7 days to help eliminate parasites and improve gut health.
Benefits: Supports the removal of parasites, enhances digestive health, and reduces microbial overgrowth.

21. Skin Detoxifying Face Mask

Ingredients: 1 tablespoon bentonite clay, 1 tablespoon raw honey, 1 teaspoon apple cider vinegar, 1 teaspoon activated charcoal powder, 1 teaspoon aloe vera gel.
Preparation: Mix all ingredients into a smooth paste. Apply evenly to clean, dry skin and leave on for 15 minutes. Rinse off with warm water.
Suggested Usage: Use once a week as part of a skin detox routine.
Benefits: Draws out impurities, reduces

inflammation, and promotes a clearer complexion.

22. Liver Flush Tincture

Ingredients: 2 tablespoons milk thistle seeds, 2 tablespoons dandelion root, 1 tablespoon artichoke leaf, 1 cup 80-proof alcohol (e.g., vodka).
Preparation: Place herbs in a glass jar and cover with alcohol. Seal tightly and store in a cool, dark place for 4-6 weeks, shaking daily. Strain and store in a dark glass bottle.
Suggested Usage: Take 20-30 drops in a small amount of water twice daily for 14 days.
Benefits: Supports liver detoxification, enhances bile flow, and protects liver cells.

23. Lymphatic System Cleanse Juice

Ingredients: 1 cup fresh watermelon, 1 cup fresh pineapple, 1 cucumber, juice of 1 lime, 1 handful mint leaves.
Preparation: Blend all ingredients until smooth. Serve immediately.
Suggested Usage: Drink once daily for 5 days to stimulate lymphatic drainage and support detoxification.
Benefits: Promotes lymphatic circulation, reduces fluid retention, and supports immune function.

24. Heavy Metal Detox Clay Mask

Ingredients: 2 tablespoons bentonite clay, 1 teaspoon activated charcoal, 1 teaspoon apple cider vinegar, 5 drops tea tree essential oil, 1 tablespoon distilled water.

Preparation: Mix all ingredients into a thick paste. Apply to the face and neck, avoiding the eyes. Leave on for 10-15 minutes, then rinse thoroughly.

Suggested Usage: Apply twice a week for 2 weeks as part of a heavy metal detox regimen.

Benefits: Draws out heavy metals from the skin, reduces inflammation, and promotes a healthy complexion.

25. Anti-Candida Detox Tea

Ingredients: 1 teaspoon pau d'arco bark, 1 teaspoon calendula flowers, 1 teaspoon chamomile flowers, 1 teaspoon licorice root.

Preparation: Steep all herbs in 3 cups of boiling water for 15 minutes. Strain and serve.

Suggested Usage: Drink 1 cup three times daily for 14 days to combat candida overgrowth and support gut health.

Benefits: Fights candida and fungal infections, supports immune health, and restores gut balance.

26. Respiratory Cleanse Steam Inhalation

Ingredients: 1 tablespoon eucalyptus leaves, 1 tablespoon peppermint leaves, 1 tablespoon thyme, 5 drops rosemary essential oil.

Preparation: Boil 4 cups of water, remove from heat, and add the herbs and essential oil. Lean over the pot, cover your head with a towel, and inhale the steam for 5-10 minutes.

Suggested Usage: Use once daily for 5 days to clear the respiratory tract and enhance lung function.

Benefits: Opens airways, clears mucus, and reduces respiratory congestion.

27. Herbal Gallbladder Flush

Ingredients: 1 tablespoon olive oil, 1 tablespoon lemon juice, 1 tablespoon fresh ginger juice, 1 clove of garlic (minced), pinch of cayenne pepper.

Preparation: Mix all ingredients and consume immediately. Follow with a glass of warm water.

Suggested Usage: Take once daily for 7 days to promote gallbladder health and reduce bile stagnation.

Benefits: Stimulates bile flow, supports gallbladder function, and helps dissolve small gallstones.

28. Hormonal Balance Detox Tea

Ingredients: 1 teaspoon vitex (chaste tree berry), 1 teaspoon red raspberry leaf, 1 teaspoon licorice root, 1 teaspoon ashwagandha root.

Preparation: Steep all ingredients in 3 cups of hot water for 15 minutes. Strain and serve.

Suggested Usage: Drink 1 cup twice daily for 14 days to support hormonal balance and detoxification.

Benefits: Balances hormone levels, reduces symptoms of hormonal imbalance, and supports reproductive health.

29. Herbal Detox Foot Soak

Ingredients: 1 cup Epsom salt, ½ cup baking soda, 1 teaspoon ground ginger, 10 drops lavender essential oil, 1 teaspoon dried rosemary.

Preparation: Mix all ingredients thoroughly and add to a basin of warm water. Soak feet for 20-30 minutes.

Suggested Usage: Use twice a week to promote detoxification through the feet.

Benefits: Draws out toxins, reduces inflammation, and relaxes muscles.

30. Adrenal Detox Adaptogen Smoothie

Ingredients: 1 tablespoon ashwagandha powder, 1 teaspoon maca powder, 1 banana, 1 cup almond milk, 1 teaspoon cinnamon, 1 tablespoon almond butter.

Preparation: Blend all ingredients until smooth. Serve immediately.

Suggested Usage: Consume once daily in the morning for 14 days to support adrenal health and stress resilience.

Benefits: Balances adrenal function, reduces fatigue, and promotes overall energy and vitality.

Book 3: Nutrition for Optimal Health

Whole Foods and Their Benefits

A diet centered around whole foods is the foundation of vibrant health, delivering nutrients in their purest and most balanced forms. Whole foods—such as fresh fruits and vegetables, whole grains, nuts, seeds, and lean proteins—are minimally processed and free from the artificial additives, preservatives, and unhealthy fats often found in packaged foods. These nutrient-rich foods contain a variety of essential vitamins, minerals, phytonutrients, and antioxidants that work together to support every function of the body. The natural synergy between these nutrients in whole foods enhances their bioavailability, meaning the body can more easily absorb and utilize them for optimal function and health.

Whole foods are particularly powerful because they offer a balanced combination of macronutrients (proteins, fats, and carbohydrates) along with an abundance of micronutrients (vitamins and minerals). For example, a simple serving of quinoa provides high-quality protein, complex carbohydrates, and fiber, along with magnesium, iron, and B vitamins, making it a superior choice compared to refined grains like white rice. Similarly, a handful of nuts like almonds or walnuts delivers healthy fats, plant-based protein, vitamin E, and magnesium, promoting heart health and satiety. This natural balance not only nourishes the body but also prevents the spikes and crashes in energy that are commonly experienced with refined carbohydrates and sugary foods.

The wide array of phytochemicals in whole foods adds another dimension to their health benefits. Phytochemicals are naturally occurring compounds found in plant foods that have been shown to have protective effects against disease. For example, cruciferous vegetables like broccoli, kale, and Brussels sprouts contain sulforaphane, a potent compound that supports the body's detoxification pathways and has been linked to a reduced risk of certain cancers. Citrus fruits such as oranges and grapefruits are rich in flavonoids, which have anti-inflammatory properties and support cardiovascular health.

The fiber content in whole foods is another critical component of their health benefits. Dietary fiber, found in abundance in vegetables, fruits, legumes, and whole grains, is essential for maintaining a healthy digestive system. Fiber adds bulk to the stool, aiding in regular bowel movements and preventing constipation. It also serves as a prebiotic, feeding the beneficial bacteria in the gut and supporting a balanced microbiome, which is vital for immunity and overall health. Additionally, fiber helps regulate blood sugar levels by slowing down the absorption of sugar into the bloodstream, making it a key player in managing and preventing type 2 diabetes.

Whole foods also play a significant role in reducing inflammation, a root cause of many chronic diseases. Inflammation is the body's natural response to injury or illness, but when it becomes chronic due to factors such as poor diet, stress, or environmental toxins, it can lead to conditions like heart disease, arthritis, and neurodegenerative disorders. Whole foods like leafy greens, berries, and fatty fish are packed with anti-inflammatory nutrients such as omega-3 fatty acids, flavonoids, and carotenoids, which help modulate the body's inflammatory response and protect against disease.

Incorporating a diverse range of whole foods into your diet ensures that the body receives a spectrum of nutrients that support everything from cellular repair and growth to immune function and hormonal balance. For instance, dark, leafy greens like spinach and Swiss chard are excellent sources of folate, a B-vitamin that is crucial for DNA synthesis and repair. Berries such as blueberries and strawberries are high in anthocyanins, which support brain health and protect against cognitive decline. Sweet potatoes, rich in beta-carotene, support skin health and vision.

The benefits of whole foods extend beyond just physical health—they also promote mental and emotional well-being. A diet rich in fruits, vegetables, and whole grains has been linked to a lower risk of depression and anxiety, likely due to the anti-inflammatory and antioxidant effects of these foods, which protect the brain from oxidative stress. Nutrients like magnesium, found in abundance in whole grains and leafy greens, play a critical role in supporting the nervous system and reducing symptoms of anxiety and tension.

Incorporating a variety of colorful whole foods into daily meals not only enhances nutrient intake but also encourages a more mindful and joyful approach to eating. The vibrant colors, textures, and flavors of whole foods naturally make meals more satisfying and enjoyable, reducing the temptation to overeat or consume less nutritious options. Preparing meals with fresh ingredients also fosters a deeper connection to food and an appreciation for the natural nourishment it provides. This mindfulness around food choices can contribute to a healthier relationship with eating, making it easier to maintain a balanced diet in the long term.

Ultimately, a diet rich in whole foods supports longevity and resilience by nourishing the body at a foundational level. It helps build a strong immune system, maintains stable energy levels, and reduces the risk of developing chronic diseases. By choosing whole foods, we not only prioritize our health but also contribute to sustainable food practices that honor both the environment and the body's natural wisdom.

Herbal Nutritional Supplements

Herbal supplements are derived from botanicals and are used to support various aspects of health and nutrition. While they should not replace whole foods, these supplements can provide concentrated doses of specific nutrients, antioxidants, and bioactive compounds that are not always obtainable in sufficient quantities from diet alone. In this way, they bridge potential nutritional gaps, enhance health outcomes, and offer targeted benefits for conditions ranging from stress and inflammation to digestive issues and immune function.

Herbal supplements are particularly valuable in situations where dietary limitations or increased nutrient demands are present. For instance, individuals on restrictive diets, such as vegans, may benefit from algae-based supplements like **spirulina** and **chlorella**, which are rich sources of complete protein, B-vitamins, iron, and omega-3 fatty acids. Spirulina, often referred to as a superfood, is packed with protein and essential amino acids, making it a great choice for those looking to boost their protein intake without animal products. Chlorella, on the other hand, is a potent detoxifier due to its high chlorophyll content and ability to bind to heavy metals, facilitating their elimination from the body.

Another category of herbal supplements includes **adaptogens**, which are herbs known for their ability to help the body adapt to stress and restore balance. **Ashwagandha** and **rhodiola** are two of the most popular adaptogens, valued for their capacity to modulate the adrenal response to stress and promote a state of calm focus. Ashwagandha has been used in Ayurvedic medicine for centuries to enhance resilience against both physical and mental stressors. It helps lower cortisol levels, supports thyroid health, and improves energy and endurance. Rhodiola, native to arctic regions, is particularly effective in combating fatigue and enhancing cognitive function, making it a popular supplement for those facing burnout or mental exhaustion.

Herbs like **turmeric** are celebrated for their potent anti-inflammatory properties. The active compound in turmeric, **curcumin**, has been extensively studied for its role in reducing inflammation, supporting joint health, and protecting against chronic diseases such as heart disease and Alzheimer's. Because curcumin's bioavailability is relatively low on its own, herbal supplements often include it in combination with black pepper extract (piperine) to enhance absorption. Adding a turmeric supplement to the diet is especially beneficial for individuals dealing with chronic inflammation or those seeking natural support for healthy aging.

Maca root is another adaptogenic herb that has gained popularity due to its energizing effects and ability to balance hormones. Grown in the high Andes of Peru, maca is rich in minerals like calcium, potassium, and iron, and has been traditionally used to boost stamina, increase libido, and support reproductive health. Its adaptogenic properties make it ideal for individuals looking to improve resilience to stress and restore hormonal equilibrium. Maca is available in powder or capsule form and can easily be incorporated into smoothies or snacks.

For digestive health, herbal supplements such as **ginger** and **peppermint** are highly effective. Ginger, with its warming and anti-nausea properties, has been used for centuries to relieve digestive discomfort, stimulate appetite, and support nutrient absorption. Peppermint, known for its soothing effects on the gastrointestinal tract, helps relax the muscles of the stomach and intestines, reducing symptoms of bloating, gas, and indigestion. These herbs can be taken in capsule form or as teas to complement a balanced diet and improve digestive function.

Milk thistle is another widely recognized herbal supplement, primarily used to support liver health. It contains a group of active compounds known as silymarins, which have powerful antioxidant and anti-inflammatory properties. Milk thistle protects liver cells from toxins, promotes regeneration, and is often recommended for individuals undergoing detoxification protocols or those with liver-related health concerns. Regular use of milk thistle can help the liver process and eliminate toxins more efficiently, supporting overall detoxification and metabolic health.

In addition to these individual herbs, there are herbal blends that combine multiple ingredients to target specific health concerns. For example, **immune-boosting formulas** often include a mix of echinacea, elderberry, and astragalus, each known for their ability to strengthen the immune system and fight off infections. Echinacea stimulates the production of white blood cells, elderberry is rich in antioxidants and supports the body's defense mechanisms, and astragalus enhances the body's resistance to stress and illness. Together, these herbs create a synergistic effect that is more potent than using each herb individually.

When selecting herbal supplements, it's essential to choose high-quality products that are free from contaminants and standardized to ensure consistent potency. Opt for organic and non-GMO options whenever possible, and look for third-party certifications to verify purity and quality. It is also advisable to consult with a healthcare professional, especially if you are taking medications or have existing health conditions, as some herbs can interact with conventional drugs.

Integrating herbal supplements into a daily health regimen can significantly amplify the benefits of a nutritious diet. They offer a targeted approach to health support, providing nutrients that are difficult to obtain through food alone, and can be tailored to address specific health concerns. Whether it's boosting energy levels, enhancing cognitive function, supporting detoxification, or promoting hormonal balance, herbal supplements provide a versatile and natural way to optimize health and well-being.

Balancing Diet with Herbal Remedies

Integrating herbs into daily meals is a powerful way to enhance both nutrition and flavor while reaping the medicinal benefits that many herbs provide. Culinary herbs such as basil, oregano, rosemary, and thyme are more than just seasonings; they are rich in phytochemicals, antioxidants, and essential oils that can help combat inflammation, support digestion, and promote overall wellness. Unlike synthetic supplements, herbs are easily incorporated into meals and work synergistically with other whole foods to enhance nutrient absorption and optimize health benefits. For example, adding a handful of fresh basil to a salad or sprinkling dried oregano over a roasted vegetable dish not only enhances taste but also provides polyphenols that can protect against oxidative stress.

A key strategy for maximizing the benefits of herbs in the diet is to pair them with foods that increase their bioavailability. **Turmeric**, a well-known anti-inflammatory herb, is a prime example. While it is often used in curry dishes and golden milk, its primary active compound, curcumin, is poorly absorbed on its own. However, when turmeric is combined with a small amount of black pepper, the piperine in black pepper boosts curcumin absorption by up to 2,000%, making the blend significantly more effective. Similarly, adding a source of healthy fat, such as olive oil or coconut milk, further enhances curcumin's bioavailability, making dishes like a coconut curry or turmeric-infused hummus both delicious and nutritionally potent.

Herbs can also be used in various forms to create nutrient-dense beverages. For example, a **green smoothie** made with fresh spinach, spirulina, and a dash of moringa powder is a nutrient powerhouse that supplies a concentrated dose of vitamins, minerals, and chlorophyll. Moringa, known as the "miracle tree," is particularly rich in vitamins A and C, calcium, and iron, making it an excellent addition to smoothies for boosting energy and supporting immune health. Another option is to include **herbal teas** like nettle, red raspberry leaf, or oat straw in your daily routine. These herbs are packed with bioavailable minerals such as magnesium, calcium, and potassium, which help support bone health, regulate muscle function, and maintain electrolyte balance. Sipping these teas throughout the day not only supports hydration but also provides a gentle and ongoing infusion of essential nutrients.

Incorporating herbs into broths and soups is another effective way to integrate them into a balanced diet. **Herbal infusions and decoctions** made from roots and barks, such as ginger, garlic, or astragalus, can be used as the base for cooking grains, legumes, and soups. For example, a rice dish cooked in a ginger-garlic broth takes on a rich, aromatic flavor while delivering digestive and immune-boosting properties. Astragalus, a traditional Chinese herb, is often used in broths to support immune function and is ideal for making nourishing soups during cold and flu season. Similarly, combining **shiitake mushrooms** and **reishi mushrooms** in a broth not only enhances the umami flavor but also provides adaptogenic benefits that help the body adapt to stress and strengthen the immune system.

Herbs are versatile ingredients that can also be added to snacks and desserts, providing therapeutic benefits without compromising taste. **Adaptogenic herbs** like ashwagandha, maca, and eleuthero can be mixed into energy balls, homemade granola, or protein bars. Ashwagandha, for example, is known for its calming effects and ability to support adrenal health, making it a great addition to a bedtime snack. Maca, a Peruvian root, has a slightly sweet and malty flavor that blends well in smoothies, oatmeal, or even baked goods. It is traditionally used to support stamina, endurance, and hormonal balance, making it ideal for anyone looking to boost energy levels naturally. Incorporating these adaptogens into nutrient-dense snacks provides an easy way to nourish the body while keeping stress levels in check.

Beyond their culinary use, herbs can be integrated into homemade condiments, dressings, and marinades to enhance the flavor profile of everyday dishes. A simple **lemon-tahini dressing** with freshly chopped parsley and dill not only brightens a salad but also delivers a dose of chlorophyll and beneficial enzymes that support detoxification. Freshly minced **garlic** combined with oregano, lemon, and olive oil makes a delicious marinade for fish or chicken while providing antibacterial and antifungal properties. Using herbs in this way allows you to subtly elevate the nutritional value of even the simplest meals.

In the realm of traditional herbal practices, there is a concept known as "**food as medicine**," where herbs and spices are used intentionally not just to flavor food, but to support specific health outcomes. For instance, **cinnamon** can be added to morning oatmeal or coffee to help regulate blood sugar levels and reduce insulin resistance. **Fenugreek**, commonly used in Middle Eastern cuisine, can be sprinkled into soups or stews to support lactation in nursing mothers and aid in digestion. Similarly, **rosemary** is often paired with roasted meats and vegetables for its carminative and antioxidant properties, which aid in digestion and reduce the formation of harmful compounds during high-heat cooking.

Incorporating herbs into daily meals also offers psychological benefits. The act of preparing food with intention and care, knowing that the ingredients are chosen for their healing properties, fosters a mindful approach to eating. This mindfulness can transform mealtimes into a form of self-care, where each meal is an opportunity to nourish the body, mind, and spirit. By experimenting with different herbs and culinary techniques, individuals can discover new flavors and health benefits, making it easier and more enjoyable to maintain a balanced, nutrient-rich diet.

In conclusion, balancing a diet with herbal remedies is about more than just adding flavor; it's about harnessing the power of nature's pharmacy to create a diet that is both healing and delicious. Whether it's sprinkling fresh herbs over a salad, stirring adaptogens into a smoothie, or brewing a nourishing herbal tea, integrating herbs into everyday meals offers a practical and enjoyable way to support long-term health and well-being.

Book 4: Mind-Body Connection

Understanding the Mind-Body Relationship

The mind-body connection refers to the profound interplay between our mental and emotional states and our physical health. Modern science and ancient healing systems both recognize that thoughts, emotions, and stress levels can significantly impact the body's physiological processes. Chronic stress, for instance, is known to trigger a cascade of hormonal changes, including elevated levels of cortisol and adrenaline, which can contribute to conditions like hypertension, digestive disorders, and weakened immunity. Similarly, unresolved emotions such as grief, anger, or anxiety may manifest as physical symptoms, ranging from tension headaches to chronic fatigue and muscle pain.

The mind-body connection emphasizes that true health extends beyond the absence of disease. When the mind is calm and emotions are balanced, the body tends to function more harmoniously, enhancing resilience and vitality. Conversely, when the mind is distressed or overwhelmed, it can lead to physiological imbalances that disrupt sleep patterns, metabolism, and the immune system's ability to ward off illness. Therefore, nurturing mental and emotional well-being is just as crucial as taking care of the physical body. Practices that foster this connection—such as mindfulness, meditation, and yoga—help regulate the nervous system, promote relaxation, and allow the body's natural healing mechanisms to work more effectively.

Herbs for Mental and Emotional Balance

Herbal medicine offers a gentle yet powerful way to support mental and emotional well-being. Various herbs have been traditionally used to alleviate anxiety, lift mood, and enhance cognitive function, making them valuable allies in managing the mind-body relationship. One such herb is **Ashwagandha (Withania somnifera)**, a renowned adaptogen used in Ayurveda for its ability to modulate the stress response. Ashwagandha helps reduce cortisol levels, improves resilience to stress, and promotes a sense of calm without causing sedation. It is particularly effective in balancing the nervous system and supporting adrenal health.

St. John's Wort (Hypericum perforatum) is another well-known herb for emotional balance. Often used to alleviate mild to moderate depression, it works by increasing the availability of serotonin and dopamine, neurotransmitters that regulate mood. However, due to its interactions with various medications, it should be used under the guidance of a healthcare professional. For those dealing with anxiety, **Lemon Balm (Melissa officinalis)** is an excellent choice. It has mild sedative properties and is known to soothe the nervous system, promoting relaxation and mental clarity without causing drowsiness.

Rhodiola (Rhodiola rosea), another adaptogenic herb, is prized for its ability to enhance cognitive function, improve mental stamina, and reduce the effects of fatigue and burnout. It is particularly beneficial for individuals experiencing emotional exhaustion or struggling to maintain focus under stress. **Passionflower (Passiflora incarnata)**, with its calming properties, is often used to relieve anxiety and promote restful sleep, making it a perfect evening tea for those who have trouble winding down. By incorporating these herbs into daily routines, individuals can create a more balanced emotional state, supporting both mental health and overall well-being.

Practices to Enhance Holistic Health

Integrating holistic practices into daily life can significantly strengthen the mind-body connection, complementing the benefits of herbal remedies. **Meditation** is one of the most effective ways to calm the mind, reduce stress, and improve emotional resilience. Regular meditation practice has been shown to lower blood pressure, reduce anxiety, and increase feelings of well-being. Mindfulness meditation, in particular, encourages present-moment awareness and helps individuals observe their thoughts and emotions without judgment. This practice fosters a deeper understanding of oneself and cultivates a sense of inner peace.

Yoga is another holistic practice that aligns body, mind, and spirit. The combination of physical postures (asanas), breath control (pranayama), and meditation creates a powerful system for balancing mental and physical health. Yoga stretches and strengthens the body, while the focus on breathwork calms the nervous system and reduces the physiological impact of stress. It is particularly effective in releasing tension stored in the body, improving flexibility, and promoting a sense of emotional equilibrium.

Breathing exercises, such as diaphragmatic breathing and alternate nostril breathing (Nadi Shodhana), are simple yet profound techniques that can quickly shift the body from a state of stress to one of relaxation. Diaphragmatic breathing, which involves deep breathing into the lower abdomen, activates the parasympathetic nervous system, promoting a state of rest and digestion. Nadi Shodhana, on the other hand, balances the left and right hemispheres of the brain, enhancing mental clarity and focus.

For those seeking to integrate these practices with herbal remedies, drinking a cup of calming herbal tea like chamomile or passionflower before meditation can deepen relaxation, while using adaptogenic herbs like ashwagandha before a yoga session can enhance stamina and focus. These holistic practices, when combined with supportive herbs, create a comprehensive approach to nurturing the mind-body connection, fostering a state of harmony and vibrant health.

Book 5: Building a Natural Medicine Cabinet

Essential Herbs for Every Home

Creating a natural medicine cabinet begins with selecting a collection of versatile, easy-to-use herbs that address a range of common ailments and support overall health. These herbs can be used to make teas, tinctures, salves, and other remedies for various purposes, from boosting immunity to easing digestive discomfort or reducing inflammation. A well-stocked herbal medicine cabinet should include herbs that have a broad spectrum of uses and are suitable for both acute and long-term health support.

Chamomile is a must-have herb for its gentle yet effective calming properties. Known for its ability to ease anxiety, promote restful sleep, and soothe digestive upsets, chamomile can be used in teas, compresses, and baths. Its anti-inflammatory properties also make it useful for treating skin irritations and minor wounds. **Peppermint** is another versatile herb that should be in every home. It is excellent for relieving digestive issues such as gas, bloating, and nausea, and its refreshing aroma can help clear the sinuses and alleviate headaches. Peppermint tea or diluted essential oil can be used to soothe muscle aches or as a cooling rub for fevers.

Ginger is indispensable for digestive health and immune support. Its warming, anti-inflammatory properties make it effective for treating colds, easing nausea, and promoting circulation. Ginger can be made into teas, used in cooking, or even applied topically as a poultice for sore muscles and joints. For respiratory and immune health, **Echinacea** is an essential herb. Echinacea stimulates the immune system, helping to fend off infections and reduce the duration of colds and flu. It can be used as a tea or tincture, making it a go-to remedy for seasonal illnesses.

Lavender is widely known for its calming properties and is ideal for reducing stress, promoting sleep, and soothing minor burns and skin irritations. It can be used as an essential oil, in teas, or in topical salves. **Calendula** is another staple for skin health. Its anti-inflammatory and antimicrobial properties make it perfect for treating cuts, scrapes, rashes, and other skin issues. Calendula is commonly used in salves, ointments, and infused oils.

For pain relief and inflammation, **Turmeric** is a powerful ally. Its active compound, curcumin, has been extensively studied for its anti-inflammatory and antioxidant effects. Turmeric can be used in teas, added to foods, or taken as a supplement. Lastly, **Garlic** is a natural antibiotic and immune booster, effective against a variety of infections. It can be taken raw, infused in honey, or used in cooking for its powerful health benefits.

Tools and Supplies for Herbal Preparation

Having the right tools and supplies is essential for preparing herbal remedies effectively and safely. The basics of an herbal preparation toolkit include items for measuring, grinding, heating, and storing herbs. A **digital kitchen scale** is necessary for accurately measuring herbs, particularly when creating tinctures or salves that require precise ratios. Similarly, **measuring spoons** and **small glass beakers** are helpful for exact measurements when blending multiple herbs or essential oils.

For grinding dried herbs, a **mortar and pestle** or **electric herb grinder** can be used, depending on the quantity and texture of the herbs. A mortar and pestle is ideal for small batches and delicate herbs, while an electric grinder is more efficient for preparing larger quantities. When making infusions, decoctions, or syrups, **stainless steel saucepans** and **non-reactive cookware** (such as glass or ceramic) are preferred to prevent any unwanted reactions between the herbs and the cooking materials. A **double boiler** is particularly useful for making salves and ointments, as it allows for gentle heating of oils and waxes without burning.

Glass jars with airtight lids are essential for storing dried herbs, tinctures, and infused oils. Mason jars work well for larger batches, while amber or cobalt blue bottles are recommended for tinctures and oils, as they protect the contents from light exposure, which can degrade potency. For straining, **fine mesh strainers** or **cheesecloth** can be used to separate plant material from liquids. Additionally, a **small funnel** is helpful for transferring liquids into storage containers without spills.

For making herbal capsules, a **capsule machine** and empty vegetable capsules are needed. These machines make filling capsules with powdered herbs quick and easy. If creating herbal teas or loose blends, **tea infusers** or **muslin bags** are useful for steeping herbs without the mess. Labeling tools, such as **waterproof labels** and **permanent markers**, are also essential for keeping track of different preparations and their dates.

Storing and Maintaining Your Herbal Collection

Proper storage of herbs and herbal preparations is crucial to preserving their potency and extending their shelf life. The three primary factors that degrade the quality of herbs are light, heat, and moisture. To protect your herbal collection, always store dried herbs in **dark glass jars** or **opaque containers** that block out light. If using clear glass jars, keep them in a dark cabinet or drawer to minimize exposure. Label each jar with the name of the herb, the date of purchase or harvest, and any other pertinent details to ensure that you can monitor freshness.

Herbs should be stored in a **cool, dry place** away from direct sunlight and humidity. High temperatures can cause volatile oils in the herbs to evaporate, diminishing their medicinal properties. A temperature range of 60-70°F (15-21°C) is ideal for most herbs. Avoid storing herbs near ovens, stoves, or other heat sources. Humidity is another enemy of dried herbs, as it can cause mold growth and spoilage. To prevent this, always ensure that jars are tightly sealed and consider adding **silica gel packets** to storage areas, especially in humid climates.

When it comes to **tinctures and oils**, the rules are similar: keep them in dark glass bottles in a cool, dark place. Tinctures, which are alcohol-based extracts, typically have a long shelf life of 2-5 years if stored properly. Infused oils, however, are more susceptible to rancidity and should be stored in the refrigerator to extend their shelf life, usually lasting 6-12 months. Salves and creams, which contain oils and waxes, should also be kept in cool, dry conditions and used within 6-12 months.

To maintain the integrity of your herbal collection, conduct regular checks for signs of spoilage. Dried herbs should retain their natural color, aroma, and texture. If you notice any discoloration, loss of fragrance, or mold, it's best to discard the affected herbs. For tinctures, a change in smell or cloudiness may indicate contamination. Oils and salves that have developed an off smell or have separated should also be discarded. Keeping your herbal supplies well-organized and clearly labeled will make it easier to monitor freshness and ensure that you are using herbs at their peak potency.

By carefully selecting essential herbs, equipping yourself with the right tools, and maintaining proper storage practices, you can build a robust natural medicine cabinet that supports health and wellness for years to come.

Book 6: Understanding Body Systems

Overview of Major Body Systems

The human body is a complex network of systems that work together to maintain health and function. Each system plays a unique role in regulating the body's physiology, and any disruption in one system can have a ripple effect on others. Understanding these systems and how they interconnect is fundamental to holistic health, as it provides insight into the root causes of health imbalances and informs the use of herbs and natural remedies to restore harmony. This chapter will provide an overview of the major body systems, including the digestive, respiratory, circulatory, immune, nervous, endocrine, musculoskeletal, and urinary systems, highlighting their primary functions and how they contribute to overall wellness.

The **digestive system** is responsible for breaking down food into nutrients that the body can absorb and utilize for energy, growth, and cellular repair. It consists of the mouth, esophagus, stomach, intestines, liver, pancreas, and gallbladder. This system not only handles nutrient absorption but also plays a significant role in immunity, as the gut houses approximately 70% of the body's immune cells. An imbalance in the digestive system, such as dysbiosis (an imbalance in gut bacteria) or poor nutrient absorption, can lead to conditions like inflammation, autoimmune disorders, and nutrient deficiencies.

The **respiratory system** includes the nose, trachea, bronchi, lungs, and diaphragm. Its primary function is to supply oxygen to the blood and remove carbon dioxide, a waste product of metabolism. Proper respiratory function is essential for cellular energy production and overall vitality. The respiratory system also serves as a barrier against airborne pathogens and environmental toxins. Issues such as asthma, chronic obstructive pulmonary disease (COPD), or infections like bronchitis can severely impair this system's ability to function, leading to diminished oxygen supply and increased susceptibility to illness.

The **circulatory system**, which comprises the heart, blood vessels, and blood, is responsible for transporting oxygen, nutrients, hormones, and waste products throughout the body. This system also plays a vital role in regulating body temperature, maintaining pH balance, and supporting immune function. Proper circulation ensures that all cells receive the nutrients they need and that toxins are efficiently removed. Conditions such as hypertension, atherosclerosis, and poor circulation can lead to serious health issues, including cardiovascular disease and metabolic dysfunction.

The **immune system** is a complex network of organs, tissues, and cells that work together to protect the body from harmful invaders like bacteria, viruses, and fungi. Key components include the thymus, spleen, bone marrow, lymph nodes, and a variety of immune cells (e.g., T-cells, B-cells, and macrophages). The immune system not only defends against infections but also plays a role in identifying and eliminating cancerous cells. When the immune system is weakened or overactive, it can lead to infections, allergies, or autoimmune disorders.

The **nervous system**, consisting of the brain, spinal cord, and a vast network of nerves, regulates every function in the body, from voluntary movements to involuntary actions like breathing and heartbeat. It is also the center of mental and emotional health, influencing mood, cognition, and stress response. The nervous system is divided into the central nervous system (CNS) and the peripheral nervous system (PNS). Any disruption in nervous system function, such as chronic stress, trauma, or neurodegenerative diseases, can affect the entire body and lead to physical, mental, and emotional imbalances.

The **endocrine system** is a collection of glands that produce and secrete hormones to regulate metabolism, growth, reproduction, and stress response. Major endocrine glands include the pituitary, thyroid, adrenals, pancreas, and gonads (ovaries and testes). Hormones act as chemical messengers that coordinate a wide range of physiological processes. Imbalances in the endocrine system, such as hypothyroidism, adrenal fatigue, or insulin resistance, can disrupt multiple body systems, leading to conditions like metabolic syndrome, infertility, or chronic fatigue.

The **musculoskeletal system** provides structural support, enables movement, and protects vital organs. It includes bones, muscles, tendons, ligaments, and connective tissues. This system also plays a role in producing blood cells and storing minerals like calcium and phosphorus. Musculoskeletal health is influenced by factors such as nutrition, physical activity, and inflammation. Conditions like arthritis, osteoporosis, and muscle atrophy can impair mobility and reduce quality of life.

The **urinary system**, consisting of the kidneys, ureters, bladder, and urethra, is responsible for filtering blood, removing waste products, and maintaining electrolyte balance. The kidneys are vital organs that regulate blood pressure, produce hormones, and control water balance. Issues like kidney stones, urinary tract infections (UTIs), or chronic kidney disease can disrupt the body's ability to eliminate toxins and maintain fluid balance, leading to systemic imbalances.

Herbal Support for Each System

Herbs have been used for centuries to support and enhance the health of each body system. When used correctly, they can help restore balance, alleviate symptoms, and promote overall well-being. Understanding which herbs are most beneficial for each system allows for more targeted and effective use of herbal medicine.

For the **digestive system**, herbs like **ginger**, **peppermint**, and **fennel** are excellent choices. Ginger is a warming herb that stimulates digestion, reduces nausea, and enhances nutrient absorption. Peppermint soothes the digestive tract, reduces gas and bloating, and helps alleviate irritable bowel syndrome (IBS) symptoms. Fennel, with its carminative properties, is used to relieve digestive spasms, ease indigestion, and improve appetite. **Slippery elm** and **marshmallow root** are mucilaginous herbs that protect and heal the mucous membranes, making them ideal for conditions like gastritis and acid reflux.

For the **respiratory system**, **mullein**, **thyme**, and **eucalyptus** are commonly used. Mullein acts as an expectorant, helping to clear mucus from the lungs and soothe inflamed tissues. Thyme has powerful antimicrobial properties, making it effective against respiratory infections such as bronchitis and colds. Eucalyptus, often used as an essential oil, helps open up the airways, reduce congestion, and relieve sinus pressure. These herbs can be used in teas, tinctures, or steam inhalations to support respiratory health.

For the **circulatory system**, **hawthorn**, **garlic**, and **ginger** are beneficial. Hawthorn strengthens the heart, improves circulation, and helps regulate blood pressure. Garlic is a natural blood thinner and cholesterol-lowering agent, making it valuable for preventing atherosclerosis and improving cardiovascular health. Ginger enhances circulation, reduces blood clot formation, and helps prevent the buildup of plaque in the arteries. These herbs can be taken as teas, tinctures, or incorporated into daily meals to support heart health.

For the **immune system**, **echinacea**, **elderberry**, and **astragalus** are key herbs. Echinacea stimulates the production of white blood cells, enhancing the body's ability to fight infections. Elderberry is rich in antioxidants and antiviral compounds, making it effective against colds and flu. Astragalus is an adaptogen that boosts immune function, reduces fatigue, and increases the body's resistance to stress. These herbs are often used in immune-boosting teas, syrups, or tinctures.

For the **nervous system**, **skullcap**, **passionflower**, and **valerian** are popular choices. Skullcap is a nervine that calms the nervous system, alleviates anxiety, and supports mental clarity. Passionflower is known for its sedative properties, making it effective for treating insomnia and restlessness. Valerian, often used as a sleep aid, relaxes the muscles and promotes deep, restful sleep. These herbs can be used in teas, tinctures, or capsules for nervous system support.

For the **endocrine system**, **ashwagandha**, **maca**, and **holy basil** are commonly recommended. Ashwagandha helps balance cortisol levels, reduce stress, and support thyroid and adrenal health. Maca, rich in minerals and phytonutrients, supports hormonal balance, fertility, and energy levels. Holy basil, also known as tulsi, is an adaptogen that regulates stress hormones and supports overall endocrine function. These herbs can be taken in powder, capsule, or tea form to support hormonal health.

For the **musculoskeletal system**, **turmeric**, **boswellia**, and **comfrey** are highly effective. Turmeric's anti-inflammatory properties help reduce pain and inflammation in conditions like arthritis. Boswellia, also known as frankincense, is used to relieve joint pain and improve mobility. Comfrey is a powerful healer for bones and tissues, traditionally used in poultices and salves for sprains, strains, and fractures.

For the **urinary system**, **corn silk**, **nettle**, and **uva ursi** are beneficial. Corn silk is a diuretic that supports kidney health and reduces inflammation in the urinary tract. Nettle is a gentle diuretic and anti-inflammatory herb that helps flush out toxins and reduce fluid retention. Uva ursi is a powerful antimicrobial herb used to treat UTIs and support overall urinary health.

Integrative Approaches to Health

Combining herbal remedies with other natural therapies provides a comprehensive approach to supporting the body's systems and enhancing overall health. Integrative health involves using multiple modalities, such as nutrition, exercise, stress management, and lifestyle changes, alongside herbal medicine to address health concerns holistically.

For example, integrating herbs with **nutritional therapy** can amplify their benefits. Using herbs like dandelion or milk thistle in conjunction with a diet rich in leafy greens and cruciferous vegetables enhances liver detoxification and overall metabolic health. Adding adaptogenic herbs like ashwagandha to a diet that includes healthy fats, whole grains, and proteins supports adrenal function and energy balance.

Incorporating **exercise and movement therapies** can further enhance the effects of herbs on the musculoskeletal and cardiovascular systems. Using anti-inflammatory herbs like turmeric and ginger in tandem with yoga or gentle stretching routines can help reduce joint pain and improve flexibility. Similarly, combining circulation-boosting herbs like cayenne or ginger with aerobic exercises supports cardiovascular health and stamina.

Incorporating **stress management techniques** such as meditation, breathing exercises, and mindfulness practices can complement the use of herbs for the nervous and endocrine systems. For instance, using calming herbs like skullcap and chamomile before meditation can deepen relaxation, while adaptogens like rhodiola or holy basil can support mental clarity and resilience during stressful periods.

Integrative health also involves **lifestyle modifications**, such as improving sleep hygiene, optimizing hydration, and reducing exposure to environmental toxins. Herbs like passionflower and valerian can be used as part of a bedtime routine to support restful sleep, while detoxifying herbs like chlorella and cilantro can be incorporated into meals to support the body's natural elimination pathways.

By combining herbal medicine with these complementary therapies, a more holistic and personalized approach to health can be achieved, addressing not just the symptoms of imbalance but also the underlying causes. This integrative strategy fosters a deeper sense of well-being, supports long-term health, and empowers individuals to take charge of their wellness journey.

Book 7: Principles of Holistic Health

Core Principles of Holistic Healing

Holistic health is based on the idea that true wellness comes from nurturing the body, mind, and spirit as interconnected parts of a whole. This approach emphasizes the importance of understanding the root causes of health issues rather than simply treating symptoms. The core principles of holistic healing involve supporting the body's natural healing processes, promoting balance and harmony, and addressing lifestyle factors such as diet, stress, and emotional health.

One of the primary tenets of holistic healing is that **prevention is better than cure**. This means taking proactive steps to maintain health and prevent disease through proper nutrition, regular physical activity, stress management, and adequate rest. Holistic health also views the individual as an active participant in their own wellness journey, encouraging personal responsibility and self-care. This perspective contrasts with conventional medicine's often reactive approach, which focuses on treating illness after it arises. By adopting preventive strategies and embracing healthy habits, individuals can build a strong foundation for lifelong wellness.

Another key principle is the **individualized nature of health and healing**. Holistic health recognizes that each person has unique needs, influenced by factors such as genetics, lifestyle, environment, and personal history. As a result, holistic practitioners tailor their recommendations to fit the individual's specific constitution and circumstances. This personalized approach often includes customized herbal protocols, dietary adjustments, and targeted lifestyle interventions designed to address the root causes of imbalance. By honoring the uniqueness of each person, holistic health practices aim to provide more effective and sustainable outcomes.

Balance and harmony are central themes in holistic health. Imbalances in one area, such as chronic stress or poor diet, can create a cascade of effects that disrupt the health of other systems. For example, chronic stress can weaken the immune system, disrupt digestion, and contribute to hormonal imbalances. Holistic health seeks to restore balance through a variety of means, including herbal support, nutritional guidance, and mind-body techniques like meditation and yoga. Restoring harmony allows the body's innate healing mechanisms to function optimally, promoting resilience and vitality.

Finally, holistic health places a strong emphasis on the **mind-body connection**. Thoughts, emotions, and mental states can significantly impact physical health, and vice versa. For instance, chronic anxiety can manifest as physical symptoms like digestive disturbances, muscle tension, or sleep issues. Conversely, physical ailments can affect emotional well-being, leading to feelings of frustration, sadness, or anxiety. Addressing mental and emotional health alongside physical health is crucial for achieving true wellness. Techniques such as mindfulness, visualization, and stress management are integrated with herbal and dietary therapies to support overall healing.

Integrating Herbs with Lifestyle Practices

Incorporating herbs into daily routines is a cornerstone of holistic health. Herbs can be used to support specific body systems, promote relaxation, boost energy, and maintain overall health. When combined with lifestyle practices such as a balanced diet, regular exercise, and stress management, herbs can enhance the benefits of these practices and create a synergistic effect that promotes long-term well-being. The key to integrating herbs with lifestyle practices is to use them intentionally and consistently in a way that fits seamlessly into daily life.

For example, a morning routine can be enhanced with **adaptogenic herbs** like ashwagandha or rhodiola, which help modulate the body's response to stress and increase energy and stamina. These herbs can be added to smoothies, taken as capsules, or enjoyed in herbal teas to start the day with mental clarity and resilience. Similarly, incorporating a **calming herbal tea** like chamomile, lemon balm, or passionflower into an evening wind-down routine can promote relaxation and improve sleep quality. Adding a few drops of a **lavender essential oil** to a diffuser or using an herbal pillow spray can further deepen the relaxation response.

Herbs can also be integrated into meal preparation. Adding **culinary herbs** such as basil, oregano, and rosemary to dishes not only enhances flavor but also delivers potent antioxidants and anti-inflammatory compounds. Incorporating herbs like **turmeric and ginger** into soups, stews, and marinades supports digestion and boosts immunity. For those with busy schedules, creating **herbal meal prep blends**—such as pre-mixed spice blends or herbal-infused oils—can make it easy to include herbs in meals without extra effort.

Herbs can be used in conjunction with **exercise and movement practices** as well. Using **ginger or cayenne** before a workout can stimulate circulation and enhance physical performance, while **turmeric and boswellia** can be used post-workout to reduce inflammation and support muscle recovery. Herbal baths infused with **epsom salts, lavender, and rosemary** are also beneficial for relaxing sore muscles and promoting recovery.

For mental and emotional support, herbs can be combined with **mindfulness practices** such as meditation, deep breathing, or journaling. Taking herbs like **holy basil** or **skullcap** before a meditation session can help calm the mind and reduce anxiety, making it easier to focus and achieve a state of inner peace. Using **adaptogenic herbs** like **maca or eleuthero** can support mental stamina and resilience during periods of high stress or emotional turmoil. These practices, when paired with herbal support, can create a powerful foundation for emotional health and mental clarity.

Incorporating herbs into skincare routines is another effective way to benefit from their healing properties. Using herbal-infused oils like **calendula, chamomile,** or **lavender** can soothe and nourish the skin, while **herbal face masks** with ingredients like **turmeric** and **neem** can reduce inflammation and promote a clear complexion. Adding herbs to **self-care rituals**, such as foot soaks, body scrubs, or herbal compresses, provides an opportunity to nurture both body and spirit.

Creating a Personalized Health Plan

Creating a personalized health plan involves tailoring diet, herbs, and lifestyle practices to meet the unique needs of the individual. This process begins with a thorough assessment of current health status, lifestyle, and wellness goals. The key to a successful plan is to address the root causes of any imbalances while supporting overall health and vitality. Start by identifying the primary health concerns and prioritizing which areas need the most attention.

Begin by evaluating **dietary habits**. Are there any nutrient deficiencies or imbalances that need to be addressed? A nutrient-dense, whole-food diet should be the foundation of the health plan. Incorporate a variety of fruits, vegetables, whole grains, lean proteins, and healthy fats. Consider adding specific herbs that support digestion and nutrient absorption, such as **ginger** or **peppermint**, to meals. For those with blood sugar imbalances, incorporating **cinnamon** or **fenugreek** can help regulate glucose levels.

Next, consider **herbal support**. Choose herbs based on the individual's health needs and goals. For example, someone dealing with chronic stress may benefit from adaptogens like **ashwagandha** or **rhodiola**, while someone focused on immune health might incorporate **elderberry** and **echinacea**. If hormonal balance is a concern, herbs like **vitex** and **maca** can be integrated. Determine the best form of each herb—whether it be teas, tinctures, capsules, or topical applications—based on the individual's preferences and lifestyle.

Incorporate **mind-body practices** such as yoga, tai chi, or meditation to support mental and emotional well-being. Pair these practices with appropriate herbs to enhance their effects. For instance, using calming herbs like **lemon balm** or **passionflower** before a meditation session can deepen relaxation, while using stimulating herbs like **ginseng** before a morning workout can increase energy and stamina.

A personalized health plan should also address **sleep and stress management**. Ensure that the individual is getting adequate, restorative sleep each night. If sleep is an issue, consider using herbs like **valerian, hops,** or **skullcap** as part of an evening routine.

Incorporate stress management techniques such as journaling, breathing exercises, or time in nature to reduce overall stress levels.

Finally, set realistic, achievable goals and establish a timeline for implementing changes. Regularly reassess and adjust the plan as needed to accommodate changes in health status, lifestyle, or wellness goals. By creating a personalized health plan that integrates herbs, nutrition, and lifestyle practices, individuals can take a proactive approach to health and build a strong foundation for long-term wellness.

Book 8: Energy Healing and Vitality

Concepts of Energy in Healing

Energy healing is based on the principle that the body is not just a physical entity but also a dynamic energy system, and maintaining balance within this system is key to health and vitality. This concept is deeply rooted in various traditional healing practices, including Traditional Chinese Medicine (TCM), Ayurveda, and indigenous healing traditions, where the flow of energy is considered fundamental to well-being. In these systems, energy is often referred to by specific names—**Qi (Chi)** in TCM, **Prana** in Ayurveda, or **Vital Force** in Western herbalism. The balance and flow of this energy through pathways or channels, such as meridians or nadis, are believed to influence both physical and mental health.

When the body's energy is flowing harmoniously, it supports all bodily functions, from cellular repair to mental clarity and emotional balance. Conversely, blockages, stagnation, or deficiencies in energy can manifest as physical illness, fatigue, emotional instability, or mental fog. These disruptions in energy flow may be caused by various factors, including poor diet, lack of exercise, chronic stress, emotional trauma, or environmental toxins. For example, in TCM, stagnant Qi can manifest as digestive issues, while deficient Qi may present as chronic fatigue and weakened immunity.

Energy healing seeks to restore balance and optimize the flow of energy throughout the body. This can be achieved through a variety of modalities, such as acupuncture, Reiki, Qigong, yoga, and herbal therapies. Herbs, in particular, play a unique role in supporting energy balance. Certain herbs are known to tonify Qi, while others clear heat, dispel dampness, or invigorate circulation. Similarly, adaptogenic herbs help the body adapt to stress and restore balance, making them ideal for supporting vitality and energy.

Understanding the body's energy systems also means recognizing the connection between the physical and the subtle body. In energy healing, it is believed that the physical body is intertwined with an energy field, often referred to as the aura, which surrounds and penetrates the body. Disruptions in this energy field can precede physical symptoms, making energy-based practices effective not only for treating existing conditions but also for preventing imbalances from developing into illness. Techniques like Reiki or Pranic Healing work to clear blockages in this energy field, while yoga and breathwork practices enhance the flow of Prana, promoting overall vitality.

In addition to restoring energy flow, energy healing also focuses on replenishing the body's **vital energy reserves**. Vital energy, also called **Jing** in TCM or **Ojas** in Ayurveda, represents the body's core energy that governs growth, reproduction, and longevity. This deep, foundational energy can be depleted by overwork, chronic stress, poor diet, and lack of rest. Herbal remedies, along with lifestyle practices that nurture the body and mind, are essential for rebuilding these reserves, ensuring long-term health and vitality.

Herbs to Boost Vital Energy

Herbs that boost energy and vitality are often classified into two categories: **stimulants** and **tonics**. Stimulants, like **ginseng** and **guarana**, provide a quick boost of energy and mental alertness by stimulating the nervous system. However, they should be used in moderation, as overuse can lead to burnout and energy crashes. Tonics, on the other hand, work more gently and support the body's energy production at a foundational level, building resilience over time. These include adaptogens like **ashwagandha**, **rhodiola**, and **eleuthero**, which help the body cope with stress and restore balance.

Ashwagandha (Withania somnifera) is one of the most revered herbs for enhancing vitality. As an adaptogen, it supports adrenal health, reduces cortisol levels, and promotes restful sleep—all of which are essential for sustaining energy levels. It is particularly effective for individuals experiencing burnout or chronic stress, as it replenishes depleted energy reserves and promotes a sense of calm focus. Ashwagandha can be taken as a powder mixed into warm milk, in capsule form, or as a tincture.

Rhodiola (Rhodiola rosea) is another powerful adaptogen known for its energizing effects. It helps combat mental fatigue, enhances cognitive function, and improves stamina, making it ideal for those who need a mental and physical boost without the jitteriness associated with stimulants. Rhodiola is particularly beneficial for individuals who experience fatigue and lack of motivation, as it enhances mental clarity and resilience.

Eleuthero (Eleutherococcus senticosus), also known as Siberian ginseng, is a tonic herb that enhances endurance and physical performance. It is often used by athletes to increase stamina and by individuals recovering from illness or chronic fatigue. Eleuthero works by supporting the hypothalamic-pituitary-adrenal (HPA) axis, helping the body adapt to stress and recover more quickly from exertion.

Maca (Lepidium meyenii), a root native to the high Andes, is valued for its ability to boost energy, endurance, and libido. It is rich in essential nutrients, including iron, calcium, and amino acids, which support overall vitality. Maca is also considered a hormonal balancer, making it useful for both men and women experiencing hormonal imbalances. It can be added to smoothies, oatmeal, or taken as a capsule.

Cordyceps (Cordyceps sinensis) is a medicinal mushroom that has long been used in Traditional Chinese Medicine to enhance stamina, support respiratory health, and boost overall energy levels. Cordyceps is particularly beneficial for those experiencing lung weakness or diminished physical capacity, as it increases oxygen utilization in the body and improves endurance. It can be taken as a powder, capsule, or added to broths and soups.

Ginseng (Panax ginseng) is perhaps the most famous energy-boosting herb. It has been used for centuries to enhance physical and mental performance, reduce fatigue, and promote longevity. Ginseng's energizing effects are due to its ability to modulate the stress response, improve circulation, and increase energy production at the cellular level. It is ideal for individuals who need a quick boost of energy, but it should be used in moderation to avoid overstimulation.

Holy Basil (Ocimum sanctum), also known as Tulsi, is revered in Ayurveda for its ability to balance energy and promote mental clarity. It acts as both a calming and energizing herb, making it suitable for reducing stress while enhancing focus and vitality. Holy Basil supports adrenal health and can be used in teas, tinctures, or capsules to promote a sense of grounded energy throughout the day.

Remedies to Enhance Vitality Naturally

31. Ashwagandha Vitality Tonic

Ingredients: 1 teaspoon ashwagandha powder, 1 cup warm milk (or plant-based milk), 1 teaspoon raw honey, a pinch of cinnamon.

Preparation: Warm the milk gently over low heat. Remove from heat and whisk in the ashwagandha powder, honey, and a pinch of cinnamon until well blended. Pour into a cup and stir again if necessary.

Suggested Usage: Drink once daily, preferably in the evening, to promote relaxation, restore energy levels, and support restful sleep.

Benefits: Replenishes depleted energy, balances cortisol levels, supports adrenal health, and promotes a sense of calm focus.

32. Rhodiola Energy Elixir

Ingredients: 1 teaspoon rhodiola root powder, 1 cup hot water, 1 teaspoon raw honey, juice of ½ lemon.

Preparation: Steep the rhodiola powder in hot water for 10-15 minutes. Strain if using whole rhodiola root or leave it as is if using powder. Add the honey and lemon juice, and stir well.

Suggested Usage: Consume in the morning or early afternoon for sustained energy and mental clarity.

Benefits: Enhances stamina, reduces mental fatigue, improves resilience to stress, and boosts mood and cognitive function.

33. Eleuthero Endurance Brew

Ingredients: 1 tablespoon eleuthero root, 1 tablespoon dried licorice root, 4 cups water.

Preparation: Combine eleuthero and licorice root in a saucepan with water. Bring to a boil, then reduce heat and simmer for 30 minutes. Strain and store the brew in a glass jar.

Suggested Usage: Drink 1 cup twice daily, in the morning and early afternoon, for enhanced physical endurance and recovery.

Benefits: Supports adrenal health, improves physical performance, increases stamina, and helps the body adapt to stress.

34. Cordyceps Power Tea

Ingredients: 1 teaspoon cordyceps powder, 1 cup hot water, 1 teaspoon raw honey (optional).

Preparation: Mix the cordyceps powder into hot water and stir until fully dissolved. Add honey for sweetness if desired.

Suggested Usage: Drink once daily to enhance respiratory health and stamina, especially before exercise or periods of physical exertion.

Benefits: Boosts energy, increases oxygen utilization, enhances respiratory health, and supports overall vitality.

35. Maca Energizing Smoothie

Ingredients: 1 teaspoon maca powder, 1 banana, 1 cup almond milk (or other plant-based milk), 1 tablespoon almond butter, 1 teaspoon honey or maple syrup.

Preparation: Blend all ingredients until smooth and creamy. Adjust the consistency by adding more almond milk if needed. Serve immediately.

Suggested Usage: Enjoy in the morning or as a midday snack for a natural energy boost and hormonal support.

Benefits: Balances hormones, supports stamina and endurance, enhances overall vitality, and improves mood and energy levels.

36. Ginseng Revitalizing Shot

Ingredients: ½ teaspoon ginseng powder (Panax ginseng), 1 teaspoon fresh lemon juice, 1 teaspoon raw honey, ¼ cup warm water.

Preparation: Mix the ginseng powder with warm water until fully dissolved. Add lemon juice and honey, and stir until combined.

Suggested Usage: Take once daily in the morning for a quick energy boost and mental alertness.

Benefits: Enhances energy levels, improves cognitive function, supports stress management, and promotes overall vitality.

37. Holy Basil Adaptogen Tea

Ingredients: 1 tablespoon dried holy basil (Tulsi) leaves, 1 cup hot water, 1 teaspoon raw honey (optional).

Preparation: Steep the holy basil leaves in hot water for 10 minutes. Strain and add honey if desired.

Suggested Usage: Drink twice daily to support adrenal health and reduce stress.

Benefits: Balances energy levels, reduces anxiety, improves mental clarity, and promotes a sense of calm.

38. Golden Milk with Turmeric and Ashwagandha

Ingredients: 1 cup coconut milk (or other plant-based milk), 1 teaspoon turmeric powder, ½ teaspoon ashwagandha powder, ¼ teaspoon cinnamon, a pinch of black pepper, 1 teaspoon raw honey or maple syrup.

Preparation: Gently heat the milk over

low heat. Add turmeric, ashwagandha, cinnamon, and black pepper. Whisk until smooth and well blended. Remove from heat and stir in honey or maple syrup.

Suggested Usage: Drink in the evening for relaxation and to promote a restful night's sleep.

Benefits: Reduces inflammation, balances cortisol levels, supports immune function, and enhances overall vitality.

39. Licorice Root Adrenal Support Tea

Ingredients: 1 teaspoon dried licorice root, 1 teaspoon dried ginger root, 1 cup hot water.

Preparation: Steep licorice root and ginger root in hot water for 15 minutes. Strain before drinking.

Suggested Usage: Drink 1 cup daily in the morning to support adrenal health and reduce fatigue.

Benefits: Balances adrenal function, supports hormonal health, and reduces stress-related exhaustion.

40. Astragalus Immunity Tonic

Ingredients: 1 tablespoon dried astragalus root, 2 cups water, 1 teaspoon raw honey (optional).

Preparation: Simmer astragalus root in water for 20 minutes. Strain and add honey if desired.

Suggested Usage: Drink 1 cup twice daily to strengthen the immune system and boost energy.

Benefits: Enhances immune function, promotes resilience, and helps the body adapt to physical and mental stress.

41. Schisandra Berry Adaptogen Elixir

Ingredients: 1 tablespoon dried schisandra berries, 2 cups water, 1 teaspoon goji berries (optional), 1 teaspoon raw honey (optional).

Preparation: Simmer schisandra berries in water for 20 minutes. Add goji berries in the last 5 minutes. Strain and add honey if desired.

Suggested Usage: Drink 1 cup in the morning for increased energy, mental clarity, and overall vitality.

Benefits: Enhances physical stamina, supports mental focus, and boosts liver health.

42. Ginger and Lemon Detox Tea

Ingredients: 1 tablespoon fresh grated ginger, juice of 1 lemon, 1 teaspoon raw honey, 1 cup hot water.

Preparation: Steep the grated ginger in hot water for 10 minutes. Strain and add lemon juice and honey. Stir well.

Suggested Usage: Drink first thing in the morning on an empty stomach to support digestion and detoxification.

Benefits: Promotes digestion, reduces inflammation, and supports liver detoxification.

43. Reishi Mushroom Vitality Brew

Ingredients: 1 tablespoon dried reishi mushroom slices, 3 cups water, 1 teaspoon raw honey.

Preparation: Simmer the reishi slices in water for 30 minutes. Strain and add honey.

Suggested Usage: Drink 1 cup daily to support immune health and reduce stress.
Benefits: Strengthens immune function, promotes relaxation, and enhances overall vitality.

44. Shatavari Hormonal Balance Tonic

Ingredients: 1 teaspoon shatavari powder, 1 cup warm milk (or plant-based milk), 1 teaspoon raw honey, a pinch of cardamom.
Preparation: Mix the shatavari powder into warm milk. Add honey and cardamom, and stir until smooth.
Suggested Usage: Drink once daily to support hormonal balance and reproductive health.
Benefits: Balances hormones, supports reproductive health, and enhances vitality in both men and women.

45. Nettle Leaf Mineral Tea

Ingredients: 1 tablespoon dried nettle leaf, 2 cups hot water, 1 teaspoon lemon juice.
Preparation: Steep the nettle leaf in hot water for 15 minutes. Strain and add lemon juice.
Suggested Usage: Drink 1 cup twice daily to boost mineral intake and support overall health.
Benefits: Provides a rich source of vitamins and minerals, supports bone health, and promotes healthy hair and skin.

46. Gotu Kola Brain Boost Tea

Ingredients: 1 teaspoon dried gotu kola leaves, 1 cup hot water, 1 teaspoon raw honey.
Preparation: Steep gotu kola leaves in hot water for 10 minutes. Strain and add honey.
Suggested Usage: Drink 1 cup in the morning to support mental clarity and cognitive function.
Benefits: Improves memory, enhances focus, reduces anxiety, and promotes overall brain health.

47. Hibiscus and Rosehip Vitality Tea

Ingredients: 1 tablespoon dried hibiscus flowers, 1 tablespoon dried rosehips, 2 cups hot water, 1 teaspoon raw honey (optional).
Preparation: Steep hibiscus flowers and rosehips in hot water for 10-15 minutes. Strain and add honey if desired.
Suggested Usage: Drink 1-2 cups daily to boost antioxidant levels and support cardiovascular health.
Benefits: Rich in vitamin C and antioxidants, supports heart health, reduces inflammation, and promotes overall vitality.

48. Lemon Balm Calming Elixir

Ingredients: 1 tablespoon dried lemon balm leaves, 1 cup hot water, 1 teaspoon raw honey, a squeeze of fresh lemon juice.
Preparation: Steep the lemon balm leaves in hot water for 10 minutes. Strain and add honey and lemon juice. Stir until combined.
Suggested Usage: Drink in the evening or during stressful times to promote

relaxation and reduce anxiety.

Benefits: Calms the nervous system, reduces anxiety and stress, and supports restful sleep.

49. Tulsi Ginger Chai

Ingredients: 1 tablespoon dried tulsi leaves, 1 teaspoon freshly grated ginger, 1 cup water, ½ cup milk (or plant-based milk), ½ teaspoon cinnamon, 1 teaspoon raw honey.

Preparation: Simmer tulsi leaves and ginger in water for 10 minutes. Add milk and cinnamon, then simmer for another 5 minutes. Strain and stir in honey.

Suggested Usage: Drink in the morning or afternoon to boost energy and reduce stress.

Benefits: Balances energy, supports the immune system, reduces stress, and enhances digestion.

50. Yerba Mate Energy Tea

Ingredients: 1 tablespoon yerba mate leaves, 1 cup hot water, 1 teaspoon lemon juice, 1 teaspoon raw honey.

Preparation: Steep yerba mate leaves in hot water for 5-7 minutes. Strain and add lemon juice and honey.

Suggested Usage: Drink in the morning or as a midday pick-me-up for sustained energy and mental focus.

Benefits: Provides natural caffeine, improves mental alertness, and boosts energy without jitters.

51. Guarana Stamina Drink

Ingredients: ½ teaspoon guarana powder, 1 cup cold water, 1 teaspoon raw honey, 1 tablespoon fresh orange juice.

Preparation: Mix guarana powder into cold water. Add honey and orange juice, and stir well.

Suggested Usage: Consume in the morning or before exercise for an energy and stamina boost.

Benefits: Increases energy levels, enhances physical performance, and reduces mental fatigue.

52. Moringa Superfood Smoothie

Ingredients: 1 teaspoon moringa powder, 1 banana, 1 cup coconut milk, 1 tablespoon chia seeds, 1 teaspoon raw honey.

Preparation: Blend all ingredients until smooth and creamy. Serve immediately.

Suggested Usage: Enjoy in the morning for a nutrient-packed start to your day.

Benefits: Rich in vitamins and minerals, boosts energy, supports immune function, and promotes overall vitality.

53. Ginkgo Biloba Memory Boost Tea

Ingredients: 1 teaspoon dried ginkgo biloba leaves, 1 cup hot water, 1 teaspoon honey.

Preparation: Steep the ginkgo leaves in hot water for 10 minutes. Strain and add honey.

Suggested Usage: Drink once daily to support cognitive function and mental clarity.

Benefits: Enhances memory, improves focus, and supports overall brain health.

54. Dandelion Root Detox Coffee

Ingredients: 1 tablespoon roasted dandelion root, 1 cup hot water, a splash of milk (optional), 1 teaspoon raw honey.
Preparation: Simmer roasted dandelion root in hot water for 10 minutes. Strain and add milk and honey if desired.
Suggested Usage: Drink in the morning as a caffeine-free alternative to coffee that supports liver detoxification.
Benefits: Supports liver health, promotes detoxification, and provides a rich, coffee-like flavor without caffeine.

55. Beetroot Circulation Elixir

Ingredients: 1 small beet (peeled and chopped), 1 apple, 1 tablespoon fresh lemon juice, 1 cup water, a pinch of cayenne pepper.
Preparation: Blend all ingredients until smooth. Strain if desired and serve immediately.
Suggested Usage: Drink in the morning or before exercise to boost circulation and energy.
Benefits: Increases blood flow, supports heart health, and enhances physical performance.

56. Bacopa Brain Tonic

Ingredients: 1 teaspoon dried bacopa leaves, 1 cup hot water, 1 teaspoon raw honey.
Preparation: Steep bacopa leaves in hot water for 10 minutes. Strain and add honey.
Suggested Usage: Drink in the morning or early afternoon to support memory and mental clarity.
Benefits: Enhances cognitive function, improves memory, and reduces anxiety and stress.

57. Peppermint Digestive Energy Tea

Ingredients: 1 tablespoon dried peppermint leaves, 1 teaspoon grated ginger, 1 cup hot water, 1 teaspoon honey.
Preparation: Steep peppermint leaves and grated ginger in hot water for 10 minutes. Strain and add honey.
Suggested Usage: Drink after meals to support digestion and boost energy.
Benefits: Eases digestive discomfort, reduces bloating, and promotes energy and mental clarity.

58. Siberian Ginseng Resilience Tonic

Ingredients: 1 tablespoon dried Siberian ginseng (Eleutherococcus) root, 2 cups water, 1 teaspoon raw honey.
Preparation: Simmer the Siberian ginseng root in water for 20 minutes. Strain and add honey.
Suggested Usage: Drink 1 cup twice daily to support energy, resilience, and stress management.
Benefits: Enhances stamina, supports adrenal health, boosts immune function, and improves the body's response to stress.

59. Fenugreek Hormonal Balance Brew

Ingredients: 1 teaspoon fenugreek seeds, 1 cup hot water, 1 teaspoon lemon juice, 1 teaspoon raw honey.

Preparation: Crush the fenugreek seeds slightly, then steep in hot water for 10-15 minutes. Strain and add lemon juice and honey.

Suggested Usage: Drink once daily to support hormonal balance, especially for women.

Benefits: Supports hormonal health, enhances digestion, and promotes balanced blood sugar levels.

60. Milk Thistle Liver Support Tea

Ingredients: 1 tablespoon milk thistle seeds, 1 teaspoon dried dandelion root, 2 cups hot water.

Preparation: Crush the milk thistle seeds slightly. Steep the seeds and dandelion root in hot water for 20 minutes. Strain before drinking.

Suggested Usage: Drink 1 cup twice daily to support liver health and detoxification.

Benefits: Protects liver cells, promotes detoxification, and enhances liver function.

61. Burdock Root Detox Tea

Ingredients: 1 tablespoon dried burdock root, 2 cups water, 1 teaspoon fresh lemon juice.

Preparation: Simmer the burdock root in water for 15-20 minutes. Strain and add lemon juice.

Suggested Usage: Drink once daily for a gentle detoxifying effect.

Benefits: Cleanses the blood, supports liver health, and promotes clear skin.

62. Calendula Immune Support Tea

Ingredients: 1 tablespoon dried calendula flowers, 1 cup hot water, 1 teaspoon raw honey.

Preparation: Steep calendula flowers in hot water for 10 minutes. Strain and add honey.

Suggested Usage: Drink 1 cup daily to support immune function and reduce inflammation.

Benefits: Enhances immune health, reduces inflammation, and supports skin healing.

63. Suma Root Vitality Elixir

Ingredients: 1 teaspoon suma root powder, 1 cup warm water, 1 teaspoon raw honey.

Preparation: Mix suma root powder into warm water until dissolved. Add honey and stir well.

Suggested Usage: Drink once daily in the morning to boost energy and enhance overall vitality.

Benefits: Enhances energy, supports stamina, and balances hormones.

64. Cacao Rejuvenation Smoothie

Ingredients: 1 tablespoon raw cacao powder, 1 banana, 1 cup almond milk, 1 tablespoon chia seeds, 1 teaspoon maca powder.

Preparation: Blend all ingredients until smooth. Serve immediately.

Suggested Usage: Enjoy as a morning or midday snack for a natural energy and mood boost.

Benefits: Provides antioxidants, boosts energy, supports mood, and enhances overall vitality.

65. Oatstraw Nervine Tea

Ingredients: 1 tablespoon dried oatstraw, 1 cup hot water, 1 teaspoon raw honey (optional).
Preparation: Steep the oatstraw in hot water for 15 minutes. Strain and add honey if desired.
Suggested Usage: Drink 1-2 cups daily to calm the nervous system and reduce stress.
Benefits: Nourishes the nervous system, reduces anxiety, supports restful sleep, and promotes overall relaxation.

66. Matcha Green Energy Tea

Ingredients: 1 teaspoon matcha green tea powder, 1 cup hot water, 1 teaspoon raw honey.
Preparation: Whisk the matcha powder into hot water until frothy. Add honey if desired.
Suggested Usage: Drink in the morning or early afternoon for a natural energy boost and mental clarity.
Benefits: Provides sustained energy, enhances focus, boosts metabolism, and supplies antioxidants.

67. Damiana Libido Enhancing Elixir

Ingredients: 1 teaspoon dried damiana leaves, 1 cup hot water, 1 teaspoon lemon juice, 1 teaspoon raw honey.
Preparation: Steep the damiana leaves in hot water for 10-15 minutes. Strain and add lemon juice and honey.
Suggested Usage: Drink once daily to enhance libido and support hormonal balance.

Benefits: Enhances libido, balances hormones, and supports reproductive health.

68. Cat's Claw Immune Boost Tea

Ingredients: 1 teaspoon dried cat's claw bark, 1 teaspoon ginger root, 2 cups water.
Preparation: Simmer cat's claw and ginger root in water for 20 minutes. Strain before drinking.
Suggested Usage: Drink 1 cup twice daily to support immune health and reduce inflammation.
Benefits: Boosts immune function, reduces inflammation, and supports joint health.

69. Goji Berry Energy Infusion

Ingredients: 1 tablespoon dried goji berries, 1 teaspoon dried schisandra berries (optional), 2 cups hot water.
Preparation: Steep the goji berries and schisandra berries in hot water for 15 minutes. Strain and serve.
Suggested Usage: Drink once daily to enhance energy, support eye health, and improve stamina.
Benefits: Increases energy, supports eye health, and boosts immune function.

70. Hawthorn Heart Tonic Tea

Ingredients: 1 tablespoon dried hawthorn berries, 1 teaspoon dried hibiscus flowers, 2 cups water, 1 teaspoon raw honey.
Preparation: Simmer hawthorn berries in water for 20 minutes. Remove from heat, add hibiscus flowers, and steep for 10 minutes. Strain and add honey if desired.

Suggested Usage: Drink 1 cup daily to support heart health and circulation.
Benefits: Strengthens the cardiovascular system, supports healthy blood pressure, and enhances circulation.

71. Echinacea Immune Defense Brew

Ingredients: 1 tablespoon dried echinacea root, 1 teaspoon dried elderberries, 2 cups water, 1 teaspoon raw honey.
Preparation: Simmer echinacea root and elderberries in water for 20 minutes. Strain and add honey.
Suggested Usage: Drink 1 cup twice daily during cold and flu season to strengthen the immune system.
Benefits: Boosts immune function, reduces the duration of colds, and supports respiratory health.

72. Thyme Respiratory Health Elixir

Ingredients: 1 tablespoon fresh thyme leaves (or 1 teaspoon dried thyme), 1 cup hot water, juice of ½ lemon, 1 teaspoon raw honey.
Preparation: Steep the thyme leaves in hot water for 10 minutes. Strain and add lemon juice and honey.
Suggested Usage: Drink 1-2 cups daily to support respiratory health and reduce congestion.
Benefits: Eases respiratory discomfort, relieves congestion, and has antimicrobial properties.

73. Cinnamon Blood Sugar Balance Tea

Ingredients: 1 cinnamon stick (or 1 teaspoon ground cinnamon), 1 teaspoon dried ginger root, 2 cups water, 1 teaspoon lemon juice.
Preparation: Simmer cinnamon and ginger in water for 15 minutes. Remove from heat and add lemon juice.
Suggested Usage: Drink 1 cup before meals to support healthy blood sugar levels.
Benefits: Balances blood sugar, enhances digestion, and supports metabolic health.

74. Rosemary Cognitive Support Tea

Ingredients: 1 teaspoon dried rosemary leaves, 1 cup hot water, 1 teaspoon raw honey.
Preparation: Steep rosemary leaves in hot water for 10 minutes. Strain and add honey.
Suggested Usage: Drink 1 cup in the morning or afternoon to promote focus and cognitive function.
Benefits: Enhances memory, improves mental clarity, and supports overall brain health.

75. Passionflower Relaxation Tonic

Ingredients: 1 teaspoon dried passionflower, 1 teaspoon dried chamomile, 1 cup hot water, 1 teaspoon raw honey.
Preparation: Steep the passionflower and chamomile in hot water for 10 minutes. Strain and add honey.
Suggested Usage: Drink in the evening to promote relaxation and reduce anxiety.
Benefits: Calms the nervous system,

reduces anxiety, and supports restful sleep.

76. Mugwort Dream Clarity Tea

Ingredients: 1 teaspoon dried mugwort, 1 teaspoon dried peppermint, 1 cup hot water.
Preparation: Steep the mugwort and peppermint in hot water for 10 minutes. Strain before drinking.
Suggested Usage: Drink before bedtime to enhance dream clarity and support restful sleep.
Benefits: Promotes vivid dreams, supports restful sleep, and may enhance dream recall.

77. Lemon Verbena Uplifting Tea

Ingredients: 1 tablespoon dried lemon verbena leaves, 1 cup hot water, 1 teaspoon raw honey.
Preparation: Steep lemon verbena leaves in hot water for 10 minutes. Strain and add honey.
Suggested Usage: Drink in the morning or afternoon to promote mood elevation and relaxation.
Benefits: Uplifts the mood, reduces anxiety, and promotes a sense of calm.

78. Kava Kava Stress Relief Brew

Ingredients: 1 teaspoon dried kava root powder, 1 cup warm water, 1 teaspoon raw honey.
Preparation: Mix the kava root powder into warm water until dissolved. Add honey and stir well.
Suggested Usage: Drink once daily to reduce stress and promote relaxation.
Benefits: Reduces anxiety, promotes relaxation, and helps relieve muscle tension.

79. Valerian Root Sleep Support Tea

Ingredients: 1 teaspoon dried valerian root, 1 teaspoon dried lemon balm, 1 cup hot water.
Preparation: Steep valerian root and lemon balm in hot water for 15 minutes. Strain before drinking.
Suggested Usage: Drink 30 minutes before bedtime to support restful sleep and reduce insomnia.
Benefits: Calms the nervous system, reduces anxiety, and promotes deep, restful sleep.

80. Chamomile and Lavender Calming Tea

Ingredients: 1 teaspoon dried chamomile flowers, 1 teaspoon dried lavender buds, 1 cup hot water, 1 teaspoon raw honey.
Preparation: Steep chamomile and lavender in hot water for 10 minutes. Strain and add honey.
Suggested Usage: Drink in the evening or during stressful times to promote relaxation and calm.

Benefits: Calms the nervous system, reduces stress and anxiety, and supports restful sleep.

Book 9: The Science of Herbal Remedies

Research and Studies on Herbal Efficacy

Scientific research on herbal remedies has grown significantly in recent years, providing valuable insights into the effectiveness of many traditional herbs. Studies have examined the biochemical properties, therapeutic effects, and mechanisms of action of various herbs, often validating long-held traditional uses. One well-documented example is the research on turmeric (Curcuma longa) and its active compound, curcumin, which has been shown to possess potent anti-inflammatory and antioxidant properties. Multiple clinical trials have highlighted curcumin's potential to reduce inflammation in conditions such as osteoarthritis, rheumatoid arthritis, and even certain cancers. It has also been found to support cardiovascular health by improving endothelial function and reducing oxidative stress.

Another widely researched herb is ginseng (Panax ginseng), often referred to as an adaptogen due to its ability to enhance resilience to stress. Ginseng has been studied for its effects on energy, cognitive function, and immunity. A meta-analysis of randomized controlled trials revealed that ginseng significantly improves cognitive performance and reduces mental fatigue, making it an effective natural remedy for enhancing mental clarity and stamina. Additionally, ginseng's immunomodulatory effects have been observed in several studies, suggesting its ability to enhance the immune system's response to infections and reduce the risk of illness.

Echinacea (Echinacea purpurea) is another herb that has undergone extensive research, particularly for its role in supporting immune health. Clinical trials have demonstrated that echinacea can reduce the duration and severity of the common cold by stimulating the production of white blood cells and enhancing the activity of the immune system. The herb's efficacy in preventing respiratory infections has been confirmed by numerous studies, making it a popular choice during cold and flu season.

The adaptogenic herb ashwagandha (Withania somnifera) has also garnered scientific attention for its ability to reduce stress and anxiety. A double-blind, placebo-controlled study found that participants who took ashwagandha extract experienced a significant reduction in cortisol levels and perceived stress compared to the placebo group. The herb was also shown to improve sleep quality and overall well-being, supporting its traditional use as a rejuvenative tonic.

In the realm of cardiovascular health, hawthorn (Crataegus monogyna) has been studied for its benefits in improving heart function. Research has shown that hawthorn can enhance the strength and efficiency of the heart's contractions, improve blood flow, and reduce symptoms of heart failure. Its bioactive flavonoids, such as quercetin and procyanidins, contribute to its cardioprotective effects by reducing oxidative stress and improving circulation.

These examples represent just a fraction of the growing body of scientific evidence supporting the efficacy of herbal remedies. While many herbs still require further research to fully understand their mechanisms and optimal dosages, current findings highlight the therapeutic potential of herbs as safe and effective tools for promoting health and treating a range of conditions.

Understanding Herbal Interactions

Understanding how herbs interact with each other and with conventional medications is crucial for ensuring safe and effective use. Herbal interactions can be classified into two main categories: synergistic interactions, where herbs enhance each other's effects, and antagonistic interactions, where one herb may reduce or counteract the effects of another. Additionally, herbs can interact with pharmaceutical drugs through various mechanisms, including altering drug metabolism, enhancing or inhibiting absorption, or competing for receptor sites.

One example of a synergistic interaction is the combination of turmeric and black pepper. The active compound in black pepper, piperine, significantly enhances the bioavailability of curcumin in turmeric by inhibiting its rapid breakdown in the liver. This combination is commonly used to increase the efficacy of turmeric for reducing inflammation and managing pain.

Conversely, an antagonistic interaction may occur when combining stimulant herbs, such as caffeine-containing guarana, with sedative herbs like valerian root. While guarana stimulates the central nervous system and increases alertness, valerian promotes relaxation and reduces anxiety, potentially diminishing the desired effects of either herb when taken together.

When it comes to herb-drug interactions, certain herbs can influence the metabolism of medications by affecting the activity of cytochrome P450 (CYP) enzymes in the liver. St. John's Wort (Hypericum perforatum) is a well-known example, as it induces CYP3A4, a major enzyme responsible for metabolizing many drugs. This induction can lead to a reduced concentration of medications such as oral contraceptives, anticoagulants, and immunosuppressants, potentially decreasing their effectiveness.

Similarly, herbs like ginkgo biloba and garlic have blood-thinning properties and can increase the risk of bleeding when combined with anticoagulant or antiplatelet medications such as warfarin or aspirin. It's essential for individuals taking such medications to consult with a healthcare provider before adding these herbs to their regimen.

To minimize the risk of interactions, it is recommended to follow guidelines such as consulting a healthcare professional, starting with low doses, spacing out doses when combining herbs with medications, and monitoring for adverse effects. Understanding these interactions is key to integrating herbal remedies safely and effectively into health practices.

Evidence-Based Herbal Practices

Evidence-based herbal practices are those that are supported by scientific research and clinical data, ensuring that herbal remedies are used in a safe and effective manner. This approach involves selecting herbs based on their proven efficacy, standardized dosages, and safety profiles. For example, using ginger to alleviate nausea is a well-established evidence-based practice, supported by multiple studies demonstrating its effectiveness in reducing symptoms of morning sickness, motion sickness, and chemotherapy-induced nausea.

To implement evidence-based herbal practices, it's essential to choose herbs with strong research backing, use standardized extracts when available, follow recommended dosages, and consider individual factors such as health status, age, and existing conditions to ensure optimal safety and efficacy.

Some of the best-documented herbs for evidence-based practices include milk thistle (Silybum marianum), which is used for liver support. Milk thistle's active compound, silymarin, has been shown to protect liver cells, promote regeneration, and reduce liver enzyme levels in conditions like fatty liver disease and hepatitis. Valerian Root (Valeriana officinalis) is supported by numerous studies for its effectiveness in promoting sleep and reducing anxiety. It is often used in evidence-based protocols for managing insomnia and stress. Peppermint (Mentha piperita) has been confirmed in clinical trials for relieving symptoms of irritable bowel syndrome (IBS) by reducing spasms in the gastrointestinal tract.

By adhering to evidence-based practices, herbalists and health practitioners can ensure that they are providing safe and effective herbal recommendations that are grounded in scientific research, ultimately promoting better health outcomes for those seeking natural remedies.

Book 10: Preparing and Using Herbal Remedies

Techniques for Herbal Extraction

Extracting the active compounds from herbs is a foundational skill in herbal medicine. Each extraction technique targets specific plant constituents, depending on the desired effect and application of the remedy. The primary methods include infusions, decoctions, tinctures, glycerites, and oil infusions. Understanding these techniques allows for a more effective and tailored use of herbs to support health and well-being.

Infusions are one of the simplest and most commonly used methods for extracting the medicinal properties of herbs, especially those rich in volatile oils, vitamins, and delicate compounds. They are typically used for leaves, flowers, and other soft plant parts. To prepare an infusion, boil water and pour it over the herb, allowing it to steep for a designated period, usually 10-15 minutes for leaves and flowers. The resulting tea can be consumed hot or cold, depending on preference. Infusions are ideal for herbs such as chamomile, peppermint, and nettle, which release their active constituents effectively in hot water. For more concentrated infusions, a longer steeping time or a higher herb-to-water ratio may be used, though this can alter the flavor profile.

Decoctions are used for tougher plant materials like roots, barks, and seeds, which require a more robust method to release their medicinal properties. Unlike infusions, decoctions involve simmering the herb in water for 20-40 minutes, allowing the heat to break down the tougher cell walls and release the beneficial compounds. Herbs like dandelion root, burdock root, and cinnamon bark are commonly prepared as decoctions. This method extracts not only water-soluble compounds but also more resilient active ingredients, making it particularly useful for creating potent herbal remedies for conditions requiring deeper support.

Tinctures are concentrated herbal extracts made by steeping herbs in alcohol or a mix of alcohol and water. Alcohol serves as a powerful solvent that extracts both water-soluble and alcohol-soluble constituents, creating a shelf-stable remedy with a long lifespan. To make a tincture, combine dried or fresh herbs with an alcohol like vodka (for general use) or brandy (for a milder flavor), typically in a 1:4 ratio for dried herbs or 1:2 for fresh herbs. The mixture is stored in a glass jar for 4-6 weeks, shaken daily to ensure even extraction, and then strained and stored in dark glass bottles. Tinctures are ideal for potent herbs like echinacea, valerian, and hawthorn, allowing for easy dosage adjustments and convenient use.

Glycerites are a non-alcoholic alternative to tinctures, using vegetable glycerin as the solvent. Glycerin is sweeter and gentler than alcohol, making it suitable for children, individuals sensitive to alcohol, or those seeking a sweeter herbal extract. While glycerites may not extract as broad a spectrum of constituents as alcohol-based tinctures, they are still effective for many herbs. To prepare a glycerite, mix the herb with a blend of glycerin and water, usually in a 3:1 ratio, and steep for 4-6 weeks in a similar manner to tinctures.

Oil infusions involve steeping herbs in a carrier oil, such as olive, coconut, or jojoba oil, to extract fat-soluble constituents. This method is often used for creating massage oils, salves, and skincare products. To make an oil infusion, gently heat the herb and oil mixture using a double boiler, maintaining a low temperature to prevent degradation of the delicate compounds. After several hours, the oil is strained and stored in a glass jar. Calendula, lavender, and comfrey are popular herbs for oil infusions due to their skin-healing properties.

Making Teas, Tinctures, and Salves

Creating different types of herbal preparations at home can be a rewarding experience, allowing for personalized remedies tailored to specific needs. The three most common preparations are teas, tinctures, and salves, each suited to a variety of health concerns.

To make a **herbal tea** (infusion), begin by selecting the appropriate herbs based on their therapeutic properties. Use 1-2 teaspoons of dried herbs per cup of water, or double the amount if using fresh herbs. Boil water and pour over the herbs, covering the cup or teapot to retain volatile oils. Steep for 10-15 minutes for leaves and flowers, or up to 30 minutes for roots and seeds if preparing a stronger infusion. Strain and drink immediately, or refrigerate for up to 24 hours. Herbal teas are ideal for daily use to support digestion, relaxation, and hydration.

For a **decoction**, use 1 tablespoon of dried root or bark per 2 cups of water. Place the herbs and water in a saucepan, bring to a boil, then reduce heat and simmer for 20-30 minutes. Strain and consume warm or cold. Decoctions are beneficial for extracting the deep-healing properties of tough plant materials and are often used for tonic herbs that build health over time.

Creating a **tincture** requires combining dried herbs with alcohol in a glass jar. For a 1:5 ratio tincture (1 part dried herb to 5 parts alcohol), fill a jar one-fifth full of the dried herb and cover completely with alcohol. Seal tightly and shake daily. After 4-6 weeks, strain the mixture through cheesecloth or a fine strainer and store in dark glass bottles. Tinctures are highly concentrated and typically dosed in drops rather than teaspoons. This makes them a powerful option for herbs that may need to be taken in smaller amounts, such as adaptogens and nervines.

Salves are topical preparations made by combining herbal oils with beeswax to create a semi-solid product that is easily applied to the skin. Start by creating a herbal oil infusion using a gentle heating method to extract the properties of herbs like calendula, comfrey, or plantain. Once the oil is infused, strain it and measure out 1 cup of herbal oil to ¼ cup of beeswax. Melt the beeswax in a double boiler, then slowly add the herbal oil, stirring until fully blended. Pour into tins or glass jars and allow to cool before sealing. Salves are excellent for skin healing, reducing inflammation, and providing a protective barrier.

Safe Usage and Dosage Guidelines

Using herbal remedies safely and effectively requires a good understanding of dosage, potential interactions, and individual tolerance. While herbs are generally safe when used correctly, some can cause adverse effects if misused. The first step in determining safe dosage is to consider the form of the herb (e.g., dried herb, tincture, or essential oil) and its potency. Generally, herbal teas and infusions are the mildest forms, while tinctures and concentrated extracts are more potent.

For **herbal teas**, a standard dose is 1-2 cups daily for general health maintenance. For stronger therapeutic effects, 3-4 cups may be used, but only under guidance from a healthcare provider if the herb has a strong action or potential side effects. In the case of **tinctures**, dosages are typically measured in drops, with a common starting point being 20-30 drops (about 1-1.5 ml) up to three times per day. However, some herbs require smaller doses, such as 5-10 drops, depending on their potency and intended use.

When using **essential oils**, it's important to remember that they are highly concentrated and should never be taken internally without professional guidance. For topical use, essential oils must be diluted in a carrier oil at a safe concentration, usually 1-3% (approximately 5-15 drops of essential oil per ounce of carrier oil).

Individuals with preexisting conditions, those taking medications, pregnant or breastfeeding women, and children should consult a healthcare professional before using any herbal remedy. Some herbs, such as St. John's Wort, can interact with medications like antidepressants, while others, such as licorice root, can affect blood pressure. Understanding potential contraindications and adjusting dosages accordingly is crucial for safe and effective use.

Ultimately, starting with low dosages and gradually increasing while monitoring for any adverse reactions is a prudent approach. Documenting the use of herbal remedies, including the type of preparation, dosage, and response, can also provide valuable insights into what works best for each individual's unique constitution and health needs. By following these guidelines, herbal enthusiasts can safely and confidently use natural remedies to support overall health and well-being.

Section II: Immune System Support

Book 11: Boosting Immunity Naturally

Herbs to Strengthen the Immune System

Herbal medicine has a long history of use for enhancing immune function and providing protection against various infections. Certain herbs, known as immunomodulators and immune tonics, are particularly effective at strengthening the immune system, balancing its activity, and preventing illness. These herbs work by stimulating the production of immune cells, enhancing the body's natural defenses, and supporting the overall vitality of the immune system.

One of the most well-known herbs for immune support is **Echinacea (Echinacea purpurea)**. Traditionally used by Native Americans, echinacea is widely recognized for its ability to boost the activity of white blood cells, which are essential for fighting off infections. It also increases the body's production of interferon, a protein that helps block viral replication. Echinacea is most effective when taken at the onset of a cold or flu, helping to reduce the severity and duration of symptoms. The root and aerial parts of the plant can be used to create teas, tinctures, or capsules, making it a versatile herb for daily immune support or acute use.

Elderberry (Sambucus nigra) is another powerful herb for immune health. Rich in antioxidants, particularly anthocyanins, elderberry enhances immune function by increasing the production of cytokines, proteins that regulate the immune response. Studies have shown that elderberry extract can reduce the severity and duration of influenza by inhibiting the ability of the virus to penetrate and replicate in host cells. Elderberry syrup is a popular preparation, often taken daily during the cold and flu season for prevention and at higher doses during illness to aid recovery.

Astragalus (Astragalus membranaceus) is a staple herb in Traditional Chinese Medicine, known for its adaptogenic and immune-enhancing properties. It strengthens the immune system by stimulating the production of white blood cells, particularly T-cells, which play a crucial role in adaptive immunity. Astragalus also supports the spleen and lymphatic system, enhancing the body's ability to filter out toxins and pathogens. It can be used long-term as a preventive measure and is often included in immune-boosting teas and soups.

Garlic (Allium sativum) is not only a culinary staple but also a potent medicinal herb with broad-spectrum antimicrobial properties. Its active compound, allicin, has been shown to have antibacterial, antiviral, and antifungal effects. Garlic stimulates the immune system by activating macrophages and natural killer cells, which help destroy foreign invaders. Regular consumption of garlic, whether raw, cooked, or in supplement form, can help prevent infections and support overall immune health.

Ginger (Zingiber officinale) is another versatile herb that supports immune function. It has antimicrobial and anti-inflammatory properties, making it effective for treating respiratory infections and soothing a sore throat. Ginger enhances circulation, promoting better delivery of immune cells throughout the body, and has a warming effect that helps expel pathogens. It is commonly used in teas, syrups, and decoctions to support the body's defenses, particularly during colder months.

Reishi mushroom (Ganoderma lucidum) is revered as a "superior tonic" in Traditional Chinese Medicine, known for its ability to modulate and strengthen the immune system. It contains beta-glucans, polysaccharides that enhance the activity of macrophages and natural killer cells, which play a key role in detecting and destroying pathogens. Reishi also acts as an adaptogen, reducing stress and supporting overall vitality. It can be taken as a tea, tincture, or capsule for long-term immune support.

Tulsi (Ocimum sanctum), also known as Holy Basil, is considered a sacred herb in Ayurveda for its ability to enhance resilience and support immunity. It has antioxidant, antimicrobial, and adaptogenic properties, making it useful for preventing illness and reducing stress, which can weaken the immune response. Tulsi is commonly prepared as a tea and can be taken daily to support immune health, reduce inflammation, and promote mental clarity.

Andrographis (Andrographis paniculata), often referred to as the "King of Bitters," is a powerful herb used in both Ayurvedic and Traditional Chinese Medicine. It has been shown to reduce the severity and duration of colds and flu by enhancing immune cell activity and inhibiting viral replication. Andrographis is particularly effective for respiratory infections and can be used preventively or at the first sign of illness.

By incorporating these herbs into daily routines, individuals can build a strong foundation for immune health. Whether taken as teas, tinctures, capsules, or syrups, these herbs work synergistically to support the immune system, providing a natural and effective way to prevent illness and enhance overall health.

Daily Practices for Immune Health

Supporting a robust immune system requires more than just taking herbs; it involves adopting a holistic approach that includes daily habits and routines to nourish and protect the body. Implementing simple lifestyle practices can create a strong foundation for immune resilience, making it easier to ward off illness and maintain optimal health.

One of the most important daily practices for immune health is maintaining a **nutrient-rich diet**. The immune system relies on a steady supply of vitamins and minerals, such as vitamin C, vitamin D, zinc, and selenium, to function properly. Consuming a variety of colorful fruits and vegetables ensures that the body receives a wide range of antioxidants and phytonutrients that protect cells from oxidative stress. Citrus fruits, berries, leafy greens, and cruciferous vegetables are particularly beneficial for boosting immunity. Additionally, incorporating immune-supporting herbs like garlic, ginger, and turmeric into daily meals can further enhance the body's defenses.

Staying hydrated is another key practice for immune health. Water is essential for flushing out toxins, maintaining mucosal barriers in the respiratory tract, and ensuring the proper circulation of immune cells. Aim to drink at least 8-10 cups of water daily, and consider adding herbal teas, such as ginger or lemon balm, for added immune support. Warm liquids, in particular, can soothe the throat and support respiratory health.

Regular **physical activity** is also crucial for maintaining a healthy immune system. Exercise promotes the circulation of immune cells, reduces inflammation, and enhances the body's ability to respond to pathogens. Activities such as brisk walking, yoga, or light strength training for 30 minutes a day can support immune function. However, it's important to avoid overtraining, as excessive exercise can suppress immune function.

Stress management is essential for immune resilience. Chronic stress can suppress the immune system by increasing cortisol levels, making the body more susceptible to infections. Incorporating stress-reduction techniques such as mindfulness meditation, deep breathing exercises, or yoga into daily routines can lower stress hormones and support immune health. Additionally, adaptogenic herbs like ashwagandha and holy basil can be used to enhance the body's stress response and protect against the negative effects of chronic stress.

Getting **adequate sleep** is perhaps the most critical factor for a healthy immune system. During sleep, the body repairs tissues, produces immune cells, and releases growth hormones that support overall health. Aim for 7-9 hours of quality sleep each night. If sleep is disrupted, consider using calming herbs such as valerian root, chamomile, or passionflower to promote relaxation and improve sleep quality.

Good hygiene practices are also essential for preventing the spread of infections. Regular handwashing, avoiding touching the face, and maintaining a clean living environment can reduce exposure to pathogens. Incorporating antimicrobial herbs like tea tree or eucalyptus in cleaning solutions or personal care products can provide additional protection.

By combining these daily habits with herbal support, individuals can create a comprehensive approach to immune health. This integrative strategy not only strengthens the body's natural defenses but also promotes overall vitality, making it easier to stay healthy and resilient throughout the year.

Remedies for Boosting Immunity

81. Echinacea Immune Support Tincture

Ingredients: 1 cup dried Echinacea root, 2 cups vodka or brandy (40% alcohol), 1 glass jar with lid.

Preparation: Place the dried Echinacea root in a glass jar and cover with alcohol. Seal the jar and store it in a cool, dark place for 4-6 weeks, shaking daily. After 6 weeks, strain and store in a dark glass bottle.

Suggested Usage: Take 20-30 drops (about 1-1.5 ml) up to 3 times daily at the onset of a cold or flu.

Benefits: Boosts immune function, reduces the duration and severity of colds and flu, and supports respiratory health.

82. Elderberry Syrup

Ingredients: 1 cup dried elderberries, 4 cups water, 1 cup raw honey, 1 cinnamon stick, 1 tablespoon fresh ginger root, grated.

Preparation: Combine elderberries, water, cinnamon, and ginger in a saucepan. Bring to a boil, then simmer for 30-45 minutes until the liquid is reduced by half. Remove from heat, strain, and stir in honey. Store in a glass jar.

Suggested Usage: Take 1 tablespoon daily for immune support, or up to 3 times daily when sick.

Benefits: Rich in antioxidants, supports immune health, and helps reduce the severity and duration of cold and flu symptoms.

83. Astragalus Root Immune Tea

Ingredients: 1 tablespoon dried astragalus root, 2 cups water.

Preparation: Simmer the dried astragalus root in water for 20-30 minutes. Strain and serve warm.

Suggested Usage: Drink 1-2 cups daily for long-term immune support, particularly during the cold and flu season.

Benefits: Enhances immune function, supports the spleen and lymphatic system, and promotes overall vitality.

84. Garlic and Honey Immune Booster

Ingredients: 1 cup raw honey, 10-12 garlic cloves, peeled.

Preparation: Place peeled garlic cloves in a glass jar and cover with raw honey. Seal the jar and let it sit for 1-2 weeks, shaking occasionally. The garlic will infuse the honey with its antimicrobial properties.

Suggested Usage: Take 1 teaspoon daily for immune support, or 3-4 times daily when experiencing cold or flu symptoms.

Benefits: Combines the antimicrobial properties of garlic with the soothing and immune-supporting effects of honey, making it an effective remedy for fighting infections.

85. Ginger and Turmeric Golden Milk

Ingredients: 1 cup coconut milk, 1 teaspoon turmeric powder, ½ teaspoon fresh grated ginger, ¼ teaspoon cinnamon, a pinch of black pepper, 1 teaspoon raw honey.

Preparation: Heat the coconut milk over low heat. Add turmeric, ginger, cinnamon, and black pepper, whisking until smooth. Remove from heat and stir in honey. Serve warm.

Suggested Usage: Drink once daily, preferably in the evening, to support immune health and reduce inflammation.

Benefits: Combines anti-inflammatory and immune-boosting herbs to support overall health, reduce inflammation, and promote restful sleep.

86. Reishi Mushroom Vitality Brew

Ingredients: 1 tablespoon dried reishi mushroom slices, 3 cups water, 1 teaspoon raw honey.

Preparation: Simmer reishi mushroom slices in water for 30 minutes. Strain and add honey. Serve warm.

Suggested Usage: Drink 1 cup daily to support immune health and reduce stress.

Benefits: Strengthens immune function, supports liver health, and acts as an adaptogen to promote resilience.

87. Andrographis Cold and Flu Defense Tea

Ingredients: 1 teaspoon dried andrographis leaves, 1 cup hot water, 1 teaspoon raw honey, juice of ½ lemon.

Preparation: Steep the dried andrographis leaves in hot water for 10-15 minutes. Strain and add honey and lemon juice. Serve warm.

Suggested Usage: Drink 1-2 cups daily at the first sign of cold or flu symptoms.

Benefits: Reduces the severity and duration of colds and flu, supports immune function, and enhances the body's defenses.

88. Tulsi and Lemon Balm Adaptogen Tea

Ingredients: 1 tablespoon dried tulsi leaves, 1 tablespoon dried lemon balm leaves, 2 cups hot water, 1 teaspoon raw honey.

Preparation: Steep the tulsi and lemon balm leaves in hot water for 10-15 minutes. Strain and add honey if desired. Serve warm.

Suggested Usage: Drink 1-2 cups daily to support immune health and reduce stress.

Benefits: Balances energy, supports the immune system, and promotes relaxation and mental clarity.

89. Fire Cider Tonic

Ingredients: 1 cup raw apple cider vinegar, ¼ cup grated fresh horseradish root, ¼ cup grated fresh ginger, 1-2 garlic cloves (crushed), 1 tablespoon cayenne pepper, 1 tablespoon raw honey.

Preparation: Combine all ingredients in a glass jar, seal tightly, and store in a cool, dark place for 4-6 weeks. Shake daily. Strain and store in a glass bottle.

Suggested Usage: Take 1-2 tablespoons daily as a preventive measure, or up to 4 times daily when sick.

Benefits: Combines potent antimicrobial, anti-inflammatory, and immune-supporting ingredients to boost immunity, support respiratory health, and reduce inflammation.

90. Olive Leaf Antiviral Tincture

Ingredients: 1 cup dried olive leaves, 2 cups vodka or brandy (40% alcohol), 1 glass jar with lid.

Preparation: Place dried olive leaves in a glass jar and cover with alcohol. Seal the jar and store in a cool, dark place for 4-6 weeks, shaking daily. After 6 weeks, strain and store in a dark glass bottle.

Suggested Usage: Take 20-30 drops up to 3 times daily for immune support and viral protection.

Benefits: Potent antiviral and immune-boosting properties, supports the body's defense against viral infections.

91. Oregano Oil Immune Elixir

Ingredients: 1 cup fresh oregano leaves, 1 cup olive oil, 1 glass jar.

Preparation: Gently heat the olive oil and add the fresh oregano leaves. Simmer on low heat for 30 minutes. Remove from heat and allow to cool, then strain and store in a glass jar.

Suggested Usage: Take 1 teaspoon daily or add to meals for immune support.

Benefits: Contains powerful antimicrobial and antiviral properties, enhances immune function, and fights infections.

92. Licorice Root Antiviral Tea

Ingredients: 1 tablespoon dried licorice root, 2 cups water.

Preparation: Simmer the licorice root in water for 15-20 minutes. Strain and serve warm.

Suggested Usage: Drink 1 cup twice daily to support respiratory health and enhance immune function.

Benefits: Soothes the respiratory tract, provides antiviral properties, and supports adrenal health.

93. Cat's Claw Immune Strengthening Decoction

Ingredients: 1 tablespoon dried cat's claw bark, 2 cups water.

Preparation: Simmer cat's claw bark in water for 20-30 minutes. Strain and serve warm.

Suggested Usage: Drink 1 cup daily for long-term immune support and to reduce inflammation.

Benefits: Enhances immune function, reduces inflammation, and promotes overall vitality.

94. Calendula and Chamomile Antimicrobial Tea

Ingredients: 1 tablespoon dried calendula flowers, 1 tablespoon dried chamomile flowers, 2 cups hot water, 1 teaspoon raw honey.

Preparation: Steep calendula and chamomile flowers in hot water for 10-15 minutes. Strain and add honey if desired.

Suggested Usage: Drink 1-2 cups daily to support immune health and reduce inflammation.

Benefits: Combines gentle antimicrobial

and anti-inflammatory herbs to support immune function and promote relaxation.

95. Mullein and Thyme Respiratory Support Tea

Ingredients: 1 tablespoon dried mullein leaves, 1 teaspoon dried thyme, 1 cup hot water.
Preparation: Steep mullein and thyme in hot water for 10 minutes. Strain before drinking.
Suggested Usage: Drink 1-2 cups daily to support respiratory health and soothe the lungs.
Benefits: Helps clear mucus, supports lung function, and provides antimicrobial effects.

96. Holy Basil and Peppermint Immune Tea

Ingredients: 1 tablespoon dried holy basil leaves, 1 tablespoon dried peppermint leaves, 2 cups hot water.
Preparation: Steep holy basil and peppermint in hot water for 10-15 minutes. Strain and serve warm.
Suggested Usage: Drink 1-2 cups daily to reduce stress and support immune health.
Benefits: Combines adaptogenic and immune-boosting properties to balance energy, reduce stress, and enhance immunity.

97. Lemon and Ginger Immune Shot

Ingredients: 1 tablespoon fresh grated ginger, juice of 1 lemon, 1 tablespoon raw honey, ½ cup warm water.

Preparation: Mix ginger, lemon juice, honey, and warm water until well blended.
Suggested Usage: Take 1 shot daily for immune support and to boost digestion.
Benefits: Combines the anti-inflammatory and immune-boosting effects of ginger and lemon for a potent immune shot.

98. Rosehip and Hibiscus Vitamin C Tea

Ingredients: 1 tablespoon dried rosehips, 1 tablespoon dried hibiscus flowers, 2 cups hot water, 1 teaspoon raw honey.
Preparation: Steep rosehips and hibiscus flowers in hot water for 15 minutes. Strain and add honey if desired.
Suggested Usage: Drink 1-2 cups daily to boost vitamin C levels and support immune function.
Benefits: Provides a rich source of vitamin C and antioxidants to strengthen the immune system and protect against free radical damage.

99. Nettle and Elderflower Immune Tonic

Ingredients: 1 tablespoon dried nettle leaves, 1 tablespoon dried elderflowers, 2 cups hot water.
Preparation: Steep nettle leaves and elderflowers in hot water for 10-15 minutes. Strain and serve warm.
Suggested Usage: Drink 1-2 cups daily to support overall immune health and reduce inflammation.
Benefits: Combines nutrient-rich nettle with elderflower's antiviral properties to support immune health and reduce seasonal allergies.

100. Shiitake Mushroom and Ginger Broth

Ingredients: 1 cup dried shiitake mushrooms, 1 tablespoon fresh grated ginger, 4 cups vegetable broth, 2 garlic cloves (crushed), 1 tablespoon tamari or soy sauce.

Preparation: Combine all ingredients in a saucepan and simmer for 30-40 minutes. Strain and serve warm.

Suggested Usage: Drink 1 cup daily to support immune function and enhance vitality.

Benefits: Rich in beta-glucans, shiitake mushrooms enhance immune health, while ginger and garlic provide additional antimicrobial and anti-inflammatory support.

101. Dandelion Root and Burdock Detox Tea

Ingredients: 1 tablespoon dried dandelion root, 1 tablespoon dried burdock root, 3 cups water, 1 teaspoon lemon juice.

Preparation: Simmer dandelion and burdock roots in water for 20-30 minutes. Strain and add lemon juice. Serve warm.

Suggested Usage: Drink 1 cup twice daily to support detoxification and overall immune health.

Benefits: Promotes liver and kidney health, supports the body's natural detox pathways, and boosts immunity by reducing toxic load.

102. Sage and Eucalyptus Steam Inhalation

Ingredients: 1 tablespoon dried sage, 1 tablespoon dried eucalyptus leaves, 4 cups boiling water.

Preparation: Place sage and eucalyptus in a large bowl and pour boiling water over the herbs. Lean over the bowl with a towel draped over your head, creating a tent to trap the steam. Inhale deeply for 5-10 minutes.

Suggested Usage: Use 1-2 times daily during colds or respiratory congestion.

Benefits: Clears nasal passages, soothes irritated respiratory tissues, and provides antimicrobial support for the respiratory system.

103. Golden Milk Paste with Ashwagandha

Ingredients: 1 cup coconut oil, 1 cup turmeric powder, 1 tablespoon ashwagandha powder, 2 teaspoons ground black pepper, 2 tablespoons raw honey.

Preparation: Combine coconut oil, turmeric, ashwagandha, and black pepper in a small saucepan. Heat gently, stirring until a paste forms. Remove from heat and stir in honey. Store in a glass jar.

Suggested Usage: Add 1 teaspoon of paste to warm milk (or plant-based milk) once daily for immune support and anti-inflammatory benefits.

Benefits: Combines the immune-boosting properties of ashwagandha with the anti-inflammatory effects of turmeric for overall health support.

104. Propolis and Honey Throat Spray

Ingredients: 1 tablespoon propolis tincture, ½ cup raw honey, ¼ cup warm

water, 10 drops peppermint essential oil, 1 spray bottle.
Preparation: Combine all ingredients and mix thoroughly. Pour into a spray bottle.
Suggested Usage: Spray 1-2 times directly onto the throat up to 4 times daily to soothe and protect against infections.
Benefits: Propolis is a powerful antimicrobial that soothes the throat and helps fight infections, while honey coats and protects irritated tissues.

105. Yarrow and Peppermint Fever-Reducing Tea

Ingredients: 1 tablespoon dried yarrow, 1 tablespoon dried peppermint, 2 cups hot water.
Preparation: Steep yarrow and peppermint in hot water for 10-15 minutes. Strain and serve warm.
Suggested Usage: Drink 1-2 cups daily at the first sign of fever to reduce temperature and promote sweating.
Benefits: Yarrow induces sweating to break fevers, while peppermint cools the body and soothes the digestive system.

106. Maitake Mushroom Immunity Soup

Ingredients: 1 cup fresh maitake mushrooms (or ½ cup dried), 4 cups vegetable broth, 1 tablespoon grated fresh ginger, 2 garlic cloves (crushed), 1 tablespoon miso paste, 2 green onions (chopped).
Preparation: Combine all ingredients except miso paste and green onions in a pot and simmer for 20-30 minutes. Remove from heat and stir in miso paste. Top with green onions before serving.

Suggested Usage: Eat 1 cup daily to boost immunity and enhance vitality.
Benefits: Maitake mushrooms support immune health, while ginger and garlic provide additional antimicrobial and anti-inflammatory benefits.

107. Chaga Mushroom and Cacao Elixir

Ingredients: 1 tablespoon dried chaga mushroom powder, 1 cup hot water, 1 tablespoon raw cacao powder, 1 teaspoon coconut oil, 1 teaspoon raw honey.
Preparation: Steep chaga powder in hot water for 15 minutes. Strain if needed, then blend with cacao, coconut oil, and honey until frothy.
Suggested Usage: Drink once daily for immune support and enhanced energy.
Benefits: Chaga is rich in antioxidants and immune-supporting polysaccharides, while cacao provides mood-boosting and cardiovascular benefits.

108. Black Seed Oil Immune Booster

Ingredients: 1 teaspoon black seed oil, 1 teaspoon raw honey.
Preparation: Mix black seed oil and honey until well combined.
Suggested Usage: Take 1 teaspoon daily for immune support and to reduce inflammation.
Benefits: Black seed oil is known for its potent anti-inflammatory and immune-boosting properties, making it an excellent choice for overall health.

109. Thyme and Sage Herbal Gargle

Ingredients: 1 tablespoon dried thyme, 1 tablespoon dried sage, 2 cups boiling water, 1 teaspoon salt.

Preparation: Steep thyme and sage in boiling water for 15 minutes. Strain and add salt. Allow to cool to a comfortable temperature.

Suggested Usage: Gargle with ½ cup of the solution up to 3 times daily to soothe a sore throat and fight infection.

Benefits: Combines powerful antimicrobial herbs to soothe the throat, reduce inflammation, and fight bacterial and viral infections.

110. Marshmallow Root and Licorice Throat Soother

Ingredients: 1 tablespoon dried marshmallow root, 1 tablespoon dried licorice root, 2 cups hot water, 1 teaspoon raw honey.

Preparation: Steep marshmallow and licorice roots in hot water for 15-20 minutes. Strain and add honey if desired.

Suggested Usage: Drink 1 cup twice daily to soothe a sore throat and support respiratory health.

Benefits: Marshmallow root coats and soothes irritated tissues, while licorice root provides antiviral and anti-inflammatory support.

111. Elderflower and Linden Cold Relief Tea

Ingredients: 1 tablespoon dried elderflowers, 1 tablespoon dried linden flowers, 2 cups hot water, 1 teaspoon raw honey.

Preparation: Steep elderflower and linden in hot water for 10-15 minutes. Strain and add honey if desired.

Suggested Usage: Drink 1-2 cups daily at the onset of cold symptoms to reduce congestion and support recovery.

Benefits: Elderflower and linden work together to reduce fever, relieve congestion, and support the immune system during illness.

112. Rosemary and Lavender Nasal Steam

Ingredients: 1 tablespoon dried rosemary, 1 tablespoon dried lavender, 4 cups boiling water.

Preparation: Place rosemary and lavender in a large bowl and pour boiling water over the herbs. Lean over the bowl with a towel draped over your head, creating a tent to trap the steam. Inhale deeply for 5-10 minutes.

Suggested Usage: Use once or twice daily during colds or respiratory congestion.

Benefits: Opens nasal passages, soothes respiratory tissues, and provides calming effects for both mind and body.

113. Cinnamon and Clove Immune Chai

Ingredients: 1 cinnamon stick, 4-5 whole cloves, 2 cups water, 1 cup milk (or plant-based milk), 1 teaspoon raw honey, 1 teaspoon grated fresh ginger.

Preparation: Combine cinnamon, cloves, and ginger with water in a saucepan. Bring to a boil, reduce heat, and simmer for 10 minutes. Add milk and simmer for another

5 minutes. Strain and add honey before serving.

Suggested Usage: Drink once daily during the winter season for immune support and warmth.

Benefits: Combines antimicrobial and warming herbs to support immune function, improve circulation, and reduce inflammation.

114. Fenugreek and Fennel Immune Tea

Ingredients: 1 teaspoon fenugreek seeds, 1 teaspoon fennel seeds, 2 cups hot water.

Preparation: Crush fenugreek and fennel seeds slightly, then steep in hot water for 10-15 minutes. Strain and serve warm.

Suggested Usage: Drink 1 cup twice daily to support respiratory health and reduce mucus.

Benefits: Fenugreek and fennel help clear mucus, soothe the digestive system, and provide immune support, making this tea beneficial for colds and respiratory congestion.

115. Turmeric and Black Pepper Anti-Inflammatory Capsules

Ingredients: ¼ cup turmeric powder, 1 teaspoon ground black pepper, empty vegetable capsules.

Preparation: Mix turmeric powder and black pepper thoroughly. Fill each capsule with the mixture using a small spoon or capsule machine. Store capsules in a cool, dry place.

Suggested Usage: Take 1-2 capsules daily to reduce inflammation and support immune health.

Benefits: Combines the potent anti-inflammatory effects of turmeric with black pepper's ability to enhance absorption, making this remedy ideal for reducing chronic inflammation.

116. Garlic and Cayenne Immunity Fire Tonic

Ingredients: 1 cup apple cider vinegar, 5-6 garlic cloves (crushed), 1 tablespoon grated fresh ginger, 1 teaspoon cayenne pepper, 1 tablespoon raw honey.

Preparation: Combine all ingredients in a glass jar, seal tightly, and store in a cool, dark place for 4 weeks. Shake daily. Strain and store in a glass bottle.

Suggested Usage: Take 1 tablespoon daily as a preventive measure, or up to 4 times daily when sick.

Benefits: Potent antimicrobial, anti-inflammatory, and immune-boosting properties, making it effective for fighting infections and boosting circulation.

117. Siberian Ginseng Immune-Boosting Tea

Ingredients: 1 tablespoon dried Siberian ginseng root, 2 cups water.

Preparation: Simmer Siberian ginseng root in water for 20 minutes. Strain and serve warm.

Suggested Usage: Drink 1 cup daily to support immune function, energy levels, and overall vitality.

Benefits: Enhances immune resilience, supports adrenal health, and improves stamina, making it a powerful adaptogen for overall health.

118. Eucalyptus and Peppermint Chest Rub

Ingredients: ¼ cup coconut oil, 10 drops eucalyptus essential oil, 5 drops peppermint essential oil, 5 drops rosemary essential oil.
Preparation: Melt the coconut oil and stir in essential oils. Mix thoroughly and transfer to a small glass jar. Allow to solidify.
Suggested Usage: Apply a small amount to the chest and throat area before bedtime or when experiencing respiratory congestion.
Benefits: Opens up the airways, relieves congestion, and soothes irritated respiratory tissues with potent, aromatic herbs.

119. Lemon Balm and Passionflower Stress-Reducing Tea

Ingredients: 1 tablespoon dried lemon balm leaves, 1 tablespoon dried passionflower, 2 cups hot water, 1 teaspoon raw honey.
Preparation: Steep lemon balm and passionflower in hot water for 10-15 minutes. Strain and add honey if desired.
Suggested Usage: Drink 1-2 cups daily to reduce stress, promote relaxation, and support the immune system.
Benefits: Combines calming and nervine herbs to reduce anxiety, promote restful sleep, and strengthen immunity.

120. Ginger and Lemon Immune Gummy

Ingredients: 1 cup fresh lemon juice, 2 tablespoons grated fresh ginger, ¼ cup raw honey, 2 tablespoons gelatin powder.
Preparation: Heat lemon juice and grated ginger in a small saucepan until warm. Remove from heat and stir in honey and gelatin powder until fully dissolved. Pour into silicone molds and refrigerate for 1-2 hours until set.
Suggested Usage: Take 1-2 gummies daily for immune support and to soothe the digestive system.
Benefits: Combines the immune-boosting and digestive-soothing properties of ginger and lemon in a delicious, easy-to-consume gummy form.

121. Cayenne and Ginger Sinus-Clearing Elixir

Ingredients: 1 cup hot water, ½ teaspoon cayenne pepper, 1 teaspoon grated fresh ginger, juice of ½ lemon, 1 teaspoon raw honey.
Preparation: Combine all ingredients and stir until well blended.
Suggested Usage: Drink 1-2 times daily during sinus congestion for relief.
Benefits: Clears nasal passages, supports circulation, and provides antimicrobial support for respiratory health.

122. Burdock and Yellow Dock Root Liver Tonic

Ingredients: 1 tablespoon dried burdock root, 1 tablespoon dried yellow dock root, 3 cups water.
Preparation: Simmer burdock and yellow dock roots in water for 20-30 minutes. Strain and serve warm.
Suggested Usage: Drink 1 cup twice daily

to support liver health and detoxification.
Benefits: Promotes liver detoxification, supports digestion, and enhances overall immune health by reducing toxin load.

123. Osha Root Respiratory Relief Tea

Ingredients: 1 tablespoon dried osha root, 2 cups water, 1 teaspoon raw honey.
Preparation: Simmer osha root in water for 15-20 minutes. Strain and add honey if desired.
Suggested Usage: Drink 1 cup up to twice daily to support respiratory health and relieve congestion.
Benefits: Osha root helps clear mucus, soothes the respiratory tract, and provides antimicrobial support.

124. Honey, Lemon, and Thyme Cough Syrup

Ingredients: 1 cup raw honey, ½ cup fresh lemon juice, 1 tablespoon dried thyme.
Preparation: Combine honey, lemon juice, and thyme in a small saucepan. Heat gently over low heat for 10-15 minutes, stirring occasionally. Remove from heat, strain, and store in a glass jar.
Suggested Usage: Take 1 teaspoon every 2-3 hours to soothe a sore throat and reduce coughing.
Benefits: Combines the antimicrobial and soothing effects of honey and thyme with the immune-boosting properties of lemon.

125. Astragalus and Goji Berry Immunity Soup

Ingredients: 2 tablespoons dried astragalus root, ¼ cup dried goji berries, 6 cups vegetable broth, 1 cup chopped mushrooms, 1 cup diced carrots, 1 cup chopped celery, 2 garlic cloves (minced).
Preparation: Combine all ingredients in a large pot and simmer for 30-40 minutes. Remove astragalus root before serving.
Suggested Usage: Consume 1 cup daily for long-term immune support and nourishment.
Benefits: Astragalus and goji berries work synergistically to enhance immune function, support vitality, and nourish the body.

126. Eleuthero and Schisandra Adaptogen Blend

Ingredients: 1 tablespoon dried eleuthero root, 1 tablespoon dried schisandra berries, 2 cups water.
Preparation: Simmer eleuthero and schisandra in water for 20-30 minutes. Strain and serve warm.
Suggested Usage: Drink 1 cup daily to support immune function, reduce stress, and enhance resilience.
Benefits: Combines the adaptogenic properties of eleuthero and schisandra to balance energy, support the adrenal system, and boost immunity.

127. Herbal Vinegar Infusion with Sage and Thyme

Ingredients: 1 cup raw apple cider vinegar, 1 tablespoon dried sage, 1 tablespoon dried thyme, 1 glass jar with lid.
Preparation: Combine all ingredients in a glass jar, seal, and let sit in a cool, dark

place for 4-6 weeks, shaking occasionally. Strain and store in a glass bottle.

Suggested Usage: Use 1 tablespoon diluted in water or as a salad dressing to support immune health and digestion.

Benefits: Sage and thyme provide potent antimicrobial and antioxidant properties, while vinegar enhances nutrient absorption.

128. Elderberry and Rosehip Vinegar Tonic

Ingredients: 1 cup raw apple cider vinegar, ¼ cup dried elderberries, ¼ cup dried rosehips, 1 glass jar with lid.

Preparation: Combine all ingredients in a glass jar, seal tightly, and store in a cool, dark place for 4-6 weeks, shaking daily. Strain and store in a glass bottle.

Suggested Usage: Take 1-2 teaspoons daily for immune support, or use as a base for salad dressings.

Benefits: Elderberries and rosehips are rich in vitamin C and antioxidants, providing a powerful boost to immune function.

129. Garlic and Mullein Ear Oil

Ingredients: 4-5 garlic cloves (crushed), 1 tablespoon dried mullein flowers, ½ cup olive oil.

Preparation: Gently heat garlic and mullein in olive oil over low heat for 30 minutes. Allow to cool, strain, and store in a glass dropper bottle.

Suggested Usage: Apply 2-3 drops in the affected ear up to twice daily to relieve earaches and fight infections.

Benefits: Garlic and mullein provide antimicrobial and anti-inflammatory effects, helping to soothe ear infections and reduce pain.

130. Herbal Chest Rub with Peppermint and Eucalyptus

Ingredients: ¼ cup shea butter, ¼ cup coconut oil, 10 drops peppermint essential oil, 10 drops eucalyptus essential oil, 5 drops rosemary essential oil.

Preparation: Melt shea butter and coconut oil together using a double boiler. Remove from heat and stir in essential oils. Transfer to

a small glass jar and let solidify.

Suggested Usage: Apply a small amount to the chest and back area before bedtime or during respiratory congestion.

Benefits: The aromatic herbs open airways, reduce congestion, and soothe the respiratory system, providing relief during colds and coughs.

Book 12: Natural Cold and Flu Remedies

Herbal Treatments for Cold Symptoms

Herbal remedies have been used for centuries to alleviate the uncomfortable symptoms of colds and flu, such as congestion, sore throat, fever, and body aches. Many of these herbs possess potent antiviral, antibacterial, and anti-inflammatory properties, making them effective at easing symptoms and promoting faster recovery. Some herbs are soothing, helping to reduce throat irritation and inflammation, while others work by breaking up mucus and congestion in the respiratory system.

One of the most popular herbs for colds is **ginger (Zingiber officinale)**, which is widely known for its warming, anti-inflammatory, and antiviral effects. Ginger helps relieve congestion, ease sore throats, and reduce fever by promoting sweating. It can be consumed as a hot tea, combined with honey and lemon, or used in steam inhalations. Its warming properties also help to stimulate circulation and support overall immune function.

Echinacea (Echinacea purpurea) is another excellent herb for combating cold symptoms. It works by stimulating the activity of white blood cells, enhancing the body's ability to fight off infections. Echinacea is most effective when taken at the first sign of illness, helping to reduce the severity and duration of symptoms. The herb can be used in tincture form, capsules, or as an infusion with other immune-boosting herbs like elderberry and ginger.

For sore throats, **licorice root (Glycyrrhiza glabra)** is a soothing remedy that provides immediate relief. Licorice is naturally sweet and has demulcent properties, which means it coats and soothes irritated mucous membranes. It also has antiviral and anti-inflammatory properties, making it ideal for sore throats and coughs associated with colds. Licorice root tea or tincture can be used throughout the day to keep the throat moist and reduce discomfort.

Thyme (Thymus vulgaris) is an herb with strong antimicrobial and expectorant properties, making it effective for treating congestion and coughs. Thyme works by thinning mucus and promoting its expulsion, making it easier to breathe. Thyme tea, combined with honey, can be sipped throughout the day to reduce coughing and clear the respiratory passages. For a stronger effect, thyme can be used in steam inhalations or as an herbal gargle.

To break up congestion and support respiratory health, **mullein (Verbascum thapsus)** is a gentle yet effective herb. Mullein leaves are known for their soothing, expectorant properties, which help expel mucus from the lungs while calming irritated tissues.

Mullein tea is often combined with other respiratory herbs like hyssop, thyme, and ginger for maximum effectiveness in easing congestion and promoting clearer breathing.

Peppermint (Mentha piperita) is another popular herb for treating cold symptoms, particularly congestion and sinus issues. The menthol in peppermint acts as a natural decongestant, helping to open nasal passages and ease breathing. Peppermint tea, used as a steam inhalation, or included in herbal chest rubs, provides quick relief for stuffy noses and sinus congestion. Its antiviral and antibacterial properties also make it a valuable addition to any cold and flu remedy.

For fever management, **yarrow (Achillea millefolium)** is a traditional remedy used to induce sweating and reduce fever. Yarrow promotes circulation, reduces inflammation, and helps the body eliminate toxins through the skin. A warm yarrow tea, sipped at the onset of a fever, can help break the fever and speed up recovery. Combined with elderflower and peppermint, yarrow makes an effective fever-reducing tea blend.

In addition to these remedies, **elderflower (Sambucus nigra)** is a gentle herb that helps manage congestion and fever. Elderflower is often used in combination with yarrow and peppermint to support the body's natural fever response, reduce inflammation, and ease nasal congestion. Elderflower tea is also soothing and can be taken throughout the day to relieve discomfort and support the immune system during illness.

Preventative Herbs for Flu Season

Preventing the onset of the flu during peak seasons involves supporting the immune system with herbs that boost resilience, reduce susceptibility to infection, and create a strong barrier against pathogens. Using a combination of immune tonics, adaptogens, and antimicrobial herbs can help keep the body strong and protected during flu season.

Astragalus (Astragalus membranaceus) is one of the best-known herbs for long-term immune support and prevention of illness. It works by stimulating the production of white blood cells and enhancing the body's ability to ward off viral and bacterial infections. Astragalus is often taken as a daily tea or tincture throughout the cold and flu season to build immune resilience and reduce the likelihood of infection. It can also be added to soups and broths for a nourishing, immune-supportive meal.

Elderberry (Sambucus nigra) is a powerful herb for flu prevention, thanks to its antiviral properties and high antioxidant content. Elderberries contain compounds that inhibit viral replication, making it harder for the flu virus to establish an infection. Elderberry syrup is a popular preparation, taken daily during the flu season to boost immunity and provide an extra layer of defense. In addition to syrup, elderberries can be made into teas, tinctures, or lozenges for easy use.

Reishi mushroom (Ganoderma lucidum) is an adaptogen and immune tonic that helps modulate immune activity, making it effective for both boosting immunity and managing immune responses. Reishi strengthens the body's resistance to infections, reduces inflammation, and supports overall vitality. It can be taken in powder form, as a tea, or in capsules for long-term immune health.

Garlic (Allium sativum) is a potent antimicrobial herb that has been used for centuries to prevent and treat infections. Garlic works by stimulating the activity of immune cells and enhancing the body's ability to fight off viruses and bacteria. Consuming raw garlic daily or taking garlic capsules during flu season can provide strong protection against illness. Garlic can also be added to meals, teas, and broths for additional support.

Holy Basil (Ocimum sanctum), or Tulsi, is an adaptogen and immune-supporting herb that enhances the body's ability to cope with stress while boosting immune function. It has antimicrobial and anti-inflammatory properties, making it useful for preventing infections and reducing the impact of seasonal stress on the immune system. Holy basil tea, tincture, or capsules can be taken daily during flu season to enhance resilience and prevent illness.

Schisandra (Schisandra chinensis) is another powerful adaptogen that supports immune health and reduces susceptibility to infection. Schisandra's high antioxidant content protects against oxidative stress, and its adaptogenic properties help the body maintain balance during periods of heightened immune activity. Schisandra berries can be made into a tea, tincture, or taken in capsules as a preventive measure.

Maitake mushroom (Grifola frondosa) is a nourishing, immune-boosting herb that enhances immune cell function and protects against viral infections. Maitake can be used in soups, broths, or as a tea to provide ongoing immune support during flu season. Combined with other immune-boosting mushrooms like shiitake and reishi, maitake is an excellent addition to any herbal flu prevention protocol.

By incorporating these herbs into daily routines, individuals can strengthen their immune defenses, reduce susceptibility to infections, and create a natural barrier against colds and flu during the peak seasons.

Remedies for Cold and Flu

131. Ginger and Lemon Throat Soothing Tea

Ingredients: 1 tablespoon fresh grated ginger, juice of 1 lemon, 1 teaspoon raw honey, 1 cup hot water.

Preparation: Steep the grated ginger in hot water for 10 minutes. Strain and add lemon juice and honey.

Suggested Usage: Drink 1 cup up to 3 times daily to soothe a sore throat and reduce inflammation.

Benefits: Combines the warming, anti-inflammatory effects of ginger with the soothing properties of lemon and honey to relieve throat irritation.

132. Echinacea and Elderberry Immune Tonic

Ingredients: ½ cup dried echinacea root, ½ cup dried elderberries, 2 cups vodka or brandy, 1 glass jar with lid.
Preparation: Combine echinacea and elderberries in a glass jar and cover with alcohol. Seal the jar and store in a cool, dark place for 4-6 weeks, shaking daily. Strain and store in a dark glass bottle.
Suggested Usage: Take 1-2 teaspoons daily during cold and flu season, or 3 times daily at the onset of symptoms.
Benefits: Boosts immune function, reduces the severity and duration of colds and flu, and provides antiviral support.

133. Peppermint and Eucalyptus Steam Inhalation

Ingredients: 1 tablespoon dried peppermint leaves, 1 tablespoon dried eucalyptus leaves, 4 cups boiling water.
Preparation: Place peppermint and eucalyptus in a large bowl and pour boiling water over the herbs. Lean over the bowl with a towel draped over your head to trap the steam. Inhale deeply for 5-10 minutes.
Suggested Usage: Use 1-2 times daily during colds or congestion for relief.
Benefits: Opens up nasal passages, soothes respiratory tissues, and provides antimicrobial support.

134. Licorice and Marshmallow Root Cough Syrup

Ingredients: 1 cup dried licorice root, 1 cup dried marshmallow root, 4 cups water, 1 cup raw honey.
Preparation: Combine licorice root and marshmallow root with water in a saucepan. Bring to a boil, then simmer for 30 minutes. Strain, return liquid to the pan, and simmer until reduced by half. Remove from heat and stir in honey. Store in a glass jar.
Suggested Usage: Take 1 tablespoon every 2-3 hours to soothe a sore throat and reduce coughing.
Benefits: Soothes irritated mucous membranes, reduces throat inflammation, and calms coughing.

135. Elderflower and Yarrow Fever-Reducing Tea

Ingredients: 1 tablespoon dried elderflower, 1 tablespoon dried yarrow, 1 cup hot water.
Preparation: Steep elderflower and yarrow in hot water for 10-15 minutes. Strain and serve warm.
Suggested Usage: Drink 1-2 cups daily at the onset of fever to reduce temperature and promote sweating.
Benefits: Elderflower and yarrow promote sweating, reduce fever, and support the body's natural defenses.

136. Garlic and Honey Cold Remedy

Ingredients: 1 cup raw honey, 10-12 garlic cloves, peeled.

Preparation: Place peeled garlic cloves in a glass jar and cover with raw honey. Seal the jar and let it sit for 1-2 weeks, shaking occasionally. The garlic will infuse the honey with its antimicrobial properties.

Suggested Usage: Take 1 teaspoon daily for immune support, or 3-4 times daily at the onset of symptoms.

Benefits: Combines the antimicrobial properties of garlic with the soothing effects of honey to fight infections and soothe the throat.

137. Thyme and Sage Gargle for Sore Throats

Ingredients: 1 tablespoon dried thyme, 1 tablespoon dried sage, 2 cups hot water, 1 teaspoon sea salt.

Preparation: Steep thyme and sage in hot water for 10-15 minutes. Strain and add sea salt. Allow to cool to a comfortable temperature.

Suggested Usage: Gargle with ½ cup of the solution up to 3 times daily to soothe a sore throat and fight infection.

Benefits: Provides strong antimicrobial and anti-inflammatory properties to reduce throat irritation and kill bacteria.

138. Cinnamon and Clove Immune Chai

Ingredients: 1 cinnamon stick, 4-5 whole cloves, 1 cup hot water, ½ cup milk (or plant-based milk), 1 teaspoon raw honey, 1 teaspoon grated fresh ginger.

Preparation: Combine cinnamon, cloves, and ginger in hot water and simmer for 10 minutes. Add milk and simmer for another 5 minutes. Strain and add honey before serving.

Suggested Usage: Drink once daily during cold and flu season to support immune health.

Benefits: Combines warming, antimicrobial, and immune-boosting herbs to support immune function and reduce inflammation.

139. Turmeric and Black Pepper Anti-Inflammatory Milk

Ingredients: 1 cup milk (or plant-based milk), 1 teaspoon turmeric powder, ¼ teaspoon ground black pepper, 1 teaspoon raw honey.

Preparation: Heat the milk over low heat. Add turmeric, black pepper, and honey, stirring until well blended. Serve warm.

Suggested Usage: Drink once daily for immune support and to reduce inflammation.

Benefits: Combines the anti-inflammatory effects of turmeric with the bioavailability-enhancing properties of black pepper.

140. Oregano Oil Nasal Spray

Ingredients: 5 drops oregano essential oil, ¼ cup distilled water, 1 small spray bottle.

Preparation: Combine oregano oil and distilled water in a small spray bottle. Shake well before each use.

Suggested Usage: Spray once into each nostril up to twice daily to clear nasal passages and reduce congestion.

Benefits: Oregano oil provides strong antiviral and antibacterial properties, helping to clear nasal congestion and fight infections.

141. Astragalus and Ginger Immunity Soup

Ingredients: 2 tablespoons dried astragalus root, 1 tablespoon grated fresh ginger, 6 cups vegetable broth, 1 cup sliced shiitake mushrooms, 1 cup diced carrots, 1 cup chopped celery, 2 garlic cloves (minced).
Preparation: Combine all ingredients in a large pot and bring to a boil. Reduce heat and simmer for 30-40 minutes. Remove astragalus root before serving.
Suggested Usage: Consume 1 cup daily during the cold and flu season for immune support and nourishment.
Benefits: Astragalus enhances immune function, while ginger and shiitake mushrooms add additional anti-inflammatory and immune-boosting properties.

142. Lemon Balm and Chamomile Calming Tea

Ingredients: 1 tablespoon dried lemon balm leaves, 1 tablespoon dried chamomile flowers, 2 cups hot water, 1 teaspoon raw honey.
Preparation: Steep lemon balm and chamomile in hot water for 10-15 minutes. Strain and add honey if desired.
Suggested Usage: Drink 1 cup in the evening to promote relaxation and reduce stress during illness.
Benefits: Combines calming and nervine herbs to support restful sleep, ease anxiety, and enhance overall immune resilience.

143. Fire Cider Immune Booster

Ingredients: 1 cup raw apple cider vinegar, ¼ cup grated fresh horseradish root, ¼ cup grated fresh ginger, 2-3 garlic cloves (crushed), 1 tablespoon cayenne pepper, 1 tablespoon raw honey.
Preparation: Combine all ingredients in a glass jar, seal tightly, and store in a cool, dark place for 4-6 weeks. Shake daily. Strain and store in a glass bottle.
Suggested Usage: Take 1 tablespoon daily as a preventive measure, or up to 3 times daily when feeling ill.
Benefits: Fire cider is a potent remedy that combines antimicrobial, anti-inflammatory, and immune-supporting herbs to fight off infections and boost immunity.

144. Rosehip and Hibiscus Vitamin C Tea

Ingredients: 1 tablespoon dried rosehips, 1 tablespoon dried hibiscus flowers, 2 cups hot water, 1 teaspoon raw honey.
Preparation: Steep rosehips and hibiscus flowers in hot water for 15 minutes. Strain and add honey if desired.
Suggested Usage: Drink 1-2 cups daily to boost vitamin C levels and support immune health.
Benefits: Provides a rich source of vitamin C and antioxidants, strengthening the immune system and protecting against free radical damage.

145. Cat's Claw and Ginger Congestion Relief Tea

Ingredients: 1 tablespoon dried cat's claw bark, 1 teaspoon grated fresh ginger, 2 cups water, 1 teaspoon raw honey.
Preparation: Simmer cat's claw and

ginger in water for 15-20 minutes. Strain and add honey if desired.

Suggested Usage: Drink 1 cup twice daily to relieve congestion and support respiratory health.

Benefits: Cat's claw and ginger work together to reduce inflammation, clear mucus, and provide immune support.

146. Elderberry Gummy Immune Boosters

Ingredients: 1 cup elderberry syrup, 2 tablespoons gelatin powder, 1 tablespoon lemon juice, 1 teaspoon raw honey.

Preparation: Heat elderberry syrup and lemon juice in a small saucepan until warm. Remove from heat and stir in gelatin and honey until fully dissolved. Pour into silicone molds and refrigerate for 1-2 hours until set.

Suggested Usage: Take 1-2 gummies daily during flu season for immune support.

Benefits: Provides the immune-boosting benefits of elderberry in a convenient, delicious form, making it easy for both children and adults to use.

147. Mullein and Hyssop Respiratory Tea

Ingredients: 1 tablespoon dried mullein leaves, 1 tablespoon dried hyssop, 2 cups hot water, 1 teaspoon raw honey.

Preparation: Steep mullein and hyssop in hot water for 15 minutes. Strain and add honey if desired.

Suggested Usage: Drink 1 cup up to 3 times daily to clear congestion and support respiratory health.

Benefits: Mullein and hyssop help clear mucus, reduce congestion, and soothe irritated respiratory tissues.

148. Ginger, Garlic, and Cayenne Detox Tonic

Ingredients: 1 cup warm water, 1 teaspoon grated fresh ginger, 1 garlic clove (minced), ½ teaspoon cayenne pepper, juice of ½ lemon.

Preparation: Combine all ingredients and mix well. Drink immediately.

Suggested Usage: Take 1 shot in the morning for detox support and to boost circulation.

Benefits: Combines potent antimicrobial and detoxifying herbs to support immune health, clear congestion, and enhance overall vitality.

149. Goldenseal and Echinacea Immune Capsules

Ingredients: ¼ cup dried goldenseal root powder, ¼ cup dried echinacea root powder, empty vegetable capsules.

Preparation: Mix goldenseal and echinacea powders thoroughly. Fill each capsule with the mixture using a small spoon or capsule machine. Store capsules in a cool, dry place.

Suggested Usage: Take 1-2 capsules daily during cold and flu season for immune support.

Benefits: Combines the immune-boosting properties of echinacea with the antimicrobial effects of goldenseal to fight infections.

150. Propolis and Honey Throat Spray

The Complete Collection of Barbara O'Neill   Jacqueline Bridge

Ingredients: 1 tablespoon propolis tincture, ½ cup raw honey, ¼ cup warm water, 10 drops peppermint essential oil, 1 spray bottle.

Preparation: Combine all ingredients and mix thoroughly. Pour into a spray bottle.

Suggested Usage: Spray 1-2 times directly onto the throat up to 4 times daily to soothe and protect against infections.

Benefits: Propolis is a powerful antimicrobial that soothes the throat and helps fight infections, while honey coats and protects irritated tissues.

151. Reishi and Chaga Mushroom Tea

Ingredients: 1 tablespoon dried reishi mushroom slices, 1 tablespoon dried chaga mushroom chunks, 4 cups water.

Preparation: Simmer reishi and chaga mushrooms in water for 30-40 minutes. Strain and serve warm.

Suggested Usage: Drink 1 cup daily for immune support and overall vitality.

Benefits: Reishi and chaga mushrooms are powerful adaptogens that support immune health, reduce inflammation, and enhance resilience to stress.

152. Calendula and Licorice Throat Lozenges

Ingredients: 1 tablespoon dried calendula flowers, 1 tablespoon dried licorice root, 1 cup water, ½ cup raw honey, ½ teaspoon slippery elm powder.

Preparation: Simmer calendula and licorice root in water for 20 minutes. Strain and return liquid to the pan. Add honey and slippery elm powder, and heat gently until thickened. Pour into a silicone mold and let harden.

Suggested Usage: Take 1 lozenge as needed to soothe a sore throat and reduce coughing.

Benefits: Combines the soothing and anti-inflammatory properties of calendula with the demulcent and antiviral effects of licorice root.

153. Ginger and Lemon Immune Shot

Ingredients: 2 tablespoons fresh grated ginger, juice of 1 lemon, 1 teaspoon raw honey, ½ cup warm water.

Preparation: Combine all ingredients and mix thoroughly.

Suggested Usage: Take 1 shot in the morning for a quick immune boost and to promote circulation.

Benefits: Provides a potent immune boost, reduces inflammation, and enhances digestion.

154. Black Seed Oil and Honey Tonic

Ingredients: 1 teaspoon black seed oil, 1 teaspoon raw honey.

Preparation: Mix black seed oil and honey until well combined.

Suggested Usage: Take 1 teaspoon daily for immune support and to reduce inflammation.

Benefits: Black seed oil is known for its anti-inflammatory and immune-boosting properties, while honey provides additional antimicrobial support.

155. Rosemary and Sage Herbal Steam

81

Ingredients: 1 tablespoon dried rosemary, 1 tablespoon dried sage, 4 cups boiling water.

Preparation: Place rosemary and sage in a large bowl and pour boiling water over the herbs. Lean over the bowl with a towel draped over your head, creating a tent to trap the steam. Inhale deeply for 5-10 minutes.

Suggested Usage: Use 1-2 times daily during congestion or respiratory discomfort.

Benefits: Opens up nasal passages, soothes irritated respiratory tissues, and provides antimicrobial support for respiratory health.

156. Yarrow, Peppermint, and Elderflower Fever Tea

Ingredients: 1 tablespoon dried yarrow, 1 tablespoon dried peppermint, 1 tablespoon dried elderflower, 2 cups hot water.

Preparation: Steep yarrow, peppermint, and elderflower in hot water for 10-15 minutes. Strain and serve warm.

Suggested Usage: Drink 1-2 cups daily at the onset of a fever to promote sweating and reduce fever.

Benefits: Promotes sweating to help break fevers, reduces inflammation, and supports the body's natural immune response.

157. Garlic and Thyme Ear Oil

Ingredients: 4-5 garlic cloves (crushed), 1 tablespoon dried thyme, ½ cup olive oil.

Preparation: Gently heat garlic and thyme in olive oil over low heat for 30 minutes. Allow to cool, strain, and store in a glass dropper bottle.

Suggested Usage: Apply 2-3 drops in the affected ear up to twice daily to relieve earaches and fight infections.

Benefits: Garlic and thyme provide strong antimicrobial and anti-inflammatory properties to soothe ear pain and fight infection.

158. Linden and Lemon Verbena Relaxation Tea

Ingredients: 1 tablespoon dried linden flowers, 1 tablespoon dried lemon verbena leaves, 2 cups hot water.

Preparation: Steep linden and lemon verbena in hot water for 10-15 minutes. Strain and serve warm.

Suggested Usage: Drink 1 cup in the evening to promote relaxation and reduce stress.

Benefits: Combines the gentle calming effects of linden with the uplifting properties of lemon verbena, making it ideal for stress relief and relaxation.

159. Onion and Honey Cough Syrup

Ingredients: 1 medium onion, thinly sliced, ½ cup raw honey.

Preparation: Place the sliced onion in a glass jar and cover with honey. Let sit for 8-12 hours until the onion releases its juice and the honey is infused. Strain and store in a glass jar.

Suggested Usage: Take 1 teaspoon every 2-3 hours to soothe a cough and reduce mucus.

Benefits: Onion and honey are natural expectorants, making this remedy effective for clearing mucus and soothing the throat.

160. Peppermint Chest Rub

Ingredients: ¼ cup coconut oil, 10 drops peppermint essential oil, 5 drops eucalyptus essential oil, 5 drops rosemary essential oil.
Preparation: Melt the coconut oil and stir in essential oils. Mix thoroughly and transfer to a small glass jar. Allow to solidify.
Suggested Usage: Apply a small amount to the chest and throat area before bedtime or when experiencing respiratory congestion.
Benefits: Provides a cooling sensation that opens airways, reduces congestion, and soothes irritated respiratory tissues.

161. Miso and Shiitake Mushroom Immunity Soup

Ingredients: 2 cups vegetable broth, ¼ cup sliced fresh shiitake mushrooms, 1 tablespoon miso paste, 1 garlic clove (minced), 1 teaspoon grated fresh ginger.
Preparation: Combine all ingredients except miso in a saucepan and simmer for 20 minutes. Remove from heat and stir in miso paste until dissolved.
Suggested Usage: Eat 1 cup daily during cold and flu season for immune support.
Benefits: Shiitake mushrooms enhance immune health, while miso provides beneficial probiotics to support gut and immune function.

162. Nettle and Ginger Detox Tea

Ingredients: 1 tablespoon dried nettle leaves, 1 teaspoon grated fresh ginger, 2 cups hot water, 1 teaspoon lemon juice.
Preparation: Steep nettle leaves and grated ginger in hot water for 10-15 minutes. Strain and add lemon juice.
Suggested Usage: Drink 1-2 cups daily for detoxification and immune support.
Benefits: Nettle is rich in vitamins and minerals, supporting detox pathways, while ginger enhances circulation and boosts immunity.

163. Eucalyptus and Lavender Bath Soak

Ingredients: 1 cup Epsom salts, 1 tablespoon dried eucalyptus leaves, 1 tablespoon dried lavender flowers, 10 drops eucalyptus essential oil, 10 drops lavender essential oil.
Preparation: Mix all ingredients in a bowl and stir until well combined. Store in a glass jar.
Suggested Usage: Add ½ cup of the mixture to a warm bath and soak for 20-30 minutes.
Benefits: Eucalyptus opens up the respiratory passages, while lavender provides relaxation and stress relief. Epsom salts aid in muscle relaxation and detoxification.

164. Holy Basil and Ashwagandha Adaptogen Tea

Ingredients: 1 tablespoon dried holy basil leaves, 1 teaspoon dried ashwagandha root, 2 cups hot water, 1 teaspoon raw honey.
Preparation: Steep holy basil and ashwagandha root in hot water for 10-15 minutes. Strain and add honey if desired.
Suggested Usage: Drink 1-2 cups daily to support adrenal health and reduce stress.

Benefits: Combines two powerful adaptogens that enhance the body's response to stress, balance energy, and boost immunity.

165. Clove and Cinnamon Respiratory Tea

Ingredients: 1 cinnamon stick, 4-5 whole cloves, 1 teaspoon grated fresh ginger, 2 cups hot water, 1 teaspoon raw honey.
Preparation: Steep the cinnamon stick, cloves, and ginger in hot water for 10-15 minutes. Strain and add honey if desired.
Suggested Usage: Drink 1 cup up to twice daily to relieve respiratory congestion and soothe the throat.
Benefits: Combines warming herbs to support respiratory health, reduce congestion, and provide antimicrobial properties.

166. Lemon and Ginger Immune Gummies

Ingredients: 1 cup lemon juice, 2 tablespoons grated fresh ginger, ¼ cup raw honey, 2 tablespoons gelatin powder.
Preparation: Heat lemon juice and grated ginger in a small saucepan until warm. Remove from heat and stir in honey and gelatin powder until fully dissolved. Pour into silicone molds and refrigerate for 1-2 hours until set.
Suggested Usage: Take 1-2 gummies daily for immune support.
Benefits: Provides the immune-boosting benefits of lemon and ginger in a tasty, easy-to-consume form.

167. Burdock and Yellow Dock Root Detox Tea

Ingredients: 1 tablespoon dried burdock root, 1 tablespoon dried yellow dock root, 3 cups water, 1 teaspoon lemon juice.
Preparation: Simmer burdock and yellow dock roots in water for 20-30 minutes. Strain and add lemon juice.
Suggested Usage: Drink 1 cup twice daily to support liver health and detoxification.
Benefits: Promotes liver detoxification, supports digestion, and enhances overall immune health by reducing toxin load.

168. Apple Cider Vinegar and Garlic Sinus Tonic

Ingredients: ½ cup raw apple cider vinegar, 5-6 garlic cloves (crushed), 1 tablespoon grated fresh ginger, juice of 1 lemon, 1 teaspoon cayenne pepper.
Preparation: Combine all ingredients in a glass jar, seal tightly, and store in a cool, dark place for 1-2 weeks. Shake daily. Strain and store in a glass bottle.
Suggested Usage: Take 1-2 teaspoons daily for sinus relief and immune support.
Benefits: Combines the antimicrobial and decongestant effects of garlic and ginger with the detoxifying properties of apple cider vinegar.

169. Ginseng and Astragalus Energy Tea

Ingredients: 1 tablespoon dried ginseng root, 1 tablespoon dried astragalus root, 2 cups water.
Preparation: Simmer ginseng and astragalus roots in water for 20 minutes.

Strain and serve warm.

Suggested Usage: Drink 1 cup daily to boost energy and support immune function.

Benefits: Combines two powerful immune-boosting and adaptogenic herbs to enhance energy levels, support stamina, and build long-term resilience.

170. Osha and Wild Cherry Bark Cough Syrup

Ingredients: 1 cup dried osha root, ½ cup dried wild cherry bark, 4 cups water, 1 cup raw honey.

Preparation: Combine osha root and wild cherry bark with water in a saucepan. Bring to a boil, then simmer for 30 minutes. Strain, return liquid to the pan, and simmer until reduced by half. Remove from heat and stir in honey. Store in a glass jar.

Suggested Usage: Take 1 tablespoon every 2-3 hours to soothe coughs and clear congestion.

Benefits: Combines two powerful respiratory herbs that soothe coughs, reduce throat irritation, and promote respiratory health.

171. Schisandra Berry Adaptogen Tea

Ingredients: 1 tablespoon dried schisandra berries, 2 cups hot water, 1 teaspoon raw honey.

Preparation: Steep schisandra berries in hot water for 15 minutes. Strain and add honey if desired.

Suggested Usage: Drink 1 cup daily to support stress management and enhance immune health.

Benefits: Schisandra berries are adaptogens that support the adrenal system, reduce stress, and provide antioxidant benefits.

172. Horehound and Licorice Root Cough Drops

Ingredients: 1 cup dried horehound, 1 cup dried licorice root, 2 cups water, 1 cup raw honey, ¼ cup powdered sugar (optional).

Preparation: Simmer horehound and licorice root in water for 30 minutes. Strain and return liquid to the pan. Add honey and simmer until thickened. Pour into candy molds and let harden. Roll in powdered sugar if desired.

Suggested Usage: Take 1 lozenge as needed to soothe a sore throat and reduce coughing.

Benefits: Combines the expectorant properties of horehound with the soothing and antiviral effects of licorice root.

173. Fenugreek and Thyme Sinus-Clearing Tea

Ingredients: 1 teaspoon fenugreek seeds, 1 teaspoon dried thyme, 2 cups hot water, 1 teaspoon raw honey.

Preparation: Crush fenugreek seeds slightly, then steep with thyme in hot water for 10-15 minutes. Strain and add honey if desired.

Suggested Usage: Drink 1 cup twice daily to clear sinuses and support respiratory health.

Benefits: Fenugreek and thyme help clear mucus, soothe the digestive system, and provide antimicrobial support, making this tea beneficial for sinus congestion and respiratory discomfort.

174. Chamomile and Lavender Bedtime Tea

Ingredients: 1 tablespoon dried chamomile flowers, 1 tablespoon dried lavender buds, 2 cups hot water, 1 teaspoon raw honey.

Preparation: Steep chamomile and lavender in hot water for 10-15 minutes. Strain and add honey if desired.

Suggested Usage: Drink 1 cup 30 minutes before bedtime to promote relaxation and restful sleep.

Benefits: Combines the calming and nervine properties of chamomile and lavender, making it ideal for reducing anxiety and promoting deep, restful sleep.

175. Elderberry and Ginger Syrup

Ingredients: 1 cup dried elderberries, 4 cups water, 1 tablespoon grated fresh ginger, 1 cup raw honey.

Preparation: Combine elderberries, water, and ginger in a saucepan. Bring to a boil, then reduce heat and simmer for 30-45 minutes until the liquid is reduced by half. Remove from heat, strain, and stir in honey. Store in a glass jar.

Suggested Usage: Take 1 tablespoon daily during cold and flu season, or up to 3 times daily at the onset of symptoms.

Benefits: Provides strong antiviral and immune-boosting properties, helping to reduce the severity and duration of colds and flu.

176. Sage and Lemon Gargle

Ingredients: 1 tablespoon dried sage, 1 cup hot water, juice of ½ lemon, ½ teaspoon sea salt.

Preparation: Steep sage in hot water for 10 minutes. Strain and add lemon juice and salt. Allow to cool to a comfortable temperature.

Suggested Usage: Gargle with ¼ cup of the solution up to 3 times daily to soothe a sore throat and reduce inflammation.

Benefits: Sage and lemon combine strong astringent and antimicrobial properties to reduce throat irritation and fight infection.

177. Turmeric and Ginger Golden Paste

Ingredients: ¼ cup turmeric powder, 2 tablespoons grated fresh ginger, 1 teaspoon ground black pepper, ½ cup water, 2 tablespoons coconut oil.

Preparation: Combine turmeric, ginger, and black pepper in a small saucepan. Add water and heat gently until a thick paste forms. Remove from heat and stir in coconut oil. Store in a glass jar.

Suggested Usage: Take 1 teaspoon daily for immune support, or mix into warm milk or tea.

Benefits: Combines the potent anti-inflammatory effects of turmeric and ginger, enhanced by black pepper for improved absorption.

178. Suma Root Immune Tonic

Ingredients: 1 teaspoon dried suma root powder, 1 cup warm water, 1 teaspoon raw honey.

Preparation: Mix suma root powder into warm water until dissolved. Add honey and stir well.

Suggested Usage: Drink once daily in the morning to boost energy and enhance overall vitality.

Benefits: Enhances energy, supports stamina, and balances hormones, making it a powerful tonic for immune support and overall health.

179. Lemongrass and Ginger Immune Tea

Ingredients: 1 tablespoon dried lemongrass, 1 tablespoon grated fresh ginger, 2 cups hot water, 1 teaspoon raw honey.

Preparation: Steep lemongrass and ginger in hot water for 10-15 minutes. Strain and add honey if desired.

Suggested Usage: Drink 1-2 cups daily for immune support and to reduce inflammation.

Benefits: Combines the soothing and anti-inflammatory effects of ginger with the refreshing properties of lemongrass to support immunity and improve digestion.

180. Peppermint and Fennel Digestive Tea

Ingredients: 1 tablespoon dried peppermint leaves, 1 teaspoon fennel seeds, 2 cups hot water.

Preparation: Steep peppermint and fennel in hot water for 10-15 minutes. Strain and serve warm.

Suggested Usage: Drink 1 cup after meals to soothe digestive discomfort and reduce bloating.

Benefits: Peppermint relaxes the digestive tract, while fennel reduces gas and bloating, making this tea ideal for digestive support and relief.

181. Bay Leaf and Thyme Respiratory Steam

Ingredients: 4-5 dried bay leaves, 1 tablespoon dried thyme, 4 cups boiling water.

Preparation: Place bay leaves and thyme in a large bowl and pour boiling water over the herbs. Lean over the bowl with a towel draped over your head, creating a tent to trap the steam. Inhale deeply for 5-10 minutes.

Suggested Usage: Use 1-2 times daily during colds or congestion for respiratory relief.

Benefits: Opens up nasal passages, clears congestion, and provides antimicrobial support for the respiratory system.

182. Black Pepper and Turmeric Capsules for Congestion

Ingredients: ¼ cup turmeric powder, 1 teaspoon ground black pepper, empty vegetable capsules.

Preparation: Mix turmeric powder and black pepper thoroughly. Fill each capsule with the mixture using a small spoon or capsule machine. Store capsules in a cool, dry place.

Suggested Usage: Take 1-2 capsules daily to reduce congestion and inflammation.

Benefits: Combines the potent anti-inflammatory effects of turmeric with black pepper's ability to enhance absorption, making this remedy ideal for reducing congestion and inflammation.

Book 13: Fighting Infections with Herbs

Antibacterial and Antiviral Herbs

Herbs have been used for centuries to combat bacterial and viral infections. Unlike synthetic drugs, which often target a single pathogen or mechanism, many herbs have broad-spectrum antimicrobial properties, acting on multiple levels to inhibit the growth of harmful microbes while supporting the body's natural defenses. Some herbs work by directly killing pathogens, while others enhance the immune response, making them powerful allies in fighting infections.

One of the most well-known antibacterial herbs is **garlic (Allium sativum)**. Garlic contains the compound allicin, which has been shown to have strong antibacterial, antiviral, and antifungal properties. It is particularly effective against respiratory infections and can be used to treat conditions like bronchitis, sinusitis, and colds. Fresh garlic, crushed or chopped to release allicin, can be consumed raw, added to meals, or made into a potent garlic and honey syrup for additional immune support.

Echinacea (Echinacea purpurea) is a popular herb for both bacterial and viral infections. It enhances the activity of white blood cells, helping the body fight off infections more effectively. Echinacea is particularly useful for treating upper respiratory infections, such as the common cold and flu. Studies have shown that echinacea can reduce the severity and duration of these infections when taken at the onset of symptoms. It is commonly prepared as a tea, tincture, or capsule.

Elderberry (Sambucus nigra) is another powerful antiviral herb that has been used traditionally for colds and flu. Elderberries contain flavonoids that inhibit the replication of viruses, making it harder for the infection to spread. Clinical studies have shown that elderberry can shorten the duration of the flu and alleviate symptoms such as fever, fatigue, and congestion. Elderberry syrup, tincture, or lozenges are popular remedies taken at the first sign of illness.

Oregano (Origanum vulgare) is a potent antimicrobial herb, particularly when used in the form of oregano oil. Oregano oil contains carvacrol and thymol, compounds known for their strong antibacterial and antiviral effects. It is effective against a wide range of pathogens, including E. coli, staphylococcus, and certain viruses. Due to its potency, oregano oil should be diluted before use and can be taken internally or applied topically for skin infections.

Thyme (Thymus vulgaris) is another herb with strong antimicrobial properties. It has been shown to be effective against both bacterial and viral pathogens, making it a versatile remedy for respiratory infections and digestive issues. Thyme contains thymol, a powerful antiseptic that can kill harmful microbes and support respiratory health by thinning mucus and promoting expectoration. Thyme can be used as a tea, tincture, or in steam inhalations.

Calendula (Calendula officinalis) is a gentle yet effective herb with antibacterial and antiviral properties. It is commonly used to treat skin infections, wounds, and sore throats. Calendula's anti-inflammatory and wound-healing properties make it an excellent choice for soothing irritated tissues and promoting faster healing. It can be used topically as a salve, wash, or gargle, or taken internally as a tea.

Olive leaf (Olea europaea) is a potent antiviral herb, known for its ability to inhibit viral replication and reduce the spread of infections. Olive leaf contains oleuropein, a compound that has been shown to be effective against a range of viruses, including influenza and herpes. Olive leaf extract can be taken as a tea, tincture, or in capsule form to combat viral infections and support immune health.

Licorice root (Glycyrrhiza glabra) is a soothing herb with strong antiviral properties. It works by interfering with the replication of viruses and modulating the immune response. Licorice is commonly used to treat respiratory infections, such as colds, bronchitis, and sore throats. Due to its soothing effects, licorice is often combined with other herbs in teas and syrups for treating coughs and throat irritation.

Natural Antibiotic Alternatives

With the growing concern over antibiotic resistance, natural antibiotic alternatives are becoming increasingly popular. These herbal remedies not only fight infections effectively but also support the body's overall health, reducing the risk of side effects associated with conventional antibiotics. Herbal antibiotics typically have a broader range of action, targeting multiple pathogens simultaneously while also boosting the immune system.

Goldenseal (Hydrastis canadensis) is a well-known herbal antibiotic traditionally used to treat a variety of infections, including respiratory, digestive, and urinary tract infections. It contains the alkaloid berberine, which has been shown to inhibit the growth of many bacteria, such as staphylococcus and streptococcus. Goldenseal is often used in combination with echinacea to enhance its immune-stimulating properties.

Usnea (Usnea barbata), also known as Old Man's Beard, is a lichen with potent antibacterial and antifungal properties. It is effective against gram-positive bacteria, such as streptococcus and staphylococcus, making it useful for treating respiratory and skin infections. Usnea can be used in tincture form or as a poultice for topical infections.

Myrrh (Commiphora myrrha) is an ancient remedy with strong antibacterial and antifungal effects. It has been used traditionally to treat oral infections, digestive issues, and respiratory conditions. Myrrh is also known for its wound-healing properties, making it useful for treating skin infections and ulcers. Myrrh can be used as a tincture, mouthwash, or added to salves for topical use.

Neem (Azadirachta indica) is an Ayurvedic herb with broad-spectrum antimicrobial properties. It is effective against a wide range of bacteria, fungi, and viruses, making it useful for treating skin infections, digestive issues, and respiratory conditions. Neem can be used as a tea, tincture, or applied topically in the form of oils and salves.

Berberine-containing herbs, such as Oregon grape (Mahonia aquifolium), barberry (Berberis vulgaris), and goldenseal, are powerful natural antibiotics. Berberine is effective against a variety of bacteria, including H. pylori, E. coli, and MRSA. It works by disrupting the bacterial cell wall and inhibiting enzyme function. These herbs are commonly used for digestive and respiratory infections.

Tea tree oil (Melaleuca alternifolia) is a potent antimicrobial oil used topically for skin infections, acne, and fungal conditions. Its antibacterial and antiviral properties make it a valuable addition to natural first aid kits. Tea tree oil should always be diluted before applying to the skin to avoid irritation.

These natural alternatives can be used alone or in combination to create a comprehensive approach to fighting infections. Whether used internally as teas, tinctures, and capsules, or applied topically as salves and washes, these herbal antibiotics provide effective, holistic support for treating and preventing infections naturally.

Remedies for Fighting Infections

183. Garlic and Honey Antimicrobial Tonic

Ingredients: 1 cup raw honey, 10-12 garlic cloves (peeled and crushed).
Preparation: Place the peeled and crushed garlic cloves in a glass jar and cover with honey. Seal tightly and let it infuse for 1-2 weeks, shaking occasionally.
Suggested Usage: Take 1 teaspoon daily for immune support, or 1 teaspoon every 2-3 hours when fighting an infection.
Benefits: Combines the potent antimicrobial properties of garlic with the soothing and immune-boosting effects of honey to fight bacterial and viral infections.

184. Echinacea and Goldenseal Immune Tincture

Ingredients: ½ cup dried echinacea root, ½ cup dried goldenseal root, 2 cups vodka or brandy (40% alcohol), 1 glass jar with lid.
Preparation: Place echinacea and goldenseal roots in a glass jar and cover with alcohol. Seal the jar and store in a cool, dark place for 4-6 weeks, shaking daily. Strain and store in a dark glass bottle.

Suggested Usage: Take 1 teaspoon up to 3 times daily at the onset of illness for immune support and to fight infections.

Benefits: Echinacea boosts immune function, while goldenseal provides powerful antimicrobial effects, making this tincture effective against colds, flu, and other infections.

185. Elderberry and Ginger Immune Syrup

Ingredients: 1 cup dried elderberries, 4 cups water, 1 tablespoon grated fresh ginger, 1 cup raw honey.

Preparation: Combine elderberries, water, and ginger in a saucepan. Bring to a boil, then simmer for 30-45 minutes until the liquid is reduced by half. Remove from heat, strain, and stir in honey. Store in a glass jar.

Suggested Usage: Take 1 tablespoon daily for prevention, or up to 3 times daily at the first sign of illness.

Benefits: Elderberry and ginger combine to create a powerful immune-boosting syrup that helps reduce the duration and severity of colds and flu.

186. Thyme and Sage Throat Gargle

Ingredients: 1 tablespoon dried thyme, 1 tablespoon dried sage, 2 cups hot water, 1 teaspoon sea salt.

Preparation: Steep thyme and sage in hot water for 10 minutes. Strain and add sea salt. Allow to cool to a comfortable temperature.

Suggested Usage: Gargle with ¼ cup of the solution up to 3 times daily to soothe a sore throat and reduce inflammation.

Benefits: Combines strong antimicrobial and anti-inflammatory properties to reduce throat irritation and fight bacterial infections.

187. Oregano Oil Antiviral Capsules

Ingredients: 10-15 drops oregano essential oil, ¼ cup olive oil, empty vegetable capsules.

Preparation: Combine oregano oil with olive oil and fill capsules using a small dropper. Store in a cool, dry place.

Suggested Usage: Take 1 capsule daily for immune support, or up to 3 times daily during acute infections.

Benefits: Oregano oil is a potent antiviral and antibacterial herb, making these capsules highly effective for fighting infections and supporting respiratory health.

188. Olive Leaf Antiviral Tea

Ingredients: 1 tablespoon dried olive leaves, 2 cups hot water.

Preparation: Steep olive leaves in hot water for 10-15 minutes. Strain and serve warm.

Suggested Usage: Drink 1-2 cups daily to support immune health and combat viral infections.

Benefits: Olive leaf is a powerful antiviral herb that inhibits viral replication and strengthens the body's defenses.

189. Calendula and Chamomile Wound Wash

Ingredients: 1 tablespoon dried calendula flowers, 1 tablespoon dried chamomile flowers, 2 cups hot water.

Preparation: Steep calendula and chamomile flowers in hot water for 15 minutes. Strain and let cool.

Suggested Usage: Use as a gentle wash to cleanse wounds and promote healing.

Benefits: Calendula and chamomile provide antimicrobial and anti-inflammatory support to promote healing and prevent infection.

190. Usnea and Echinacea Throat Spray

Ingredients: ½ cup dried usnea, ½ cup dried echinacea root, 1 cup vodka or brandy (40% alcohol), 1 cup distilled water, 10 drops peppermint essential oil, 1 small spray bottle.

Preparation: Combine usnea and echinacea with alcohol in a glass jar and let steep for 4-6 weeks. Strain and dilute with an equal amount of distilled water. Add peppermint oil and pour into a spray bottle.

Suggested Usage: Spray 2-3 times directly onto the throat up to 4 times daily to reduce sore throat symptoms and fight infection.

Benefits: Usnea and echinacea work synergistically to provide antimicrobial and immune-boosting effects, while peppermint soothes and reduces inflammation.

191. Goldenseal and Myrrh Mouthwash

Ingredients: 1 tablespoon dried goldenseal root, 1 tablespoon myrrh gum powder, 1 cup boiling water, 1 teaspoon sea salt.

Preparation: Steep goldenseal and myrrh in boiling water for 20 minutes. Strain and add sea salt. Allow to cool.

Suggested Usage: Swish 1-2 tablespoons in the mouth for 1-2 minutes up to 3 times daily to treat oral infections and reduce inflammation.

Benefits: Goldenseal and myrrh have powerful antimicrobial properties, making this mouthwash effective for treating gum disease, mouth ulcers, and sore throats.

192. Licorice and Marshmallow Root Cough Syrup

Ingredients: 1 cup dried licorice root, 1 cup dried marshmallow root, 4 cups water, 1 cup raw honey.

Preparation: Combine licorice root and marshmallow root with water in a saucepan. Bring to a boil, then simmer for 30 minutes. Strain, return liquid to the pan, and simmer until reduced by half. Remove from heat and stir in honey. Store in a glass jar.

Suggested Usage: Take 1 tablespoon every 2-3 hours to soothe a sore throat and reduce coughing.

Benefits: Licorice and marshmallow root coat and soothe the throat, reduce inflammation, and provide antiviral support.

193. Ginger and Lemon Immune Shot

Ingredients: 2 tablespoons grated fresh ginger, juice of 1 lemon, 1 teaspoon raw honey, ½ cup warm water.

Preparation: Combine all ingredients and mix thoroughly.

Suggested Usage: Take 1 shot in the

morning for a quick immune boost and to promote circulation.

Benefits: Provides a potent immune boost, reduces inflammation, and enhances digestion, making it an ideal daily tonic during flu season.

194. Cinnamon and Clove Antimicrobial Chai

Ingredients: 1 cinnamon stick, 4-5 whole cloves, 2 cups water, 1 cup milk (or plant-based milk), 1 teaspoon grated fresh ginger, 1 teaspoon raw honey.

Preparation: Combine cinnamon, cloves, and ginger in water and bring to a boil. Reduce heat and simmer for 10 minutes. Add milk and simmer for another 5 minutes. Strain and add honey before serving.

Suggested Usage: Drink 1 cup daily during cold and flu season for antimicrobial support.

Benefits: Combines warming herbs with strong antimicrobial properties to support immune function, reduce inflammation, and ease respiratory congestion.

195. Fire Cider Immune Booster

Ingredients: 1 cup raw apple cider vinegar, ¼ cup grated fresh horseradish root, ¼ cup grated fresh ginger, 2 garlic cloves (crushed), 1 tablespoon cayenne pepper, 1 tablespoon raw honey.

Preparation: Combine all ingredients in a glass jar, seal tightly, and store in a cool, dark place for 4-6 weeks. Shake daily. Strain and store in a glass bottle.

Suggested Usage: Take 1 tablespoon daily as a preventive measure, or up to 4 times daily when sick.

Benefits: Potent antimicrobial, anti-inflammatory, and immune-boosting properties make this tonic effective for fighting infections, supporting digestion, and reducing inflammation.

196. Cat's Claw and Ginger Anti-Inflammatory Tea

Ingredients: 1 tablespoon dried cat's claw bark, 1 teaspoon grated fresh ginger, 2 cups water, 1 teaspoon raw honey.

Preparation: Simmer cat's claw and ginger in water for 15-20 minutes. Strain and add honey if desired.

Suggested Usage: Drink 1 cup twice daily to support immune health and reduce inflammation.

Benefits: Cat's claw and ginger work together to reduce inflammation, support the immune system, and promote overall vitality.

197. Propolis and Honey Throat Spray

Ingredients: 1 tablespoon propolis tincture, ½ cup raw honey, ¼ cup warm water, 10 drops peppermint essential oil, 1 spray bottle.

Preparation: Combine all ingredients and mix thoroughly. Pour into a spray bottle.

Suggested Usage: Spray 1-2 times directly onto the throat up to 4 times daily to soothe and protect against infections.

Benefits: Propolis is a powerful antimicrobial that soothes the throat and helps fight infections, while honey coats and protects irritated tissues.

198. Astragalus and Reishi Mushroom Tonic

Ingredients: 1 tablespoon dried astragalus root, 1 tablespoon dried reishi mushroom slices, 4 cups water.
Preparation: Simmer astragalus and reishi in water for 30-40 minutes. Strain and serve warm.
Suggested Usage: Drink 1 cup daily to support immune function, enhance energy, and reduce stress.
Benefits: Astragalus and reishi mushrooms provide immune-boosting, adaptogenic, and anti-inflammatory benefits, making this tonic ideal for long-term health support.

199. Neem Leaf Antibacterial Tincture

Ingredients: 1 cup dried neem leaves, 2 cups vodka or brandy (40% alcohol), 1 glass jar with lid.
Preparation: Place neem leaves in a glass jar and cover with alcohol. Seal and store in a cool, dark place for 4-6 weeks, shaking daily. Strain and store in a dark glass bottle.
Suggested Usage: Take 10-20 drops diluted in water up to twice daily for antibacterial support.
Benefits: Neem is a broad-spectrum antimicrobial herb that supports the body's defense against bacterial infections, while also promoting detoxification and healthy skin.

200. Holy Basil and Lemon Balm Anti-Viral Tea

Ingredients: 1 tablespoon dried holy basil leaves, 1 tablespoon dried lemon balm leaves, 2 cups hot water, 1 teaspoon raw honey.
Preparation: Steep holy basil and lemon balm in hot water for 10-15 minutes. Strain and add honey if desired.
Suggested Usage: Drink 1-2 cups daily to support immune health and fight viral infections.
Benefits: Holy basil and lemon balm combine strong antiviral properties with calming effects, making this tea ideal for reducing stress and enhancing immune function.

201. Sage and Rosemary Sinus Steam

Ingredients: 1 tablespoon dried sage, 1 tablespoon dried rosemary, 4 cups boiling water.
Preparation: Place sage and rosemary in a large bowl and pour boiling water over the herbs. Lean over the bowl with a towel draped over your head to trap the steam. Inhale deeply for 5-10 minutes.
Suggested Usage: Use 1-2 times daily during colds or congestion for sinus relief.
Benefits: Opens up nasal passages, soothes irritated respiratory tissues, and provides antimicrobial support for respiratory health.

202. Yarrow and Peppermint Fever-Reducing Tea

Ingredients: 1 tablespoon dried yarrow, 1 tablespoon dried peppermint, 2 cups hot water, 1 teaspoon raw honey.
Preparation: Steep yarrow and peppermint in hot water for 10-15

minutes. Strain and add honey if desired.

Suggested Usage: Drink 1-2 cups daily at the onset of fever to reduce temperature and promote sweating.

Benefits: Yarrow induces sweating to break fevers, while peppermint cools the body and soothes the digestive system.

203. Turmeric and Black Pepper Anti-Inflammatory Capsules

Ingredients: ¼ cup turmeric powder, 1 teaspoon ground black pepper, empty vegetable capsules.

Preparation: Mix turmeric powder and black pepper thoroughly. Fill each capsule with the mixture using a small spoon or capsule machine. Store capsules in a cool, dry place.

Suggested Usage: Take 1-2 capsules daily to reduce inflammation and support immune health.

Benefits: Combines the potent anti-inflammatory effects of turmeric with black pepper's ability to enhance absorption, making this remedy ideal for reducing chronic inflammation.

204. Elderflower and Linden Cold Relief Tea

Ingredients: 1 tablespoon dried elderflower, 1 tablespoon dried linden flowers, 2 cups hot water, 1 teaspoon raw honey.

Preparation: Steep elderflower and linden in hot water for 10-15 minutes. Strain and add honey if desired.

Suggested Usage: Drink 1-2 cups daily at the onset of cold symptoms to reduce congestion and support recovery.

Benefits: Elderflower and linden work together to reduce fever, relieve congestion, and support the immune system during illness.

205. Schisandra Berry Adaptogen Tea

Ingredients: 1 tablespoon dried schisandra berries, 2 cups hot water, 1 teaspoon raw honey.

Preparation: Steep schisandra berries in hot water for 15 minutes. Strain and add honey if desired.

Suggested Usage: Drink 1 cup daily to support stress management and enhance immune health.

Benefits: Schisandra berries are powerful adaptogens that support the adrenal system, reduce stress, and provide antioxidant benefits, making this tea ideal for long-term vitality and resilience.

206. Garlic and Mullein Ear Oil

Ingredients: 4-5 garlic cloves (crushed), 1 tablespoon dried mullein flowers, ½ cup olive oil.

Preparation: Gently heat garlic and mullein in olive oil over low heat for 30 minutes. Allow to cool, strain, and store in a glass dropper bottle.

Suggested Usage: Apply 2-3 drops in the affected ear up to twice daily to relieve earaches and fight infections.

Benefits: Garlic and mullein provide antimicrobial and anti-inflammatory properties, helping to soothe ear infections and reduce pain.

207. Bay Leaf and Eucalyptus Steam Inhalation

Ingredients: 4-5 dried bay leaves, 1 tablespoon dried eucalyptus leaves, 4 cups boiling water.

Preparation: Place bay leaves and eucalyptus in a large bowl and pour boiling water over the herbs. Lean over the bowl with a towel draped over your head, creating a tent to trap the steam. Inhale deeply for 5-10 minutes.

Suggested Usage: Use 1-2 times daily during colds or respiratory discomfort for relief.

Benefits: Opens up nasal passages, soothes irritated respiratory tissues, and provides antimicrobial support for respiratory health.

208. Chamomile and Lavender Bedtime Tea

Ingredients: 1 tablespoon dried chamomile flowers, 1 tablespoon dried lavender buds, 2 cups hot water, 1 teaspoon raw honey.

Preparation: Steep chamomile and lavender in hot water for 10-15 minutes. Strain and add honey if desired.

Suggested Usage: Drink 1 cup 30 minutes before bedtime to promote relaxation and restful sleep.

Benefits: Combines the calming and nervine properties of chamomile and lavender, making it ideal for reducing anxiety and promoting deep, restful sleep.

209. Ginger, Garlic, and Cayenne Detox Tonic

Ingredients: 1 cup warm water, 1 teaspoon grated fresh ginger, 1 garlic clove (minced), ½ teaspoon cayenne pepper, juice of ½ lemon.

Preparation: Combine all ingredients and mix well. Drink immediately.

Suggested Usage: Take 1 shot in the morning for detox support and to boost circulation.

Benefits: Combines potent antimicrobial and detoxifying herbs to support immune health, clear congestion, and enhance overall vitality.

210. Reishi and Chaga Mushroom Immune Brew

Ingredients: 1 tablespoon dried reishi mushroom slices, 1 tablespoon dried chaga mushroom chunks, 4 cups water.

Preparation: Simmer reishi and chaga mushrooms in water for 30-40 minutes. Strain and serve warm.

Suggested Usage: Drink 1 cup daily for immune support and overall vitality.

Benefits: Reishi and chaga mushrooms are powerful adaptogens that support immune health, reduce inflammation, and enhance resilience to stress.

211. Eucalyptus and Peppermint Chest Rub

Ingredients: ¼ cup shea butter, ¼ cup coconut oil, 10 drops eucalyptus essential oil, 10 drops peppermint essential oil, 5 drops rosemary essential oil.

Preparation: Melt shea butter and coconut oil together using a double boiler. Remove from heat and stir in essential oils. Transfer to a small glass jar and let solidify.

Suggested Usage: Apply a small amount to the chest and back area before bedtime or during respiratory congestion.

Benefits: Opens up airways, reduces

congestion, and soothes irritated respiratory tissues, providing relief during colds and coughs.

212. Nettle and Rosehip Vitamin C Tea

Ingredients: 1 tablespoon dried nettle leaves, 1 tablespoon dried rosehips, 2 cups hot water, 1 teaspoon raw honey.
Preparation: Steep nettle and rosehips in hot water for 10-15 minutes. Strain and add honey if desired.
Suggested Usage: Drink 1-2 cups daily to support immune health and increase vitamin C levels.
Benefits: Combines the nutrient-rich properties of nettle with the high vitamin C content of rosehips, providing a powerful immune-boosting and anti-inflammatory tea.

213. Lemon Balm and Licorice Root Antiviral Tea

Ingredients: 1 tablespoon dried lemon balm leaves, 1 tablespoon dried licorice root, 2 cups hot water, 1 teaspoon raw honey.
Preparation: Steep lemon balm and licorice root in hot water for 15 minutes. Strain and add honey if desired.
Suggested Usage: Drink 1-2 cups daily during cold and flu season to prevent and manage viral infections.
Benefits: Combines the antiviral properties of lemon balm and licorice to support immune health, soothe the respiratory tract, and reduce inflammation.

214. Onion and Honey Cough Syrup

Ingredients: 1 medium onion (thinly sliced), ½ cup raw honey.
Preparation: Place the sliced onion in a glass jar and cover with honey. Let sit for 8-12 hours until the onion releases its juice and the honey is infused. Strain and store in a glass jar.
Suggested Usage: Take 1 teaspoon every 2-3 hours to soothe a cough and reduce mucus.
Benefits: Onion and honey are natural expectorants, making this remedy effective for clearing mucus and soothing the throat.

215. Mullein and Thyme Respiratory Tea

Ingredients: 1 tablespoon dried mullein leaves, 1 teaspoon dried thyme, 1 cup hot water, 1 teaspoon raw honey.
Preparation: Steep mullein and thyme in hot water for 10 minutes. Strain and serve warm.
Suggested Usage: Drink 1-2 cups daily to clear congestion and support respiratory health.
Benefits: Mullein and thyme help clear mucus, support lung function, and provide antimicrobial effects, making this tea beneficial for colds and respiratory congestion.

216. Horehound and Licorice Cough Drops

Ingredients: 1 cup dried horehound, 1 cup dried licorice root, 2 cups water, 1 cup raw honey, ¼ cup powdered sugar (optional).

Preparation: Simmer horehound and licorice root in water for 30 minutes. Strain and return liquid to the pan. Add honey and simmer until thickened. Pour into candy molds and let harden. Roll in powdered sugar if desired.

Suggested Usage: Take 1 lozenge as needed to soothe a sore throat and reduce coughing.

Benefits: Combines the expectorant properties of horehound with the soothing and antiviral effects of licorice root, making these cough drops effective for clearing mucus and soothing the throat.

217. Burdock and Yellow Dock Detox Tea

Ingredients: 1 tablespoon dried burdock root, 1 tablespoon dried yellow dock root, 3 cups water.

Preparation: Simmer burdock and yellow dock roots in water for 20-30 minutes. Strain and serve warm.

Suggested Usage: Drink 1 cup twice daily to support liver health and detoxification.

Benefits: Burdock and yellow dock promote liver detoxification, support digestion, and enhance overall immune health by reducing toxic load.

218. Oregon Grape and Barberry Antimicrobial Tincture

Ingredients: ½ cup dried Oregon grape root, ½ cup dried barberry root, 2 cups vodka or brandy (40% alcohol), 1 glass jar with lid.

Preparation: Place Oregon grape and barberry roots in a glass jar and cover with

alcohol. Seal and store in a cool, dark place for 4-6 weeks, shaking daily. Strain and store in a dark glass bottle.

Suggested Usage: Take 20-30 drops diluted in water up to twice daily for antimicrobial support.

Benefits: Oregon grape and barberry contain berberine, a potent antimicrobial compound that supports the body's defenses against bacterial and fungal infections.

219. Ginger and Turmeric Golden Paste

Ingredients: ¼ cup turmeric powder, 2 tablespoons grated fresh ginger, 1 teaspoon ground black pepper, ½ cup water, 2 tablespoons coconut oil.

Preparation: Combine turmeric, ginger, and black pepper in a small saucepan. Add water and heat gently until a thick paste forms. Remove from heat and stir in coconut oil. Store in a glass jar.

Suggested Usage: Take 1 teaspoon daily for immune support, or mix into warm milk or tea.

Benefits: Combines the potent anti-inflammatory effects of turmeric and ginger, enhanced by black pepper for improved absorption, making this paste ideal for reducing inflammation and supporting overall health.

220. Neem and Turmeric Antimicrobial Capsules

Ingredients: ¼ cup neem leaf powder, ¼ cup turmeric powder, empty vegetable capsules.

Preparation: Mix neem and turmeric powders thoroughly. Fill each capsule with the mixture using a small spoon or capsule machine. Store capsules in a cool, dry place.

Suggested Usage: Take 1-2 capsules daily for antimicrobial support and to reduce inflammation.

Benefits: Combines the broad-spectrum antimicrobial properties of neem with the anti-inflammatory effects of turmeric, making these capsules effective for supporting immune health and fighting infections.

221. Elderberry and Hibiscus Vitamin C Syrup

Ingredients: 1 cup dried elderberries, ½ cup dried hibiscus flowers, 4 cups water, 1 cup raw honey.

Preparation: Combine elderberries and hibiscus flowers with water in a saucepan. Bring to a boil, then simmer for 30-45 minutes until the liquid is reduced by half. Remove from heat, strain, and stir in honey. Store in a glass jar.

Suggested Usage: Take 1 tablespoon daily for prevention, or up to 3 times daily at the onset of symptoms.

Benefits: Rich in vitamin C and antioxidants, this syrup strengthens the immune system and helps reduce the severity of cold and flu symptoms.

222. Sage and Lemon Gargle

Ingredients: 1 tablespoon dried sage, 1 cup hot water, juice of ½ lemon, ½ teaspoon sea salt.

Preparation: Steep sage in hot water for 10 minutes. Strain and add lemon juice and salt. Allow to cool to a comfortable temperature.

Suggested Usage: Gargle with ¼ cup of the solution up to 3 times daily to soothe a sore throat and reduce inflammation.

Benefits: Sage and lemon combine strong astringent and antimicrobial properties to reduce throat irritation and fight infection.

223. Calendula and Plantain Wound-Healing Salve

Ingredients: ½ cup dried calendula flowers, ½ cup dried plantain leaves, 1 cup olive oil, ¼ cup beeswax, 10 drops tea tree essential oil.

Preparation: Gently heat calendula and plantain in olive oil for 1 hour. Strain and return to the saucepan. Add beeswax and stir until melted. Remove from heat and stir in tea tree oil. Pour into glass jars and let solidify.

Suggested Usage: Apply a small amount to minor cuts, scrapes, and burns as needed to promote healing and prevent infection.

Benefits: Calendula and plantain provide antimicrobial, anti-inflammatory, and skin-healing properties, making this salve ideal for soothing irritated or damaged skin.

224. Pau d'Arco Antifungal Decoction

Ingredients: 2 tablespoons dried pau d'arco bark, 3 cups water.

Preparation: Simmer pau d'arco bark in water for 20-30 minutes. Strain and serve warm.

Suggested Usage: Drink 1 cup twice daily to fight fungal infections and support immune health.

Benefits: Pau d'arco is a powerful

antifungal herb that inhibits the growth of yeast and fungi, making it effective for treating candida and other fungal infections.

225. Black Seed Oil and Honey Immune Tonic

Ingredients: 1 teaspoon black seed oil, 1 teaspoon raw honey.
Preparation: Mix black seed oil and honey until well combined.
Suggested Usage: Take 1 teaspoon daily for immune support and to reduce inflammation.
Benefits: Black seed oil is known for its potent anti-inflammatory and immune-boosting properties, while honey provides additional antimicrobial support.

226. Turmeric and Honey Anti-Inflammatory Paste

Ingredients: ¼ cup turmeric powder, 2 tablespoons raw honey, 1 teaspoon ground black pepper, 1 tablespoon grated fresh ginger.
Preparation: Mix all ingredients until a smooth paste forms. Store in a glass jar.
Suggested Usage: Take 1 teaspoon daily for immune support and to reduce inflammation, or apply topically to sore joints and muscles.
Benefits: Combines the anti-inflammatory effects of turmeric and ginger with honey's soothing properties, making this paste ideal for internal and external use.

227. Fenugreek and Thyme Sinus-Clearing Tea

Ingredients: 1 teaspoon fenugreek seeds, 1 teaspoon dried thyme, 2 cups hot water, 1 teaspoon raw honey.
Preparation: Slightly crush fenugreek seeds, then steep them with thyme in hot water for 10-15 minutes. Strain and add honey if desired.
Suggested Usage: Drink 1 cup up to twice daily to clear sinuses and support respiratory health.
Benefits: Fenugreek and thyme help clear mucus, soothe the respiratory system, and provide antimicrobial support, making this tea beneficial for sinus congestion and respiratory discomfort.

228. Cinnamon, Clove, and Thyme Antibacterial Tea

Ingredients: 1 cinnamon stick, 4-5 whole cloves, 1 teaspoon dried thyme, 2 cups hot water, 1 teaspoon raw honey.
Preparation: Combine cinnamon, cloves, and thyme in hot water and steep for 10-15 minutes. Strain and add honey if desired.
Suggested Usage: Drink 1 cup daily during cold and flu season for antimicrobial support.
Benefits: Combines powerful antibacterial and warming herbs to support immune function, reduce inflammation, and provide relief for respiratory congestion.

229. Usnea and Calendula Wound Poultice

Ingredients: 1 tablespoon dried usnea, 1 tablespoon dried calendula flowers, 2 tablespoons hot water.
Preparation: Mix usnea and calendula with hot water to create a thick paste.

Allow to cool slightly.

Suggested Usage: Apply the poultice to minor wounds, cuts, or infected areas and cover with a clean cloth. Leave on for 20-30 minutes, then rinse off gently.

Benefits: Usnea and calendula provide strong antimicrobial, anti-inflammatory, and healing properties, making this poultice ideal for treating infections and promoting wound healing.

230. Elecampane and Licorice Cough Elixir

Ingredients: 1 cup dried elecampane root, 1 cup dried licorice root, 4 cups water, 1 cup raw honey.

Preparation: Combine elecampane and licorice root with water in a saucepan. Bring to a boil, then simmer for 30 minutes. Strain, return liquid to the pan, and simmer until reduced by half. Remove from heat and stir in honey. Store in a glass jar.

Suggested Usage: Take 1 tablespoon every 2-3 hours to soothe a cough and reduce mucus.

Benefits: Elecampane and licorice root work together to soothe irritated respiratory tissues, reduce inflammation, and promote expectoration, making this elixir effective for clearing stubborn coughs.

231. Bayberry and Sage Throat Gargle

Ingredients: 1 tablespoon dried bayberry root, 1 tablespoon dried sage, 2 cups hot water, ½ teaspoon sea salt.

Preparation: Steep bayberry root and sage in hot water for 10-15 minutes. Strain and add sea salt. Allow to cool to a comfortable temperature.

Suggested Usage: Gargle with ¼ cup of the solution up to 3 times daily to soothe a sore throat and reduce inflammation.

Benefits: Bayberry and sage provide strong astringent and antimicrobial properties to reduce throat irritation, fight infections, and promote healing.

232. Olive Leaf and Ginger Antiviral Tea

Ingredients: 1 tablespoon dried olive leaves, 1 teaspoon grated fresh ginger, 2 cups hot water, 1 teaspoon raw honey.

Preparation: Steep olive leaves and ginger in hot water for 15 minutes. Strain and add honey if desired.

Suggested Usage: Drink 1-2 cups daily to support immune health and fight viral infections.

Benefits: Combines the potent antiviral properties of olive leaf with the warming and anti-inflammatory effects of ginger to enhance the body's defenses and speed up recovery from viral infections.

Book 14: Allergy Relief through Natural Means

Allergies are a common concern affecting millions of people worldwide. They occur when the immune system mistakenly identifies harmless substances such as pollen, pet dander, or certain foods as threats, leading to a series of symptoms like sneezing, itching, congestion, and even severe reactions like anaphylaxis. Finding relief from allergies often involves more than just treating the symptoms; it requires a comprehensive approach that includes herbal remedies, lifestyle adjustments, and dietary considerations to strengthen the body's defenses and reduce reactivity. This chapter explores effective herbs and holistic strategies to alleviate allergy symptoms naturally, focusing on immune modulation, inflammation control, and lifestyle practices.

Herbs to Alleviate Allergic Reactions

Herbs have been used for centuries to treat various ailments, and many are particularly effective in managing allergic reactions. These herbs work by reducing histamine release, calming inflammation, and supporting the immune system. Several herbs stand out for their ability to modulate the immune response and reduce the body's reactivity to allergens. Let's explore some of the most effective herbs for allergy relief.

1. Nettle (Urtica dioica)
Nettle is a natural antihistamine that helps reduce the body's allergic response. It contains compounds that block histamine receptors, reducing symptoms such as sneezing, itching, and nasal congestion. Nettle is particularly effective for seasonal allergies like hay fever. It can be taken as a tea, tincture, or in capsule form. Regular use throughout the allergy season can help build up the body's resistance to allergens.

2. Butterbur (Petasites hybridus)
Butterbur is another herb known for its antihistamine properties. It works by inhibiting leukotrienes and histamines, which are chemicals released during an allergic reaction. Studies have shown that butterbur can be as effective as some over-the-counter antihistamines without causing drowsiness. However, it's essential to use a product labeled as PA-free, as some butterbur preparations contain pyrrolizidine alkaloids that can be harmful to the liver. Butterbur is most commonly used in capsule form for allergy relief.

3. Quercetin
While not an herb per se, quercetin is a natural flavonoid found in many plants, including apples, onions, and leafy greens. It has potent antioxidant and anti-inflammatory properties, making it highly effective in stabilizing mast cells and reducing histamine release. Quercetin is often used in combination with vitamin C to enhance its absorption and effectiveness. It can be taken as a supplement during allergy season to reduce the frequency and severity of allergic reactions.

4. Eyebright (Euphrasia officinalis)

As the name suggests, eyebright is particularly beneficial for eye-related allergy symptoms, such as redness, itching, and watering. It acts as an astringent and anti-inflammatory, reducing irritation and swelling in the mucous membranes. Eyebright can be taken as a tea or tincture and is also used in eye washes to soothe irritated eyes caused by allergens.

5. Goldenrod (Solidago canadensis)

Goldenrod is often misunderstood as an allergen itself, but it is actually a powerful herb for managing seasonal allergies. It helps reduce inflammation, supports the respiratory system, and alleviates sinus congestion. Goldenrod can be taken as a tea or tincture and is often combined with other allergy-relief herbs like nettle and elderflower.

6. Licorice Root (Glycyrrhiza glabra)

Licorice root is a soothing herb that helps reduce inflammation and modulates the immune system. It is particularly useful for individuals with asthma or respiratory allergies, as it helps soothe the mucous membranes and reduce bronchial inflammation. Licorice root is often used in teas and syrups for respiratory health, but it should be used with caution in individuals with high blood pressure, as it can cause sodium retention.

7. Astragalus (Astragalus membranaceus)

Astragalus is a traditional Chinese herb that strengthens the immune system and helps reduce the body's reactivity to allergens. It works by modulating the immune response, making it particularly effective for long-term allergy management. Astragalus can be taken as a tea, tincture, or in capsule form and is often used in combination with other immune-boosting herbs.

8. Elderflower (Sambucus nigra)

Elderflower is another herb commonly used for respiratory allergies. It helps clear mucus, reduce inflammation, and alleviate sinus congestion. Elderflower tea is particularly effective during allergy season to support respiratory health and reduce the impact of airborne allergens. Elderflower is often combined with peppermint and yarrow for a comprehensive allergy-relief tea blend.

9. Ginger (Zingiber officinale)

Ginger is a potent anti-inflammatory herb that helps reduce allergic reactions by inhibiting the production of pro-inflammatory cytokines. It is particularly effective for individuals who experience respiratory or digestive allergies. Ginger tea, taken regularly, can help reduce inflammation and improve overall immune function. It can also be added to meals or taken as a supplement to support digestive and immune health.

10. Turmeric (Curcuma longa)

Turmeric is well known for its anti-inflammatory properties, primarily due to its active compound, curcumin. It helps reduce allergic reactions by modulating the immune response and reducing histamine release. Turmeric can be taken as a tea, added to meals, or used in supplement form to support overall health and reduce allergy symptoms.

These herbs, when used individually or in combination, provide a natural approach to reducing allergic reactions. Incorporating them into daily routines, especially during allergy season, can significantly lessen the severity of symptoms and improve quality of life for those prone to seasonal and environmental allergies.

Natural Anti-Inflammatory Remedies

Allergic reactions are closely linked to inflammation, as the body's immune response to allergens often leads to swelling, redness, and discomfort in various tissues. Using herbs with strong anti-inflammatory properties can help reduce these symptoms and promote a more balanced immune response. Here are some of the most effective anti-inflammatory herbs for managing allergy symptoms:

1. Turmeric
Turmeric's anti-inflammatory effects are largely due to its curcumin content, which helps reduce the production of pro-inflammatory cytokines. Curcumin works by inhibiting the activity of the NF-κB pathway, a key regulator of the inflammatory response. For optimal absorption, turmeric is often combined with black pepper, which contains piperine—a compound that enhances curcumin's bioavailability.

2. Ginger
Ginger is another potent anti-inflammatory herb that works by inhibiting the production of pro-inflammatory molecules like prostaglandins and leukotrienes. It also has antioxidant properties that help protect tissues from damage caused by chronic inflammation. Ginger can be used in teas, tinctures, and meals, making it a versatile addition to any anti-inflammatory regimen.

3. Boswellia (Boswellia serrata)
Boswellia, also known as frankincense, is a resin extracted from the Boswellia tree and has been used for centuries to reduce inflammation. It works by inhibiting the 5-LOX enzyme, which is responsible for the production of inflammatory leukotrienes. Boswellia is particularly effective for managing respiratory inflammation and can be taken as a supplement or in tincture form.

4. Licorice Root
Licorice root has powerful anti-inflammatory effects, primarily due to its glycyrrhizin content. It helps reduce inflammation in the respiratory tract, making it ideal for individuals with asthma or chronic respiratory allergies. Licorice root is also a demulcent,

which means it soothes irritated mucous membranes and reduces coughing. It is commonly used in herbal teas, syrups, and tinctures.

5. Holy Basil (Ocimum sanctum)

Holy basil, also known as tulsi, is an adaptogenic herb that helps reduce stress and inflammation. It modulates the body's response to allergens by balancing cortisol levels and reducing oxidative stress. Holy basil tea is a popular choice for managing stress-induced inflammation and supporting immune health.

6. Green Tea (Camellia sinensis)

Green tea contains polyphenols called catechins, which have strong anti-inflammatory and antioxidant properties. These compounds help reduce histamine release and support immune balance. Drinking green tea regularly can help reduce the severity of allergic reactions and improve overall immune health.

7. Bromelain

Bromelain is an enzyme found in pineapple that has potent anti-inflammatory and mucolytic properties. It works by breaking down mucus, reducing inflammation, and promoting tissue repair. Bromelain is often used in supplement form to support respiratory health and reduce sinus congestion.

8. Marshmallow Root (Althaea officinalis)

Marshmallow root is a soothing herb that helps reduce inflammation in the mucous membranes. It works by forming a protective layer over irritated tissues, making it ideal for individuals with respiratory or digestive allergies. Marshmallow root can be used in teas, tinctures, or as a powder added to smoothies.

9. Rosemary (Rosmarinus officinalis)

Rosemary is a fragrant herb with potent anti-inflammatory properties. It contains rosmarinic acid, which has been shown to reduce allergic responses and support respiratory health. Rosemary can be used in cooking, as a tea, or as a tincture to reduce inflammation and improve overall health.

10. Chamomile (Matricaria chamomilla)

Chamomile is a gentle anti-inflammatory herb that helps reduce allergic reactions and soothe irritated tissues. It is particularly effective for managing skin allergies and soothing digestive discomfort. Chamomile tea, taken regularly, can help reduce inflammation and improve overall well-being.

Combining these anti-inflammatory herbs with those that modulate the immune response can provide comprehensive support for managing allergy symptoms and promoting a balanced immune system.

Book 15: Supporting Autoimmune Health

Autoimmune diseases present unique challenges because they involve an overactive immune response where the body mistakenly attacks its own tissues, perceiving them as harmful invaders. Conditions such as rheumatoid arthritis, lupus, multiple sclerosis, and Hashimoto's thyroiditis are just a few examples of the wide variety of autoimmune disorders. These diseases are complex, and finding effective treatment approaches often involves more than merely suppressing the immune system. Instead, the goal is to modulate and balance immune activity, allowing the body to defend itself properly without turning against its own cells. This chapter explores herbal and natural strategies to support autoimmune health by reducing inflammation, promoting immune system balance, and enhancing overall well-being.

Herbs have been used for centuries to support the body's natural healing processes, and many are particularly suited for managing autoimmune conditions due to their unique properties. By modulating the immune response and reducing chronic inflammation, these herbs can help alleviate symptoms, prevent flare-ups, and promote long-term wellness for individuals living with autoimmune diseases. One herb that stands out in this category is **Ashwagandha**. Known for its adaptogenic properties, Ashwagandha helps balance the body's response to stress and modulates immune function. It is especially useful for people with autoimmune disorders, as it reduces chronic inflammation and enhances resilience against stress. Ashwagandha supports adrenal health, lowers cortisol levels, and improves overall vitality, making it an excellent choice for managing autoimmune conditions. It is typically consumed in supplement form or as a powder that can be added to smoothies and drinks.

Turmeric is another exceptional herb for autoimmune health. Famous for its potent anti-inflammatory properties, which are largely due to its active compound, curcumin, turmeric helps regulate inflammatory enzymes and cytokines, thereby reducing tissue damage. This makes it a powerful ally in conditions like rheumatoid arthritis and lupus, where chronic inflammation causes joint pain and stiffness. Regular consumption of turmeric can help alleviate pain, improve joint health, and reduce the frequency of autoimmune flare-ups. For optimal results, turmeric is often combined with black pepper, which enhances the bioavailability of curcumin. It can be taken in teas, incorporated into meals, or used as a supplement.

One lesser-known but highly beneficial herb is the **Reishi Mushroom**, a powerful adaptogen that helps balance immune function and reduce autoimmune reactivity. Reishi works by regulating the activity of T-cells and natural killer (NK) cells, ensuring that the immune system remains vigilant against pathogens without attacking the body's own tissues. With its anti-inflammatory and antioxidant properties, Reishi is ideal for managing conditions like lupus and multiple sclerosis. It can be consumed as a tea, taken in tincture form, or used in capsules, depending on personal preference.

For individuals dealing with autoimmune diseases that affect the digestive or respiratory systems, **Licorice Root** is a soothing and supportive herb. It has a long history of use for its anti-inflammatory and immune-modulating effects, particularly in conditions like Crohn's disease and asthma. Licorice root helps reduce inflammation, soothe irritated mucous membranes, and balance cortisol levels, making it beneficial for a wide range of autoimmune disorders. However, because it can cause sodium retention and elevate blood pressure, it should be used with caution, especially in people with hypertension. Licorice root is commonly used in herbal teas, syrups, and tinctures for its therapeutic benefits.

Another potent immune-modulating herb is **Schisandra**, a berry that has been used in traditional Chinese medicine for centuries to support liver function and balance the body's response to stress. Schisandra's ability to reduce oxidative stress and improve resilience makes it particularly effective for autoimmune conditions that are worsened by stress, such as lupus or multiple sclerosis. By promoting liver detoxification and supporting adrenal health, Schisandra enhances the body's ability to maintain a balanced immune response. It is often taken as a tea, tincture, or in capsule form to support comprehensive immune health.

Boswellia, commonly known as frankincense, is another invaluable herb for autoimmune conditions characterized by inflammation. Boswellia works by inhibiting the 5-LOX enzyme, which is responsible for the production of inflammatory leukotrienes. This makes it particularly effective for managing rheumatoid arthritis, where joint inflammation is a primary concern. Boswellia's anti-inflammatory properties can help reduce pain, stiffness, and swelling, providing significant relief for people dealing with chronic joint inflammation. It is typically taken in supplement form, but can also be found in topical creams for localized relief.

Another adaptogenic herb that plays a significant role in managing autoimmune conditions is **Holy Basil**. Known for its ability to reduce stress and balance the immune response, Holy Basil offers a unique combination of anti-inflammatory and antioxidant benefits. Regular consumption of Holy Basil can help lower the frequency and intensity of autoimmune flare-ups, while also promoting a sense of calm and well-being. It is often consumed as a tea, but can also be used in tincture or capsule form.

For individuals experiencing chronic pain and inflammation, **Ginger** can be a simple yet effective remedy. Ginger's anti-inflammatory effects are primarily due to its ability to inhibit the production of pro-inflammatory cytokines and enzymes, making it a valuable addition to the diet of anyone with autoimmune conditions. It is especially effective in managing the pain and inflammation associated with rheumatoid arthritis and lupus. Ginger can be used in teas, incorporated into meals, or taken as a supplement to provide consistent anti-inflammatory support.

Another herb to consider is **Cat's Claw**, a traditional Amazonian herb with strong immune-modulating and anti-inflammatory properties. Cat's Claw is particularly effective for autoimmune conditions that affect the digestive system, such as Crohn's disease or ulcerative colitis. It helps reduce inflammation, support immune function, and protect against oxidative stress, making it a valuable addition to a comprehensive autoimmune health plan. Cat's Claw can be consumed as a tea, tincture, or in capsule form.

Finally, **Gotu Kola** is a rejuvenating herb that helps reduce inflammation, support immune health, and promote tissue repair. It is particularly beneficial for individuals with autoimmune skin conditions, such as psoriasis or eczema. Gotu Kola works by reducing the production of inflammatory cytokines and supporting the regeneration of healthy skin tissue. It can be used topically in creams or taken as a tea or tincture for internal support.

Managing autoimmune diseases requires more than just reducing symptoms—it involves achieving a balanced immune response that reduces overactivity while supporting overall health. Adaptogenic herbs like ashwagandha, holy basil, and rhodiola are essential in this process, as they help balance the body's response to stress, which is a significant factor in many autoimmune conditions. Chronic stress increases inflammation and disrupts immune function, making it crucial to regulate cortisol levels and support adrenal health. Adaptogens help the body adapt to stress, improve resilience, and promote a balanced immune response.

Alongside adaptogens, incorporating anti-inflammatory herbs such as turmeric, ginger, and boswellia can help reduce chronic inflammation, a hallmark of autoimmune diseases. These herbs work by inhibiting pro-inflammatory enzymes and cytokines, promoting a balanced immune response, and preventing further tissue damage. When combined with immune-modulating herbs like reishi mushroom, astragalus, and cat's claw, they create a powerful synergy that supports the body's natural defenses while preventing overactivity that can lead to autoimmune reactions.

Additionally, gut health is closely linked to immune health, and many autoimmune conditions are associated with gut dysbiosis or leaky gut syndrome. Using herbs like licorice root, marshmallow root, and slippery elm to soothe and heal the gut lining can significantly reduce inflammation and support healthy digestion. A healthy gut is essential for maintaining a balanced immune system and reducing the risk of autoimmune flare-ups. For this reason, addressing gut health should be a primary focus in any autoimmune health plan.

Integrating these herbs into a holistic lifestyle approach that includes a nutrient-dense diet, stress management techniques, and adequate rest can provide comprehensive support for managing autoimmune conditions. This holistic strategy not only reduces inflammation and balances the immune response but also enhances overall health and well-being, making it a valuable approach for anyone living with autoimmune diseases.

Remedies for Chronic Inflammation

233. Turmeric and Black Pepper Anti-Inflammatory Paste

Ingredients: ¼ cup turmeric powder, 1 teaspoon ground black pepper, ½ cup coconut oil.
Preparation: Mix turmeric powder and black pepper together. Gradually add the coconut oil until a thick paste forms. Store in a glass jar in the refrigerator.
Suggested Usage: Take 1 teaspoon daily, mixed into warm milk or tea, to reduce inflammation.
Benefits: The combination of turmeric and black pepper enhances the bioavailability of curcumin, the active compound in turmeric, which helps reduce inflammation, alleviate joint pain, and improve overall immune function.

234. Ginger and Honey Immune Tonic

Ingredients: 2 tablespoons grated fresh ginger, 1 tablespoon raw honey, juice of 1 lemon, 1 cup warm water.
Preparation: Combine all ingredients in a cup and mix well until the honey is fully dissolved.
Suggested Usage: Drink 1 cup daily, preferably in the morning, to support immune health and reduce inflammation.
Benefits: Ginger has potent anti-inflammatory properties and helps reduce respiratory congestion, while honey provides antimicrobial support. The addition of lemon adds vitamin C, making

this tonic an excellent choice for boosting immunity.

235. Boswellia and Ashwagandha Anti-Inflammatory Capsules

Ingredients: ¼ cup dried Boswellia extract, ¼ cup dried Ashwagandha powder, empty vegetable capsules.
Preparation: Mix Boswellia and Ashwagandha powders thoroughly. Fill each capsule using a small spoon or capsule machine. Store in a cool, dry place.
Suggested Usage: Take 1-2 capsules daily to reduce inflammation and support overall health.
Benefits: Boswellia is known for its ability to reduce inflammation and alleviate joint pain, while Ashwagandha helps modulate the body's stress response and balance immune function, making this combination ideal for managing chronic inflammatory conditions.

236. Licorice and Marshmallow Root Soothing Tea

Ingredients: 1 tablespoon dried licorice root, 1 tablespoon dried marshmallow root, 2 cups hot water, 1 teaspoon raw honey.
Preparation: Steep licorice and marshmallow roots in hot water for 15 minutes. Strain and add honey if desired.
Suggested Usage: Drink 1 cup up to twice daily to soothe inflammation in the

digestive and respiratory tracts.
Benefits: Licorice root and marshmallow root work together to coat and soothe mucous membranes, reduce inflammation, and promote healing in irritated tissues, making this tea particularly beneficial for individuals with gastrointestinal or respiratory issues.

237. Reishi Mushroom Adaptogen Tonic

Ingredients: 1 tablespoon dried reishi mushroom slices, 3 cups water, 1 teaspoon raw honey (optional).
Preparation: Simmer reishi mushroom slices in water for 30-40 minutes. Strain and serve warm. Add honey if desired.
Suggested Usage: Drink 1 cup daily for immune support and to reduce stress-related inflammation.
Benefits: Reishi mushroom is a powerful adaptogen that helps modulate the immune response, reduce inflammation, and promote overall resilience to stress, making it ideal for supporting long-term health in individuals with autoimmune conditions.

238. Cat's Claw and Holy Basil Immune Modulating Tea

Ingredients: 1 tablespoon dried cat's claw bark, 1 tablespoon dried holy basil leaves, 2 cups hot water.
Preparation: Steep cat's claw and holy basil in hot water for 15 minutes. Strain and serve warm.
Suggested Usage: Drink 1-2 cups daily to support immune health and reduce inflammation.
Benefits: Cat's claw is known for its

powerful immune-modulating effects, while holy basil helps balance cortisol levels and reduce stress, making this tea blend effective for reducing chronic inflammation and supporting a balanced immune response.

239. Green Tea and Rosemary Anti-Inflammatory Infusion

Ingredients: 1 tablespoon dried green tea leaves, 1 teaspoon dried rosemary, 2 cups hot water, 1 teaspoon raw honey.
Preparation: Steep green tea and rosemary in hot water for 10 minutes. Strain and add honey if desired.
Suggested Usage: Drink 1 cup daily to reduce inflammation and support cognitive function.
Benefits: Green tea contains powerful antioxidants called catechins that reduce inflammation, while rosemary has been shown to support brain health and reduce oxidative stress. This infusion is ideal for individuals looking to support both immune and cognitive health.

240. Astragalus and Schisandra Berry Resilience Tonic

Ingredients: 1 tablespoon dried astragalus root, 1 tablespoon dried schisandra berries, 3 cups water.
Preparation: Simmer astragalus and schisandra berries in water for 30 minutes. Strain and serve warm.
Suggested Usage: Drink 1 cup daily for immune support and increased resilience to stress.
Benefits: Astragalus helps modulate the immune response and protect against stress-related immune suppression, while

schisandra enhances energy and supports liver function, making this tonic ideal for promoting resilience in individuals dealing with chronic inflammation.

241. Nettle and Dandelion Liver Support Tea

Ingredients: 1 tablespoon dried nettle leaves, 1 tablespoon dried dandelion root, 2 cups hot water, 1 teaspoon lemon juice.
Preparation: Steep nettle leaves and dandelion root in hot water for 15 minutes. Strain and add lemon juice.
Suggested Usage: Drink 1-2 cups daily to support liver function and promote detoxification.
Benefits: Nettle and dandelion are rich in vitamins and minerals that support liver detoxification, reduce inflammation, and promote healthy blood flow, making this tea an excellent choice for individuals looking to cleanse and support overall health.

242. Elderberry and Echinacea Immune-Boosting Syrup

Ingredients: 1 cup dried elderberries, ½ cup dried echinacea root, 4 cups water, 1 cup raw honey.
Preparation: Combine elderberries, echinacea root, and water in a saucepan. Bring to a boil, then simmer for 30 minutes. Strain, return the liquid to the pan, and reduce by half. Remove from heat and stir in honey. Store in a glass jar.
Suggested Usage: Take 1 tablespoon daily for immune support, or up to 3 times daily at the onset of symptoms.
Benefits: Elderberries and echinacea are known for their immune-boosting and

antiviral properties, making this syrup highly effective for reducing the duration and severity of colds and flu.

243. Chamomile and Lavender Calming Tea

Ingredients: 1 tablespoon dried chamomile flowers, 1 tablespoon dried lavender buds, 2 cups hot water, 1 teaspoon raw honey.
Preparation: Steep chamomile and lavender in hot water for 15 minutes. Strain and add honey if desired.
Suggested Usage: Drink 1 cup in the evening to promote relaxation and reduce stress-related inflammation.
Benefits: Chamomile and lavender are gentle, calming herbs that help reduce anxiety and inflammation, making this tea ideal for promoting restful sleep and reducing stress-induced immune dysfunction.

244. Devil's Claw and Ginger Joint Support Capsules

Ingredients: ¼ cup dried Devil's Claw root powder, ¼ cup dried ginger root powder, empty vegetable capsules.
Preparation: Mix Devil's Claw and ginger root powders thoroughly. Use a small spoon or capsule machine to fill each capsule. Store in a cool, dry place.
Suggested Usage: Take 1-2 capsules daily to reduce joint inflammation and alleviate pain.
Benefits: Devil's Claw is known for its powerful anti-inflammatory properties and ability to relieve joint pain and stiffness, while ginger enhances circulation and provides additional anti-inflammatory

support, making this combination ideal for managing arthritis and other inflammatory joint conditions.

245. Turmeric and Ginger Golden Milk

Ingredients: 1 cup unsweetened almond milk, 1 teaspoon turmeric powder, 1 teaspoon grated fresh ginger, ¼ teaspoon ground cinnamon, 1 teaspoon raw honey.
Preparation: Combine almond milk, turmeric, ginger, and cinnamon in a small saucepan. Heat gently over low heat for 5-7 minutes, stirring continuously. Remove from heat and stir in honey. Serve warm.
Suggested Usage: Drink 1 cup daily in the evening to reduce inflammation and promote relaxation.
Benefits: This golden milk combines the anti-inflammatory properties of turmeric and ginger, with the calming effects of cinnamon and honey, making it an excellent nighttime drink for reducing chronic inflammation and promoting restful sleep.

246. Gotu Kola and Licorice Anti-Inflammatory Tea

Ingredients: 1 tablespoon dried Gotu Kola leaves, 1 tablespoon dried licorice root, 2 cups hot water, 1 teaspoon lemon juice.
Preparation: Steep Gotu Kola leaves and licorice root in hot water for 15 minutes. Strain and add lemon juice.
Suggested Usage: Drink 1-2 cups daily to reduce inflammation and support immune health.
Benefits: Gotu Kola promotes wound healing and reduces inflammation, while

licorice root soothes irritated tissues and modulates the immune response, making this tea beneficial for conditions such as psoriasis and eczema.

247. Cinnamon and Clove Antioxidant Tea

Ingredients: 1 cinnamon stick, 4-5 whole cloves, 2 cups hot water, 1 teaspoon raw honey.
Preparation: Steep the cinnamon stick and cloves in hot water for 10-15 minutes. Strain and add honey if desired.
Suggested Usage: Drink 1 cup daily to reduce inflammation and support immune function.
Benefits: Cinnamon and clove are rich in antioxidants and possess strong anti-inflammatory properties, making this tea effective for reducing oxidative stress and supporting overall health.

248. Milk Thistle and Burdock Root Detox Tea

Ingredients: 1 tablespoon dried milk thistle seeds, 1 tablespoon dried burdock root, 3 cups water.
Preparation: Simmer milk thistle seeds and burdock root in water for 20-30 minutes. Strain and serve warm.
Suggested Usage: Drink 1 cup twice daily to support liver health and promote detoxification.
Benefits: Milk thistle and burdock root are renowned for their liver-supporting and detoxifying properties. This tea helps cleanse the liver, reduce inflammation, and promote healthy digestion, making it ideal for individuals dealing with chronic inflammatory conditions.

249. Fenugreek and Thyme Sinus-Clearing Tea

Ingredients: 1 teaspoon fenugreek seeds, 1 teaspoon dried thyme, 2 cups hot water, 1 teaspoon raw honey.

Preparation: Slightly crush fenugreek seeds, then steep them with thyme in hot water for 10-15 minutes. Strain and add honey if desired.

Suggested Usage: Drink 1 cup up to twice daily to clear sinuses and support respiratory health.

Benefits: Fenugreek and thyme help clear mucus, soothe the respiratory system, and provide antimicrobial support, making this tea beneficial for sinus congestion and respiratory discomfort.

250. Holy Basil and Lemon Balm Relaxation Tea

Ingredients: 1 tablespoon dried holy basil leaves, 1 tablespoon dried lemon balm leaves, 2 cups hot water, 1 teaspoon raw honey.

Preparation: Steep holy basil and lemon balm in hot water for 10-15 minutes. Strain and add honey if desired.

Suggested Usage: Drink 1 cup in the evening to reduce stress and promote relaxation.

Benefits: Holy basil is an adaptogen that helps balance cortisol levels and reduce stress, while lemon balm has calming properties that promote a sense of well-being, making this tea ideal for supporting mental and emotional health.

251. Calendula and Plantain Wound-Healing Salve

Ingredients: ½ cup dried calendula flowers, ½ cup dried plantain leaves, 1 cup olive oil, ¼ cup beeswax, 10 drops tea tree essential oil.

Preparation: Gently heat calendula and plantain in olive oil for 1 hour. Strain and return to the saucepan. Add beeswax and stir until melted. Remove from heat and stir in tea tree oil. Pour into glass jars and let solidify.

Suggested Usage: Apply a small amount to minor cuts, scrapes, and burns as needed to promote healing and prevent infection.

Benefits: Calendula and plantain are renowned for their anti-inflammatory, antimicrobial, and wound-healing properties, making this salve ideal for soothing irritated skin and promoting faster healing.

252. Passionflower and Skullcap Nerve-Soothing Tea

Ingredients: 1 tablespoon dried passionflower, 1 tablespoon dried skullcap, 2 cups hot water, 1 teaspoon raw honey.

Preparation: Steep passionflower and skullcap in hot water for 10-15 minutes. Strain and add honey if desired.

Suggested Usage: Drink 1 cup in the evening to soothe the nerves and reduce inflammation.

Benefits: Passionflower and skullcap are gentle nervine herbs that help calm the nervous system, reduce anxiety, and alleviate nerve-related inflammation, making this tea ideal for supporting emotional well-being and promoting restful sleep.

253. Aloe Vera and Peppermint Digestive Soothing Gel

Ingredients: ¼ cup fresh aloe vera gel, 5 drops peppermint essential oil.
Preparation: Mix aloe vera gel with peppermint oil until well combined. Store in a glass jar in the refrigerator.
Suggested Usage: Take 1 tablespoon before meals to soothe digestive discomfort and reduce inflammation.
Benefits: Aloe vera soothes and heals the digestive tract, while peppermint helps reduce bloating and inflammation, making this gel ideal for managing conditions like irritable bowel syndrome and acid reflux.

254. Slippery Elm and Marshmallow Root Gut-Healing Tea

Ingredients: 1 tablespoon dried slippery elm bark, 1 tablespoon dried marshmallow root, 2 cups hot water, 1 teaspoon raw honey.
Preparation: Steep slippery elm and marshmallow root in hot water for 15-20 minutes. Strain and add honey if desired.
Suggested Usage: Drink 1-2 cups daily to soothe and heal the digestive tract.
Benefits: Slippery elm and marshmallow root are demulcent herbs that form a protective layer over mucous membranes, reducing inflammation and promoting healing in conditions like gastritis, colitis, and leaky gut syndrome.

255. Sage and Lemon Gargle

Ingredients: 1 tablespoon dried sage, 1 cup hot water, juice of ½ lemon, ½ teaspoon sea salt.
Preparation: Steep sage in hot water for 10 minutes. Strain and add lemon juice and sea salt. Allow to cool to a comfortable temperature.
Suggested Usage: Gargle with ¼ cup of the solution up to 3 times daily to soothe a sore throat and reduce inflammation.
Benefits: Sage and lemon provide strong astringent and antimicrobial properties that help reduce throat irritation, clear mucus, and support respiratory health.

256. Cinnamon and Licorice Immune Support Tea

Ingredients: 1 cinnamon stick, 1 tablespoon dried licorice root, 2 cups hot water, 1 teaspoon raw honey.
Preparation: Steep cinnamon and licorice root in hot water for 15 minutes. Strain and add honey if desired.
Suggested Usage: Drink 1 cup daily to support immune health and reduce inflammation.
Benefits: Cinnamon is rich in antioxidants, while licorice root modulates the immune response and soothes irritated tissues, making this tea blend ideal for boosting immunity and reducing inflammation.

257. Ginger and Turmeric Digestive Tonic

Ingredients: 1 tablespoon grated fresh ginger, 1 teaspoon turmeric powder, juice of ½ lemon, 1 cup warm water, 1 teaspoon raw honey.
Preparation: Combine all ingredients and mix thoroughly.
Suggested Usage: Drink 1 cup before

meals to support digestion and reduce inflammation.

Benefits: Ginger and turmeric have powerful anti-inflammatory and digestive-supporting properties that help reduce bloating, support gut health, and enhance nutrient absorption.

258. Nettle and Rosehip Vitamin C Tea

Ingredients: 1 tablespoon dried nettle leaves, 1 tablespoon dried rosehips, 2 cups hot water, 1 teaspoon raw honey.

Preparation: Steep nettle leaves and rosehips in hot water for 15 minutes. Strain and add honey if desired.

Suggested Usage: Drink 1-2 cups daily to support immune health and increase vitamin C levels.

Benefits: Nettle is rich in vitamins and minerals, while rosehips provide a concentrated source of vitamin C and antioxidants, making this tea effective for boosting the immune system and reducing inflammation.

259. Lemon Balm and Peppermint Relaxation Tea

Ingredients: 1 tablespoon dried lemon balm leaves, 1 tablespoon dried peppermint leaves, 2 cups hot water.

Preparation: Steep lemon balm and peppermint in hot water for 10-15 minutes. Strain and serve warm.

Suggested Usage: Drink 1 cup in the evening to promote relaxation and reduce stress.

Benefits: Lemon balm and peppermint have calming and digestive-supporting properties that help soothe the nervous system, reduce anxiety, and promote restful sleep.

260. Ashwagandha and Rhodiola Stress-Reducing Capsules

Ingredients: ¼ cup dried Ashwagandha powder, ¼ cup dried Rhodiola root powder, empty vegetable capsules.

Preparation: Mix Ashwagandha and Rhodiola powders thoroughly. Fill each capsule using a small spoon or capsule machine. Store in a cool, dry place.

Suggested Usage: Take 1-2 capsules daily to reduce stress and support adrenal health.

Benefits: Ashwagandha and Rhodiola are adaptogens that help the body adapt to stress, balance cortisol levels, and enhance energy and focus, making these capsules ideal for supporting mental and emotional well-being.

261. Basil and Lemongrass Cooling Tea

Ingredients: 1 tablespoon dried basil leaves, 1 tablespoon dried lemongrass, 2 cups hot water.

Preparation: Steep basil and lemongrass in hot water for 10-15 minutes. Strain and serve warm or chilled.

Suggested Usage: Drink 1 cup in the afternoon to cool the body and support digestion.

Benefits: Basil and lemongrass have cooling and anti-inflammatory properties that help reduce heat and inflammation, making this tea effective for soothing digestive issues and calming the mind.

262. Goldenrod and Elderflower Sinus Relief Tea

Ingredients: 1 tablespoon dried goldenrod, 1 tablespoon dried elderflower, 2 cups hot water, 1 teaspoon raw honey.
Preparation: Steep goldenrod and elderflower in hot water for 15 minutes. Strain and add honey if desired.
Suggested Usage: Drink 1-2 cups daily to relieve sinus congestion and support respiratory health.
Benefits: Goldenrod and elderflower help clear mucus, reduce inflammation, and support the respiratory system, making this tea blend effective for relieving sinus pressure and congestion.

263. Chaga and Reishi Immune-Boosting Brew

Ingredients: 1 tablespoon dried Chaga mushroom chunks, 1 tablespoon dried Reishi mushroom slices, 4 cups water.
Preparation: Simmer Chaga and Reishi mushrooms in water for 30-40 minutes. Strain and serve warm.
Suggested Usage: Drink 1 cup daily to support immune health and reduce inflammation.
Benefits: Chaga and Reishi are powerful adaptogens that help modulate the immune response, reduce inflammation, and promote overall health and resilience, making this brew ideal for long-term immune support.

264. Sage and Rosemary Antioxidant Tea

Ingredients: 1 tablespoon dried sage, 1 tablespoon dried rosemary, 2 cups hot water.
Preparation: Steep sage and rosemary in hot water for 10-15 minutes. Strain and serve warm.
Suggested Usage: Drink 1 cup daily to reduce oxidative stress and support cognitive health.
Benefits: Sage and rosemary are rich in antioxidants and have strong anti-inflammatory properties, making this tea effective for protecting against oxidative damage and supporting brain function.

265. Eucalyptus and Peppermint Chest Rub

Ingredients: ¼ cup shea butter, ¼ cup coconut oil, 10 drops eucalyptus essential oil, 10 drops peppermint essential oil, 5 drops rosemary essential oil.
Preparation: Melt shea butter and coconut oil together using a double boiler. Remove from heat and stir in essential oils. Transfer to a small glass jar and let solidify.
Suggested Usage: Apply a small amount to the chest and back area before bedtime or during respiratory congestion.
Benefits: Eucalyptus and peppermint open up airways, reduce congestion, and soothe irritated respiratory tissues, providing relief during colds and coughs, making this rub ideal for supporting respiratory health.

266. Dandelion Root and Yellow Dock Detox Tea

Ingredients: 1 tablespoon dried dandelion root, 1 tablespoon dried yellow dock root,

3 cups water.

Preparation: Simmer dandelion root and yellow dock root in water for 20-30 minutes. Strain and serve warm.

Suggested Usage: Drink 1-2 cups daily to support liver detoxification and promote healthy digestion.

Benefits: Dandelion root and yellow dock are potent detoxifying herbs that support liver function, promote bile production, and help cleanse the blood, making this tea ideal for overall detoxification and reducing inflammation.

267. Burdock and Oregon Grape Root Liver Cleanse

Ingredients: 1 tablespoon dried burdock root, 1 tablespoon dried Oregon grape root, 3 cups water.

Preparation: Simmer burdock root and Oregon grape root in water for 30 minutes. Strain and serve warm.

Suggested Usage: Drink 1 cup twice daily to cleanse the liver and support healthy digestion.

Benefits: Burdock and Oregon grape root are known for their liver-cleansing and blood-purifying properties, making this tea highly effective for individuals looking to detoxify and reduce systemic inflammation.

268. Devil's Claw and Boswellia Joint Relief Capsules

Ingredients: ¼ cup dried Devil's Claw root powder, ¼ cup dried Boswellia powder, empty vegetable capsules.

Preparation: Mix Devil's Claw and Boswellia powders thoroughly. Fill each capsule using a small spoon or capsule machine. Store in a cool, dry place.

Suggested Usage: Take 1-2 capsules daily to reduce joint pain and inflammation.

Benefits: Devil's Claw and Boswellia are both powerful anti-inflammatory herbs that help alleviate joint pain and stiffness, making these capsules ideal for managing arthritis and other inflammatory joint conditions.

269. Fenugreek and Ginger Respiratory Tea

Ingredients: 1 tablespoon fenugreek seeds, 1 tablespoon grated fresh ginger, 2 cups hot water, 1 teaspoon raw honey.

Preparation: Slightly crush fenugreek seeds and steep them with grated ginger in hot water for 10-15 minutes. Strain and add honey if desired.

Suggested Usage: Drink 1 cup up to twice daily to support respiratory health and reduce congestion.

Benefits: Fenugreek and ginger have strong expectorant and anti-inflammatory properties, making this tea blend effective for clearing mucus, soothing the respiratory tract, and reducing respiratory inflammation.

270. Ginger, Garlic, and Cayenne Circulation Tonic

Ingredients: 1 cup warm water, 1 teaspoon grated fresh ginger, 1 minced garlic clove, ½ teaspoon cayenne pepper, juice of ½ lemon.

Preparation: Combine all ingredients in a cup and mix well. Drink immediately.

Suggested Usage: Take 1 shot daily to support circulation and reduce inflammation.

Benefits: Ginger, garlic, and cayenne are powerful circulatory stimulants that help increase blood flow, reduce inflammation, and promote cardiovascular health, making this tonic ideal for individuals with poor circulation or inflammatory conditions.

271. Lemongrass and Ginger Anti-Inflammatory Tea

Ingredients: 1 tablespoon dried lemongrass, 1 tablespoon grated fresh ginger, 2 cups hot water, 1 teaspoon raw honey.

Preparation: Steep lemongrass and ginger in hot water for 10-15 minutes. Strain and add honey if desired.

Suggested Usage: Drink 1-2 cups daily to reduce inflammation and support digestion.

Benefits: Lemongrass and ginger have strong anti-inflammatory and digestive-supporting properties, making this tea effective for reducing bloating, soothing the digestive tract, and alleviating pain.

272. Peppermint and Fennel Digestive Tea

Ingredients: 1 tablespoon dried peppermint leaves, 1 teaspoon fennel seeds, 2 cups hot water.

Preparation: Steep peppermint and fennel in hot water for 10-15 minutes. Strain and serve warm.

Suggested Usage: Drink 1 cup after meals to reduce bloating and promote healthy digestion.

Benefits: Peppermint relaxes the digestive tract, while fennel reduces gas and bloating, making this tea blend ideal for relieving digestive discomfort and promoting healthy digestion.

273. Marshmallow Root and Licorice Throat Soother

Ingredients: 1 tablespoon dried marshmallow root, 1 tablespoon dried licorice root, 2 cups hot water, 1 teaspoon raw honey.

Preparation: Steep marshmallow root and licorice root in hot water for 15 minutes. Strain and add honey if desired.

Suggested Usage: Drink 1 cup up to twice daily to soothe a sore throat and reduce inflammation.

Benefits: Marshmallow root and licorice root are both demulcent herbs that coat and soothe the throat, reducing irritation and inflammation, making this tea effective for coughs, sore throats, and other respiratory conditions.

274. St. John's Wort and Lemon Balm Nerve Support Tea

Ingredients: 1 tablespoon dried St. John's Wort, 1 tablespoon dried lemon balm leaves, 2 cups hot water, 1 teaspoon raw honey.

Preparation: Steep St. John's Wort and lemon balm in hot water for 15 minutes. Strain and add honey if desired.

Suggested Usage: Drink 1 cup daily to support nervous system health and reduce anxiety.

Benefits: St. John's Wort is known for its ability to reduce anxiety and support mood, while lemon balm has calming properties that help reduce stress and promote a sense of well-being.

275. Ginkgo Biloba and Gotu Kola Brain Boost Tea

Ingredients: 1 tablespoon dried Ginkgo Biloba leaves, 1 tablespoon dried Gotu Kola leaves, 2 cups hot water.
Preparation: Steep Ginkgo Biloba and Gotu Kola leaves in hot water for 10-15 minutes. Strain and serve warm.
Suggested Usage: Drink 1-2 cups daily to support cognitive function and improve memory.
Benefits: Ginkgo Biloba and Gotu Kola are both known for their ability to enhance cognitive function, improve circulation to the brain, and reduce mental fatigue, making this tea blend ideal for supporting brain health.

276. Shatavari and Licorice Hormone Balance Tonic

Ingredients: 1 tablespoon dried Shatavari root, 1 tablespoon dried licorice root, 3 cups water.
Preparation: Simmer Shatavari and licorice root in water for 20-30 minutes. Strain and serve warm.
Suggested Usage: Drink 1 cup daily to support hormonal balance and reduce inflammation.
Benefits: Shatavari is known for its hormone-balancing effects, particularly in women, while licorice root helps modulate cortisol levels and reduce inflammation, making this tonic ideal for supporting hormonal health and reducing stress-related inflammation.

277. Maca and Ashwagandha Vitality Elixir

Ingredients: 1 tablespoon maca powder, 1 teaspoon ashwagandha powder, 1 cup warm almond milk, 1 teaspoon raw honey, a pinch of cinnamon.
Preparation: Combine maca and ashwagandha powders in a cup. Gradually add warm almond milk while stirring continuously. Add honey and cinnamon, stirring until fully mixed. Serve warm.
Suggested Usage: Drink 1 cup in the morning to enhance energy and promote vitality.
Benefits: Maca and ashwagandha are both adaptogens that support hormonal balance, reduce stress, and boost stamina, making this elixir ideal for enhancing physical and mental resilience.

278. Oatstraw and Skullcap Nervine Tea

Ingredients: 1 tablespoon dried oatstraw, 1 tablespoon dried skullcap, 2 cups hot water, 1 teaspoon raw honey.
Preparation: Steep oatstraw and skullcap in hot water for 15 minutes. Strain and add honey if desired.
Suggested Usage: Drink 1-2 cups in the evening to soothe the nervous system and promote relaxation.
Benefits: Oatstraw and skullcap are gentle nervine herbs that help calm the nervous system, reduce anxiety, and alleviate stress, making this tea blend effective for supporting emotional well-being and promoting restful sleep.

279. Calendula and Chamomile Skin Soothing Oil

Ingredients: ½ cup dried calendula flowers, ½ cup dried chamomile flowers,

1 cup olive oil, 10 drops lavender essential oil.

Preparation: Gently heat calendula and chamomile flowers in olive oil over low heat for 1 hour. Strain and let cool. Stir in lavender essential oil and transfer to a glass jar.

Suggested Usage: Apply a small amount to irritated or inflamed skin as needed to soothe and moisturize.

Benefits: Calendula and chamomile have anti-inflammatory and skin-healing properties, making this oil ideal for soothing eczema, rashes, and dry, irritated skin.

280. Passionflower and Valerian Relaxation Tea

Ingredients: 1 tablespoon dried passionflower, 1 tablespoon dried valerian root, 2 cups hot water.

Preparation: Steep passionflower and valerian root in hot water for 10-15 minutes. Strain and serve warm.

Suggested Usage: Drink 1 cup in the evening to reduce anxiety and promote restful sleep.

Benefits: Passionflower and valerian are both powerful calming herbs that help alleviate anxiety, reduce tension, and promote deep, restful sleep, making this tea blend ideal for individuals with insomnia or high stress levels.

281. Cat's Claw and Boswellia Joint Support Capsules

Ingredients: ¼ cup dried Cat's Claw bark powder, ¼ cup dried Boswellia powder, empty vegetable capsules.

Preparation: Mix Cat's Claw and Boswellia powders thoroughly. Fill each capsule using a small spoon or capsule machine. Store in a cool, dry place.

Suggested Usage: Take 1-2 capsules daily to reduce joint inflammation and alleviate pain.

Benefits: Cat's Claw and Boswellia are both known for their strong anti-inflammatory properties and ability to reduce joint pain and stiffness, making these capsules ideal for managing conditions such as arthritis and other inflammatory joint disorders.

282. Black Seed Oil and Honey Anti-Inflammatory Tonic

Ingredients: 1 teaspoon black seed oil, 1 teaspoon raw honey.

Preparation: Mix black seed oil and honey until well combined.

Suggested Usage: Take 1 teaspoon daily to support immune health and reduce inflammation.

Benefits: Black seed oil is known for its potent anti-inflammatory and antioxidant properties, while honey provides additional antimicrobial support, making this tonic highly effective for managing chronic inflammation and boosting overall immunity.

Book 16: Natural Antivirals and Antibacterials

Our modern world is filled with a myriad of viral and bacterial threats that challenge our health, particularly during the cold and flu seasons. While conventional medicine offers a range of pharmaceutical options, these often come with side effects and, in the case of bacterial infections, the growing issue of antibiotic resistance. As a result, many people are turning to natural alternatives to support their health. Herbs have long been used for their antimicrobial properties and remain a powerful option for strengthening the body's defenses and combating infections. This chapter will explore potent herbs that offer antiviral and antibacterial benefits, highlighting their therapeutic potential and how they can be safely and effectively used to promote health and recovery.

Powerful Herbs with Antiviral Properties

Viruses are particularly challenging pathogens to combat because they infiltrate the body's cells, making them difficult to target without also harming the host. However, nature offers a variety of herbs that help support the body's own defenses against viral infections, either by inhibiting viral replication, boosting the immune system, or protecting cells from viral invasion. Many of these herbs work in harmony with the body's natural immune responses, making them valuable tools for both prevention and treatment.

One of the most renowned antiviral herbs is **Olive Leaf**. Known for its active compound oleuropein, olive leaf has been shown to disrupt viral replication and boost the immune system's response. It is particularly effective against influenza and the herpes virus. Olive leaf can be taken as a tea, tincture, or in capsule form. Regular use during flu season can significantly reduce the frequency and severity of viral infections.

Elderberry is another potent antiviral herb that has gained popularity in recent years. Studies have shown that elderberry extract can reduce the duration of flu symptoms and inhibit the binding of viruses to cells. Rich in antioxidants and flavonoids, elderberry also helps modulate the immune system, making it effective for both prevention and early treatment. Elderberry is often used in syrups and teas for its pleasant taste and high efficacy.

Another herb to consider is **Lemon Balm**, which has a long history of use as an antiviral remedy. Its active compounds, such as rosmarinic acid, have been shown to prevent the replication of herpes simplex virus and other common viruses. Lemon balm is particularly useful for topical applications in cold sore treatments, as well as in teas for general antiviral support.

Oregano Oil is one of nature's most potent antiviral and antibacterial substances. Containing high levels of carvacrol, oregano oil can inhibit viral replication and support overall immune health. It is often used in capsule form or as a diluted topical treatment. Due to its potency, caution should be taken when using oregano oil internally, and it is best used for short-term treatment during acute viral infections.

Astragalus is another herb widely recognized for its immune-boosting and antiviral properties. It enhances the body's production of interferon, a protein that signals the presence of viruses to the immune system. Astragalus is commonly used in traditional Chinese medicine as a tonic herb, making it ideal for long-term use to strengthen the body's defenses. It can be taken as a tea, tincture, or in capsules.

Cat's Claw is a powerful antiviral herb native to the Amazon rainforest. It is known for its ability to modulate the immune system, reduce inflammation, and fight viral infections, particularly those affecting the respiratory system. Its effectiveness against herpes and respiratory viruses makes it a valuable addition to any antiviral protocol. Cat's Claw is typically consumed as a tea or tincture.

Lemon Balm and **Licorice Root** also deserve mention as potent antiviral herbs. Licorice root is effective against a variety of viruses, including hepatitis and herpes, due to its glycyrrhizin content, which inhibits viral replication. It also soothes mucous membranes, making it particularly beneficial for respiratory infections. Licorice root is best used in tea or tincture form and should be used with caution in individuals with high blood pressure.

Combating Bacterial Infections Naturally

Bacterial infections pose a unique challenge in the modern era, as the overuse of conventional antibiotics has led to the rise of antibiotic-resistant strains. Fortunately, many herbs offer natural antibacterial properties without contributing to resistance. These herbs work by disrupting bacterial cell walls, inhibiting bacterial enzymes, or modulating the body's immune response to help clear infections naturally.

Garlic is one of the most well-researched natural antibacterials. Containing allicin, a compound known for its broad-spectrum antibacterial effects, garlic can fight infections ranging from respiratory issues to skin infections. It is effective against antibiotic-resistant strains like MRSA and can be used both internally and topically. Fresh garlic, garlic oil, or garlic capsules are common preparations used to harness its potent antimicrobial effects.

Goldenseal is another powerful antibacterial herb, often referred to as a natural antibiotic. Its effectiveness is largely due to its berberine content, which disrupts the enzymes necessary for bacterial replication. Goldenseal is especially useful for infections of the mucous membranes, such as sinus infections or urinary tract infections. It is most often used in tincture or capsule form.

Thyme and **Oregano** are both rich in thymol and carvacrol, respectively, compounds that are lethal to many strains of bacteria. Thyme is particularly useful for respiratory infections, and thyme tea or steam inhalation can help clear bronchial congestion and reduce bacterial growth. Oregano, as mentioned earlier, is so potent that it can even combat difficult bacterial infections like Staphylococcus aureus. It can be used in diluted oil form, capsules, or teas.

Usnea, also known as old man's beard, is a lichen with strong antibacterial and antifungal properties. It contains usnic acid, which has been shown to disrupt bacterial cell walls, making it effective against respiratory and skin infections. Usnea can be used as a tincture or infused in oils for topical applications.

Calendula is traditionally used for wound healing and fighting bacterial infections of the skin. It possesses both antimicrobial and anti-inflammatory properties, making it ideal for topical use in salves and creams. When used as a tea or tincture, calendula also helps support the immune system and fight internal infections.

Echinacea is often associated with immune support, but it also has direct antibacterial properties. It works by enhancing the activity of white blood cells, which are responsible for clearing bacterial infections. Echinacea can be used in teas, tinctures, or capsules to combat infections and speed up recovery.

Finally, **Propolis**, a resin produced by bees, is an incredibly potent antibacterial agent. It is effective against both Gram-positive and Gram-negative bacteria, making it a versatile natural antibiotic. Propolis is often used in throat sprays, tinctures, and lozenges to target respiratory and oral infections.

By incorporating these natural antivirals and antibacterials into your health regimen, you can effectively support your body in fighting infections, whether they are viral or bacterial in nature. With the right herbal approach, it is possible to enhance your immune defenses, reduce the severity of infections, and promote overall health without the risks associated with over-reliance on conventional antibiotics. These remedies, when used thoughtfully and in conjunction with a healthy lifestyle, provide a comprehensive natural strategy for combating pathogens and maintaining optimal health.

Remedies for Infection Control

283. Olive Leaf Antiviral Tincture

Ingredients: ½ cup dried olive leaves, 2 cups vodka or brandy (40% alcohol), 1 glass jar with a tight-fitting lid.

Preparation: Place the dried olive leaves in the glass jar and cover with vodka. Seal tightly and store in a cool, dark place for 4-6 weeks, shaking daily. Strain and store in a dark glass bottle.
Suggested Usage: Take 1 dropperful (about 20-30 drops) up to 3 times daily to

support immune health and fight viral infections.

Benefits: Olive leaf contains oleuropein, a powerful antiviral and antioxidant compound that inhibits viral replication and enhances the immune system's response.

284. Echinacea and Goldenseal Immune Tonic

Ingredients: 1 tablespoon dried echinacea root, 1 tablespoon dried goldenseal root, 3 cups water, 1 cup raw honey.

Preparation: Simmer echinacea and goldenseal roots in water for 30 minutes. Strain and return the liquid to the pan. Simmer until reduced by half, then remove from heat and stir in honey. Store in a glass jar.

Suggested Usage: Take 1 tablespoon daily for prevention, or up to 3 times daily at the onset of symptoms.

Benefits: Echinacea stimulates immune activity, while goldenseal acts as a natural antibiotic, making this tonic effective for supporting immune function and fighting infections.

285. Elderberry and Ginger Immune Syrup

Ingredients: 1 cup dried elderberries, ½ cup grated fresh ginger, 4 cups water, 1 cup raw honey.

Preparation: Combine elderberries, ginger, and water in a saucepan. Bring to a boil, then simmer for 30-45 minutes until the liquid is reduced by half. Strain and return to the pan. Add honey and stir until well mixed. Store in a glass jar.

Suggested Usage: Take 1 tablespoon

daily during cold and flu season, or 3 times daily at the onset of symptoms.

Benefits: Elderberries are rich in antioxidants and flavonoids, which support the immune system and reduce the duration of colds and flu, while ginger helps alleviate respiratory congestion and supports overall immune health.

286. Garlic and Thyme Antimicrobial Oil

Ingredients: 4-5 garlic cloves (crushed), 1 tablespoon dried thyme, ½ cup olive oil.

Preparation: Gently heat garlic and thyme in olive oil over low heat for 30 minutes. Allow to cool, strain, and store in a glass jar.

Suggested Usage: Apply a small amount to cuts, scrapes, or fungal infections up to twice daily.

Benefits: Garlic and thyme are powerful antimicrobials that help fight bacterial and fungal infections, reduce inflammation, and promote healing.

287. Oregano Oil Capsules

Ingredients: ¼ cup dried oregano leaves, 1 tablespoon olive oil, empty vegetable capsules.

Preparation: Blend the dried oregano leaves into a fine powder and mix with olive oil until well combined. Fill the capsules with the mixture and store in a cool, dry place.

Suggested Usage: Take 1 capsule daily for up to 2 weeks to fight infections and boost immunity.

Benefits: Oregano oil is rich in carvacrol, a compound with strong antibacterial, antifungal, and antiviral properties, making these capsules effective for combating a range of pathogens.

288. Lemon Balm and Cat's Claw Antiviral Tea

Ingredients: 1 tablespoon dried lemon balm leaves, 1 tablespoon dried cat's claw bark, 2 cups hot water, 1 teaspoon raw honey.
Preparation: Steep lemon balm and cat's claw in hot water for 15 minutes. Strain and add honey if desired.
Suggested Usage: Drink 1-2 cups daily to support immune health and reduce viral infections.
Benefits: Lemon balm has strong antiviral properties, especially against the herpes virus, while cat's claw helps modulate the immune response and reduce inflammation.

289. Usnea and Calendula Wound Wash

Ingredients: 2 tablespoons dried usnea, 2 tablespoons dried calendula, 4 cups water.
Preparation: Simmer usnea and calendula in water for 20-30 minutes. Strain and let cool. Store in a glass jar.
Suggested Usage: Use as a wash for cuts, scrapes, and minor wounds up to twice daily.
Benefits: Usnea contains usnic acid, a powerful antimicrobial agent, while calendula promotes healing and reduces inflammation, making this wash ideal for preventing infections in minor wounds.

290. Thyme and Rosemary Steam Inhalation

Ingredients: 1 tablespoon dried thyme, 1 tablespoon dried rosemary, 4 cups boiling water.
Preparation: Place thyme and rosemary in a large bowl and pour boiling water over them. Lean over the bowl with a towel draped over your head, creating a tent to trap the steam. Inhale deeply for 5-10 minutes.
Suggested Usage: Use 1-2 times daily during colds or respiratory infections to clear congestion and reduce inflammation.
Benefits: Thyme and rosemary both have powerful antimicrobial and decongestant properties, making this steam inhalation effective for clearing sinuses and soothing irritated respiratory tissues.

291. Licorice Root Antiviral Tea

Ingredients: 1 tablespoon dried licorice root, 2 cups hot water, 1 teaspoon raw honey.
Preparation: Steep licorice root in hot water for 15 minutes. Strain and add honey if desired.
Suggested Usage: Drink 1-2 cups daily to soothe the throat and reduce viral load.
Benefits: Licorice root has potent antiviral properties due to its glycyrrhizin content, which helps inhibit viral replication and soothe inflamed mucous membranes.

292. Holy Basil and Ginger Immunity Tea

Ingredients: 1 tablespoon dried holy basil leaves, 1 tablespoon grated fresh ginger, 2 cups hot water, 1 teaspoon raw honey.
Preparation: Steep holy basil and ginger in hot water for 15 minutes. Strain and add

honey if desired.

Suggested Usage: Drink 1 cup daily to reduce stress and support immune health.

Benefits: Holy basil is an adaptogen that helps balance cortisol levels and support the immune system, while ginger has strong anti-inflammatory properties, making this tea blend effective for reducing inflammation and enhancing immune function.

293. Propolis and Honey Throat Spray

Ingredients: 1 tablespoon propolis tincture, 2 tablespoons raw honey, 2 tablespoons warm water, a spray bottle.

Preparation: Combine all ingredients and mix thoroughly. Transfer to a spray bottle.

Suggested Usage: Spray directly into the throat 2-3 times daily during colds or sore throats.

Benefits: Propolis is a powerful antimicrobial and immune-supporting agent, while honey soothes the throat and provides additional antibacterial support, making this spray ideal for relieving sore throats and supporting oral health.

294. Eucalyptus and Peppermint Chest Rub

Ingredients: ¼ cup shea butter, ¼ cup coconut oil, 10 drops eucalyptus essential oil, 10 drops peppermint essential oil, 5 drops rosemary essential oil.

Preparation: Melt the shea butter and coconut oil using a double boiler. Remove from heat and stir in the essential oils. Transfer to a glass jar and allow to cool.

Suggested Usage: Apply a small amount to the chest and upper back during colds or respiratory congestion, up to 2 times daily.

Benefits: Eucalyptus and peppermint open up airways, reduce congestion, and soothe irritated respiratory tissues, providing relief from colds and coughs.

295. Cinnamon and Clove Antibacterial Gargle

Ingredients: 1 cinnamon stick, 5-6 whole cloves, 2 cups hot water, ½ teaspoon sea salt.

Preparation: Steep cinnamon and cloves in hot water for 15 minutes. Strain and let cool to a comfortable temperature. Stir in sea salt until dissolved.

Suggested Usage: Gargle with ¼ cup of the solution up to 3 times daily to reduce throat infections.

Benefits: Cinnamon and clove possess strong antibacterial and antiviral properties, making this gargle effective for soothing sore throats and preventing bacterial growth in the mouth and throat.

296. Ginger, Honey, and Lemon Cough Syrup

Ingredients: 1 cup grated fresh ginger, 1 cup raw honey, juice of 2 lemons, 2 cups water.

Preparation: Simmer ginger in water for 20 minutes. Strain and return the liquid to the pan. Add honey and lemon juice, stirring until well combined. Store in a glass jar.

Suggested Usage: Take 1 tablespoon up to 4 times daily to soothe coughs and reduce inflammation.

Benefits: Ginger helps reduce inflammation and ease respiratory discomfort, while honey coats and soothes the throat. Lemon adds a dose of vitamin C, making this syrup ideal for supporting the immune system during colds and flu.

297. Chamomile and Sage Mouth Rinse

Ingredients: 1 tablespoon dried chamomile flowers, 1 tablespoon dried sage leaves, 2 cups hot water, 1 teaspoon sea salt.

Preparation: Steep chamomile and sage in hot water for 15 minutes. Strain and stir in sea salt. Let cool to a comfortable temperature.

Suggested Usage: Use ¼ cup of the rinse to swish around the mouth and gargle up to 3 times daily.

Benefits: Chamomile and sage are both anti-inflammatory and antimicrobial, making this rinse effective for soothing gum inflammation, reducing mouth infections, and freshening breath.

298. Pau d' Arco Antifungal Decoction

Ingredients: 2 tablespoons dried Pau d'Arco bark, 4 cups water.

Preparation: Simmer Pau d'Arco bark in water for 30 minutes. Strain and serve warm.

Suggested Usage: Drink 1 cup up to twice daily to combat fungal infections and support immune health.

Benefits: Pau d'Arco contains lapachol, a compound known for its strong antifungal and antimicrobial properties, making this decoction effective for fighting yeast and fungal infections.

299. Myrrh and Goldenseal Gum Health Powder

Ingredients: 1 tablespoon dried myrrh powder, 1 tablespoon dried goldenseal powder, ½ teaspoon sea salt.

Preparation: Mix all ingredients thoroughly and store in a small glass jar.

Suggested Usage: Apply a small pinch to the gums and gently massage in, or add ¼ teaspoon to a small amount of water to swish as a mouth rinse.

Benefits: Myrrh and goldenseal are both potent antimicrobials that help reduce gum inflammation, prevent infections, and promote overall gum health.

300. Calendula and Lavender Wound-Healing Salve

Ingredients: ½ cup dried calendula flowers, ¼ cup dried lavender buds, 1 cup olive oil, ¼ cup beeswax, 10 drops tea tree essential oil.

Preparation: Gently heat calendula and lavender in olive oil for 1 hour. Strain and return to the pan. Add beeswax and stir until melted. Remove from heat and stir in tea tree oil. Pour into glass jars and let solidify.

Suggested Usage: Apply a small amount to cuts, scrapes, and burns as needed to promote healing and prevent infection.

Benefits: Calendula and lavender have anti-inflammatory, antimicrobial, and skin-healing properties, making this salve ideal for soothing irritated skin and speeding up the healing process.

301. Oregon Grape Root Antimicrobial Capsules

Ingredients: ¼ cup dried Oregon grape root powder, ¼ cup dried goldenseal powder, empty vegetable capsules.
Preparation: Mix the Oregon grape root and goldenseal powders thoroughly. Fill each capsule using a small spoon or capsule machine. Store in a cool, dry place.
Suggested Usage: Take 1 capsule up to twice daily to support the immune system and fight bacterial infections.
Benefits: Oregon grape root and goldenseal are both rich in berberine, a compound with strong antibacterial and antimicrobial properties, making these capsules effective for combating infections.

302. Sage and Thyme Antibacterial Tea

Ingredients: 1 tablespoon dried sage leaves, 1 tablespoon dried thyme, 2 cups hot water, 1 teaspoon raw honey.
Preparation: Steep sage and thyme in hot water for 15 minutes. Strain and add honey if desired.
Suggested Usage: Drink 1-2 cups daily during colds and respiratory infections.
Benefits: Sage and thyme are known for their potent antibacterial and antiviral properties, making this tea blend effective for soothing sore throats, reducing congestion, and fighting infections.

303. Elderflower and Yarrow Fever-Reducing Tea

Ingredients: 1 tablespoon dried elderflowers, 1 tablespoon dried yarrow, 2 cups hot water, 1 teaspoon raw honey.
Preparation: Steep elderflower and yarrow in hot water for 15 minutes. Strain and add honey if desired.
Suggested Usage: Drink 1-2 cups daily to reduce fever and promote sweating.
Benefits: Elderflower and yarrow have diaphoretic properties, meaning they help induce sweating and reduce fever, making this tea effective for managing fevers associated with colds and flu.

304. Black Walnut and Wormwood Parasite Cleanse

Ingredients: 1 tablespoon dried black walnut hull powder, 1 tablespoon dried wormwood powder, empty vegetable capsules.
Preparation: Mix black walnut hull and wormwood powders thoroughly. Fill each capsule using a small spoon or capsule machine. Store in a cool, dry place.
Suggested Usage: Take 1 capsule daily for up to 2 weeks to eliminate parasites.
Benefits: Black walnut and wormwood are powerful antiparasitic herbs that help expel intestinal parasites and support digestive health.

305. Peppermint and Lavender Sinus Steam

Ingredients: 1 tablespoon dried peppermint leaves, 1 tablespoon dried lavender buds, 4 cups boiling water.
Preparation: Place peppermint and lavender in a large bowl. Pour boiling water over the herbs. Lean over the bowl with a towel over your head to trap the

steam, and inhale deeply for 5-10 minutes.
Suggested Usage: Use 1-2 times daily during sinus congestion or respiratory infections.
Benefits: Peppermint opens up nasal passages and clears congestion, while lavender's calming properties reduce inflammation, making this steam effective for easing sinus pressure and respiratory discomfort.

306. Horseradish and Ginger Sinus-Clearing Tonic

Ingredients: 1 tablespoon freshly grated horseradish root, 1 tablespoon grated fresh ginger, juice of 1 lemon, 1 teaspoon raw honey, 1 cup warm water.
Preparation: Combine all ingredients in a cup and mix thoroughly until the honey is dissolved.
Suggested Usage: Drink 1 cup up to twice daily to clear nasal congestion and support respiratory health.
Benefits: Horseradish and ginger are potent decongestants that help clear sinus passages, reduce mucus, and support overall respiratory function.

307. Lemon Balm and Licorice Respiratory Tea

Ingredients: 1 tablespoon dried lemon balm leaves, 1 tablespoon dried licorice root, 2 cups hot water, 1 teaspoon raw honey.
Preparation: Steep lemon balm and licorice root in hot water for 15 minutes. Strain and add honey if desired.
Suggested Usage: Drink 1-2 cups daily to reduce respiratory inflammation and support immune health.

Benefits: Lemon balm is a calming herb that helps reduce stress and inflammation, while licorice root soothes the respiratory tract and reduces inflammation, making this tea ideal for respiratory infections and chronic coughs.

308. Cat's Claw and Astragalus Immune Support Capsules

Ingredients: ¼ cup dried Cat's Claw bark powder, ¼ cup dried Astragalus root powder, empty vegetable capsules.
Preparation: Mix Cat's Claw and Astragalus powders thoroughly. Fill each capsule using a small spoon or capsule machine. Store in a cool, dry place.
Suggested Usage: Take 1 capsule daily to support immune health and reduce inflammation.
Benefits: Cat's Claw and Astragalus are both powerful immune-modulating herbs that help balance the immune response, making these capsules ideal for supporting long-term immune health and preventing infections.

309. Garlic and Mullein Ear Oil

Ingredients: 5-6 garlic cloves (crushed), ¼ cup dried mullein flowers, ½ cup olive oil.
Preparation: Gently heat garlic and mullein in olive oil over low heat for 30 minutes. Strain and let cool. Store in a small glass bottle.
Suggested Usage: Apply 2-3 drops in the affected ear, up to twice daily, to relieve ear infections and reduce inflammation.
Benefits: Garlic is a powerful antimicrobial, while mullein soothes irritation and reduces inflammation,

making this oil highly effective for managing ear infections and reducing earache.

310. Neem and Turmeric Antimicrobial Paste

Ingredients: 1 tablespoon dried neem powder, 1 tablespoon dried turmeric powder, ¼ cup water.

Preparation: Combine neem and turmeric powders, then add water gradually to form a thick paste. Store in a glass jar.

Suggested Usage: Apply a small amount to infected or inflamed areas of the skin up to twice daily.

Benefits: Neem and turmeric are both potent antimicrobials and anti-inflammatories, making this paste ideal for treating skin infections, acne, and inflammatory skin conditions.

311. Ginger, Lemon, and Cayenne Immune Shot

Ingredients: 1 tablespoon grated fresh ginger, juice of 1 lemon, ¼ teaspoon cayenne pepper, 1 cup warm water, 1 teaspoon raw honey.

Preparation: Combine all ingredients in a cup and mix until honey is dissolved.

Suggested Usage: Take 1 shot in the morning during cold and flu season to support immune health and reduce inflammation.

Benefits: Ginger and cayenne boost circulation and reduce inflammation, while lemon and honey provide additional immune support, making this shot a powerful way to start your day and ward off infections.

312. Marshmallow Root and Licorice Soothing Tea

Ingredients: 1 tablespoon dried marshmallow root, 1 tablespoon dried licorice root, 2 cups hot water, 1 teaspoon raw honey.

Preparation: Steep marshmallow root and licorice root in hot water for 15 minutes. Strain and add honey if desired.

Suggested Usage: Drink 1-2 cups daily to soothe the digestive and respiratory tracts.

Benefits: Marshmallow root and licorice root are demulcent herbs that coat and protect mucous membranes, making this tea effective for soothing irritated tissues in the throat, stomach, and intestines.

313. Aloe Vera and Peppermint Gel for Skin Irritations

Ingredients: ½ cup fresh aloe vera gel, 5 drops peppermint essential oil.

Preparation: Mix aloe vera gel and peppermint oil until well combined. Store in a glass jar in the refrigerator.

Suggested Usage: Apply a small amount to irritated or inflamed skin up to 3 times daily to reduce itching and redness.

Benefits: Aloe vera cools and soothes the skin, while peppermint provides a mild analgesic effect, making this gel ideal for managing rashes, sunburns, and other skin irritations.

314. Rosemary and Tea Tree Antimicrobial Hand Wash

Ingredients: 1 cup liquid castile soap, 10 drops rosemary essential oil, 10 drops tea tree essential oil, 1 tablespoon fractionated coconut oil.

Preparation: Combine all ingredients in a soap dispenser and shake well.

Suggested Usage: Use as a hand wash to reduce the risk of infection and keep hands clean.

Benefits: Rosemary and tea tree have potent antimicrobial properties, making this hand wash effective for eliminating germs and maintaining hand hygiene.

315. Elderberry and Cinnamon Antiviral Tea

Ingredients: 1 tablespoon dried elderberries, 1 cinnamon stick, 2 cups hot water, 1 teaspoon raw honey.

Preparation: Steep elderberries and cinnamon in hot water for 15 minutes. Strain and add honey if desired.

Suggested Usage: Drink 1-2 cups daily during cold and flu season to support immune health and fight viral infections.

Benefits: Elderberries are known for their antiviral properties, while cinnamon has strong antioxidant and anti-inflammatory effects, making this tea blend effective for reducing the duration and severity of viral infections.

316. Echinacea and Nettle Immune Tonic

Ingredients: 1 tablespoon dried echinacea root, 1 tablespoon dried nettle leaves, 3 cups water, 1 tablespoon raw honey.

Preparation: Simmer echinacea root and nettle leaves in water for 30 minutes. Strain and return the liquid to the pan. Reduce the liquid by half, then remove from heat and stir in honey. Store in a glass jar.

Suggested Usage: Take 1 tablespoon daily to support immune health and reduce inflammation.

Benefits: Echinacea stimulates immune activity, while nettle is rich in vitamins and minerals that strengthen the body's natural defenses, making this tonic effective for enhancing immunity during cold and flu season.

317. Calendula and Chamomile Eye Wash

Ingredients: 1 tablespoon dried calendula flowers, 1 tablespoon dried chamomile flowers, 2 cups hot water.

Preparation: Steep calendula and chamomile flowers in hot water for 15 minutes. Strain and allow to cool to room temperature. Store in a clean, sterile jar.

Suggested Usage: Use a small amount as a gentle eye wash up to twice daily to relieve eye irritation and reduce inflammation.

Benefits: Calendula and chamomile are soothing and anti-inflammatory herbs that help reduce redness, swelling, and irritation in the eyes, making this wash effective for managing conjunctivitis and general eye discomfort.

318. Ginger and Oregano Cold and Flu Capsules

Ingredients: ¼ cup dried ginger powder, ¼ cup dried oregano powder, empty vegetable capsules.

Preparation: Mix the ginger and oregano powders thoroughly. Use a small spoon or capsule machine to fill each capsule. Store in a cool, dry place.

Suggested Usage: Take 1-2 capsules daily

at the onset of cold or flu symptoms.

Benefits: Ginger and oregano have strong antiviral and antimicrobial properties that help reduce inflammation, boost immune function, and fight infections, making these capsules effective for managing symptoms and speeding recovery.

319. Turmeric and Black Pepper Antimicrobial Paste

Ingredients: ¼ cup turmeric powder, 1 teaspoon ground black pepper, ¼ cup water, 1 tablespoon coconut oil.
Preparation: Combine turmeric and black pepper in a small bowl. Gradually add water until a thick paste forms. Stir in coconut oil until smooth. Store in a glass jar.
Suggested Usage: Apply a small amount to infected or inflamed areas of the skin twice daily.
Benefits: Turmeric and black pepper provide potent anti-inflammatory and antimicrobial properties, making this paste ideal for treating minor infections, acne, and skin irritations.

320. Sage, Lavender, and Rosemary Disinfectant Spray

Ingredients: 1 cup distilled water, 1 cup white vinegar, 10 drops sage essential oil, 10 drops lavender essential oil, 10 drops rosemary essential oil, a spray bottle.
Preparation: Combine all ingredients in a spray bottle and shake well.
Suggested Usage: Use as a natural disinfectant for cleaning surfaces and preventing the spread of germs.
Benefits: Sage, lavender, and rosemary are powerful antimicrobials that help eliminate bacteria, viruses, and fungi, making this spray effective for maintaining cleanliness and preventing infections in the home.

321. Usnea and Yarrow Herbal Wash for Cuts

Ingredients: 1 tablespoon dried usnea, 1 tablespoon dried yarrow, 4 cups water.
Preparation: Simmer usnea and yarrow in water for 30 minutes. Strain and allow to cool. Store in a glass jar.
Suggested Usage: Use as a wash for cuts, scrapes, and minor wounds up to twice daily.
Benefits: Usnea contains usnic acid, a powerful antimicrobial agent, while yarrow promotes wound healing and reduces inflammation, making this wash ideal for preventing infections in minor wounds and supporting tissue repair.

322. Lemon and Ginger Throat Soother

Ingredients: Juice of 1 lemon, 1 tablespoon grated fresh ginger, 1 teaspoon raw honey, 1 cup warm water.
Preparation: Combine all ingredients in a cup and mix thoroughly until honey is dissolved.
Suggested Usage: Drink 1 cup up to twice daily to soothe sore throats and reduce inflammation.
Benefits: Lemon provides vitamin C and antioxidants, while ginger and honey have anti-inflammatory and soothing properties, making this remedy effective for relieving throat irritation and supporting immune health.

323. Fennel and Peppermint Digestive Tea

Ingredients: 1 tablespoon fennel seeds, 1 tablespoon dried peppermint leaves, 2 cups hot water.

Preparation: Steep fennel seeds and peppermint in hot water for 15 minutes. Strain and serve warm.

Suggested Usage: Drink 1 cup after meals to support digestion and reduce bloating.

Benefits: Fennel helps reduce gas and bloating, while peppermint relaxes the digestive tract, making this tea blend ideal for alleviating digestive discomfort and promoting healthy digestion.

324. Olive Leaf and Echinacea Throat Gargle

Ingredients: 1 tablespoon dried olive leaf, 1 tablespoon dried echinacea root, 2 cups hot water, ½ teaspoon sea salt.

Preparation: Steep olive leaf and echinacea root in hot water for 20 minutes. Strain and let cool. Add sea salt and stir until dissolved.

Suggested Usage: Gargle with ¼ cup of the solution up to 3 times daily to reduce throat infections and soothe irritation.

Benefits: Olive leaf and echinacea have strong antimicrobial and immune-supporting properties, making this gargle effective for soothing sore throats and preventing bacterial growth in the mouth and throat.

325. Turmeric and Ginger Immune Support Elixir

Ingredients: 1 tablespoon grated fresh turmeric, 1 tablespoon grated fresh ginger, juice of 1 lemon, 1 teaspoon raw honey, 1 cup warm water.

Preparation: Combine all ingredients in a cup and mix thoroughly until honey is dissolved.

Suggested Usage: Drink 1 cup daily to boost immunity and reduce inflammation.

Benefits: Turmeric and ginger have strong anti-inflammatory and immune-boosting properties, while lemon and honey provide additional immune support, making this elixir effective for preventing infections and supporting overall health.

326. Thyme and Garlic Respiratory Tonic

Ingredients: 1 tablespoon dried thyme, 2 garlic cloves (minced), 2 cups hot water, 1 teaspoon raw honey.

Preparation: Steep thyme and garlic in hot water for 15 minutes. Strain and add honey if desired.

Suggested Usage: Drink 1-2 cups daily to reduce respiratory congestion and support lung health.

Benefits: Thyme and garlic have strong antimicrobial and expectorant properties that help clear mucus, reduce inflammation, and support respiratory health, making this tonic effective for managing colds, bronchitis, and other respiratory infections.

327. Lemon Balm and Elderflower Immune Tea

Ingredients: 1 tablespoon dried lemon balm leaves, 1 tablespoon dried elderflowers, 2 cups hot water, 1 teaspoon raw honey.

Preparation: Steep lemon balm and elderflowers in hot water for 15 minutes. Strain and add honey if desired.

Suggested Usage: Drink 1-2 cups daily to support immune health and reduce inflammation.

Benefits: Lemon balm has calming and antiviral properties, while elderflower boosts immunity and supports respiratory health. This tea is ideal for reducing the severity of colds and supporting overall immune function.

328. Clove and Cinnamon Gum Health Rinse

Ingredients: 1 cinnamon stick, 5-6 whole cloves, 2 cups hot water, ½ teaspoon sea salt.

Preparation: Steep the cinnamon stick and cloves in hot water for 15 minutes. Strain and let cool. Stir in sea salt until dissolved.

Suggested Usage: Swish ¼ cup of the rinse around the mouth up to 3 times daily to reduce gum inflammation and fight bacteria.

Benefits: Clove and cinnamon are powerful antimicrobials that help reduce oral bacteria, soothe gum inflammation, and freshen breath, making this rinse effective for supporting overall oral health.

329. Goldenrod and Elderberry Immune Tonic

Ingredients: 1 tablespoon dried goldenrod, 1 tablespoon dried elderberries, 3 cups water, 1 cup raw honey.

Preparation: Simmer goldenrod and elderberries in water for 30 minutes. Strain and return the liquid to the pan. Reduce by half, then remove from heat and stir in honey. Store in a glass jar.

Suggested Usage: Take 1 tablespoon daily to boost immune function, or up to 3 times daily during illness.

Benefits: Goldenrod and elderberries are rich in antioxidants and support immune health, making this tonic effective for preventing and reducing the severity of colds and flu.

330. Chamomile and Sage Sore Throat Tea

Ingredients: 1 tablespoon dried chamomile flowers, 1 tablespoon dried sage leaves, 2 cups hot water, 1 teaspoon raw honey.

Preparation: Steep chamomile and sage in hot water for 15 minutes. Strain and add honey if desired.

Suggested Usage: Drink 1-2 cups daily to soothe sore throats and reduce inflammation.

Benefits: Chamomile and sage have strong anti-inflammatory and antimicrobial properties that help reduce throat irritation, soothe mucous membranes, and fight infections, making this tea effective for relieving sore throats and supporting respiratory health.

331. Goldenseal and Echinacea Sinus Steam

Ingredients: 1 tablespoon dried goldenseal root, 1 tablespoon dried echinacea root, 4 cups boiling water.

Preparation: Place goldenseal and echinacea roots in a large bowl and pour boiling water over them. Lean over the bowl with a towel draped over your head to trap the steam. Inhale deeply for 5-10 minutes.

Suggested Usage: Use 1-2 times daily during sinus infections to clear congestion and reduce inflammation.

Benefits: Goldenseal and echinacea have powerful antimicrobial and immune-boosting properties that help reduce sinus congestion, fight infections, and support overall respiratory health.

332. Lemongrass and Ginger Anti-Inflammatory Tea

Ingredients: 1 tablespoon dried lemongrass, 1 tablespoon grated fresh ginger, 2 cups hot water, 1 teaspoon raw honey.

Preparation: Steep lemongrass and ginger in hot water for 15 minutes. Strain and add honey if desired.

Suggested Usage: Drink 1-2 cups daily to reduce inflammation and support digestive health.

Benefits: Lemongrass and ginger have strong anti-inflammatory and digestive-supporting properties, making this tea effective for reducing bloating, soothing the digestive tract, and alleviating pain.

Book 17: Herbal Adaptogens for Immune Balance

Adaptogens are a unique class of herbs that help the body adapt to stress, restore balance, and maintain overall homeostasis. Unlike other herbs that may target specific symptoms or bodily functions, adaptogens work holistically to promote resilience, supporting multiple body systems simultaneously. They primarily function by regulating the hypothalamic-pituitary-adrenal (HPA) axis and balancing the production of stress hormones like cortisol. This regulation helps protect the body from the detrimental effects of chronic stress, which can include suppressed immune function, increased inflammation, and hormonal imbalances. By enhancing the body's natural ability to handle physical, emotional, and environmental stressors, adaptogens promote long-term health and resilience, making them invaluable for immune support and overall well-being.

When the body is under constant stress, the immune system is one of the first areas to be compromised. Stress hormones like cortisol, when elevated over long periods, can suppress the activity of immune cells, reduce the production of essential immune molecules, and leave the body more vulnerable to infections and inflammation. Adaptogens counteract these effects by modulating the stress response, supporting adrenal function, and enhancing the efficiency of immune responses. They help the body maintain a balanced state of health, known as homeostasis, even in the face of external challenges. As such, adaptogens are not just for people dealing with high stress but are also beneficial for those looking to maintain overall immune health, improve energy levels, and support the body's natural defense mechanisms.

Understanding Adaptogens

Adaptogens have been used for centuries in traditional medicine systems, including Ayurveda and Traditional Chinese Medicine (TCM), to increase vitality, endurance, and resistance to stress. The concept of adaptogens was first defined in the mid-20th century by Russian scientists who were researching herbs that could enhance the performance and resilience of soldiers and athletes. To be classified as an adaptogen, an herb must meet three criteria: it must be non-toxic and safe for long-term use; it must help the body resist a wide range of physical, chemical, and biological stressors; and it must restore balance and normalize bodily functions, regardless of the direction of the imbalance.

Unlike stimulants, which provide a temporary boost in energy, or sedatives, which induce relaxation, adaptogens have a bidirectional effect. This means they can energize when energy is low and calm when there is excess stimulation. By supporting the endocrine system, nervous system, and immune system simultaneously, adaptogens provide a balanced, holistic approach to health. They do not push the body in one direction but instead help it achieve a state of optimal functioning.

Top Adaptogenic Herbs for Immune Support

Ashwagandha (*Withania somnifera*)

Ashwagandha is one of the most well-known adaptogens, particularly valued for its ability to reduce stress, lower cortisol levels, and promote restful sleep. It has been used for centuries in Ayurvedic medicine to enhance resilience, improve vitality, and support overall health. Ashwagandha is particularly effective for individuals dealing with chronic stress, fatigue, and immune suppression. It works by balancing cortisol levels, protecting the body from the effects of stress, and boosting the production of white blood cells, making it an excellent choice for enhancing immunity and reducing inflammation. Ashwagandha can be taken as a tincture, in capsule form, or as a powder added to warm milk or smoothies.

Rhodiola (*Rhodiola rosea*)

Rhodiola is a powerful adaptogen native to the Arctic regions of Europe and Asia. It has been traditionally used to enhance stamina, reduce fatigue, and improve mental clarity. Rhodiola is particularly effective at modulating the body's stress response and supporting cognitive function, making it ideal for individuals experiencing burnout or high levels of mental stress. It also has immune-boosting properties, as it enhances the activity of natural killer (NK) cells, which play a critical role in defending the body against infections and tumors. Rhodiola can be taken as a tea, tincture, or capsule.

Reishi Mushroom (*Ganoderma lucidum*)

Reishi is often referred to as the "Mushroom of Immortality" in Traditional Chinese Medicine due to its ability to promote longevity, balance the immune system, and protect against the effects of stress. Reishi works by modulating the activity of white blood cells, balancing inflammatory responses, and enhancing the body's natural ability to resist infections. It is particularly beneficial for individuals dealing with autoimmune conditions or chronic inflammation, as it helps bring the immune system into balance. Reishi can be taken as a tea, in capsule form, or in powdered form added to smoothies and soups.

Holy Basil (*Ocimum sanctum*)

Also known as Tulsi, Holy Basil is revered in Ayurvedic medicine as a powerful adaptogen that helps the body cope with physical and mental stress. It is known for its ability to balance cortisol levels, reduce anxiety, and promote emotional well-being. Holy Basil also has strong antimicrobial and anti-inflammatory properties, making it effective for supporting the immune system and reducing the risk of infections. It can be consumed as a tea, tincture, or capsule, or even added to culinary dishes for its aromatic and health-boosting properties.

Schisandra (*Schisandra chinensis*)

Schisandra is a berry traditionally used in Chinese medicine to improve energy, endurance, and mental performance. It is known as a "five-flavor fruit" because it contains all five basic tastes: sweet, sour, salty, bitter, and pungent, symbolizing its broad range of health benefits. Schisandra works by balancing the nervous system, enhancing liver detoxification, and supporting adrenal health. It is also a powerful antioxidant, protecting the body from oxidative stress and inflammation. Schisandra is commonly taken as a tea, tincture, or capsule and can be combined with other adaptogens for comprehensive stress support.

Eleuthero (*Eleutherococcus senticosus*)

Also known as Siberian Ginseng, Eleuthero is an adaptogen used for enhancing physical endurance, reducing fatigue, and supporting immune health. It is particularly effective for individuals recovering from illness or experiencing prolonged periods of stress. Eleuthero works by enhancing the body's resilience to stress, increasing energy levels, and supporting the function of the adrenal glands. It can also improve mental clarity and cognitive performance. Eleuthero is typically taken in capsule or tincture form, and it pairs well with other adaptogens like Rhodiola and Ashwagandha.

Astragalus (*Astragalus membranaceus*)

Astragalus is a staple in Traditional Chinese Medicine, known for its immune-boosting and anti-inflammatory properties. It works by enhancing the body's production of interferons and other immune molecules, making it effective for both preventing and treating infections. Astragalus is particularly beneficial for individuals with weakened immunity or those recovering from illness, as it helps build resilience and protect against future infections. Astragalus can be taken as a tea, tincture, or in capsule form and is often combined with Reishi and other immune-supporting adaptogens.

Cordyceps Mushroom (*Cordyceps sinensis*)

Cordyceps is a unique adaptogen that is traditionally used to enhance stamina, increase energy, and support respiratory health. It works by improving oxygen utilization, boosting ATP production, and enhancing immune function, making it ideal for individuals looking to improve physical performance and recover from fatigue. Cordyceps also has anti-inflammatory and immune-modulating properties, making it a valuable addition to any adaptogenic regimen. It can be consumed as a tea, in capsule form, or as a powder added to drinks and dishes.

These adaptogenic herbs can be incorporated into a daily routine to help balance the body's stress response, support immune function, and promote overall well-being. Adaptogens work best when used consistently over time, allowing the body to build resilience and maintain a state of equilibrium even in the face of stress and environmental challenges.

Remedies for Enhancing Resilience

333. Ashwagandha and Holy Basil Adaptogen Tea

Ingredients: 1 tablespoon dried Ashwagandha root, 1 tablespoon dried Holy Basil leaves, 2 cups hot water, 1 teaspoon raw honey.

Preparation: Steep Ashwagandha root and Holy Basil leaves in hot water for 15 minutes. Strain and add honey if desired.

Suggested Usage: Drink 1-2 cups daily to reduce stress and support overall immune health.

Benefits: Ashwagandha helps balance cortisol levels and promotes resilience to stress, while Holy Basil calms the mind and reduces anxiety, making this tea ideal for restoring balance and enhancing vitality.

334. Reishi and Astragalus Immune Support Decoction

Ingredients: 1 tablespoon dried Reishi mushroom slices, 1 tablespoon dried Astragalus root, 4 cups water.

Preparation: Simmer Reishi and Astragalus in water for 30-40 minutes. Strain and serve warm.

Suggested Usage: Drink 1 cup daily to support the immune system and enhance energy.

Benefits: Reishi modulates the immune response and reduces inflammation, while Astragalus strengthens immunity and protects against stress-related immune suppression, making this decoction effective for long-term immune health.

335. Rhodiola and Eleuthero Energy Capsules

Ingredients: ¼ cup dried Rhodiola root powder, ¼ cup dried Eleuthero root powder, empty vegetable capsules.

Preparation: Mix Rhodiola and Eleuthero powders thoroughly. Use a small spoon or capsule machine to fill each capsule. Store in a cool, dry place.

Suggested Usage: Take 1-2 capsules daily to boost energy and reduce fatigue.

Benefits: Rhodiola and Eleuthero both enhance physical and mental endurance, reduce stress, and improve cognitive performance, making these capsules ideal for boosting energy and focus.

336. Schisandra and Goji Berry Vitality Tonic

Ingredients: 1 tablespoon dried Schisandra berries, 1 tablespoon dried Goji berries, 3 cups water, 1 teaspoon raw honey.

Preparation: Simmer Schisandra and Goji berries in water for 30 minutes. Strain and serve warm. Add honey if desired.

Suggested Usage: Drink 1 cup daily to enhance energy and support immune health.

Benefits: Schisandra enhances mental clarity and resilience, while Goji berries are rich in antioxidants and support liver function, making this tonic effective for boosting vitality and promoting overall well-being.

337. Cordyceps and Ginger Stamina Tea

Ingredients: 1 tablespoon dried Cordyceps mushroom, 1 tablespoon grated fresh ginger, 2 cups hot water, 1 teaspoon lemon juice.

Preparation: Steep Cordyceps and ginger in hot water for 20 minutes. Strain and add lemon juice.

Suggested Usage: Drink 1 cup before physical activity to enhance stamina and energy.

Benefits: Cordyceps increases oxygen utilization and boosts energy levels, while ginger improves circulation and digestion, making this tea ideal for athletes and individuals looking to improve physical performance.

338. Eleuthero and Licorice Stress Relief Capsules

Ingredients: ¼ cup dried Eleuthero root powder, ¼ cup dried Licorice root powder, empty vegetable capsules.

Preparation: Mix Eleuthero and Licorice powders thoroughly. Use a small spoon or capsule machine to fill each capsule. Store in a cool, dry place.

Suggested Usage: Take 1 capsule daily to reduce stress and support adrenal health.

Benefits: Eleuthero strengthens the adrenal glands and reduces fatigue, while Licorice helps modulate cortisol levels, making these capsules ideal for managing chronic stress and supporting adrenal recovery.

339. Tulsi and Lemon Balm Calming Elixir

Ingredients: 1 tablespoon dried Tulsi leaves, 1 tablespoon dried Lemon Balm leaves, 2 cups hot water, 1 teaspoon raw honey.

Preparation: Steep Tulsi and Lemon Balm in hot water for 15 minutes. Strain

and add honey if desired.

Suggested Usage: Drink 1 cup in the evening to promote relaxation and reduce anxiety.

Benefits: Tulsi and Lemon Balm have calming and mood-enhancing properties that help soothe the nervous system, reduce stress, and promote restful sleep.

340. Maca and Ashwagandha Hormone Balance Smoothie

Ingredients: 1 teaspoon Maca powder, 1 teaspoon Ashwagandha powder, 1 cup almond milk, 1 banana, 1 teaspoon raw honey, ¼ teaspoon cinnamon.

Preparation: Blend all ingredients until smooth. Serve immediately.

Suggested Usage: Drink 1 cup daily to support hormonal balance and enhance energy.

Benefits: Maca and Ashwagandha work synergistically to balance hormone levels, improve mood, and boost energy, making this smoothie ideal for supporting overall hormonal health.

341. Reishi and Chaga Adaptogen Latte

Ingredients: 1 teaspoon Reishi mushroom powder, 1 teaspoon Chaga mushroom powder, 1 cup unsweetened almond milk, 1 teaspoon raw honey, a pinch of cinnamon.

Preparation: Heat almond milk gently and stir in Reishi, Chaga, and cinnamon until fully dissolved. Add honey and stir until mixed. Serve warm.

Suggested Usage: Drink 1 cup in the evening to reduce stress and support immune health.

Benefits: Reishi and Chaga are powerful adaptogens that help modulate the immune system, reduce inflammation, and promote relaxation, making this latte effective for supporting overall well-being.

342. Holy Basil and Ginger Anti-Inflammatory Tincture

Ingredients: ½ cup dried Holy Basil leaves, ½ cup grated fresh ginger, 2 cups vodka or brandy (40% alcohol), 1 glass jar with a tight-fitting lid.
Preparation: Place Holy Basil and ginger in the glass jar and cover with vodka. Seal tightly and store in a cool, dark place for 4-6 weeks, shaking daily. Strain and store in a dark glass bottle.
Suggested Usage: Take 1 dropperful (about 20-30 drops) up to twice daily to reduce inflammation and support immune health.
Benefits: Holy Basil and ginger are powerful anti-inflammatory herbs that reduce pain, support digestion, and enhance immune function, making this tincture ideal for managing inflammation and promoting resilience.

343. Rhodiola and Ginseng Energy Elixir

Ingredients: 1 tablespoon dried Rhodiola root, 1 tablespoon dried Ginseng root, 3 cups water, 1 teaspoon raw honey.
Preparation: Simmer Rhodiola and Ginseng roots in water for 30 minutes. Strain and add honey if desired.
Suggested Usage: Drink 1 cup daily to boost energy, focus, and endurance.
Benefits: Rhodiola and Ginseng both

enhance physical and mental stamina, improve cognitive function, and support the body's ability to cope with stress, making this elixir effective for boosting energy and resilience.

344. Adaptogen Mushroom Immune-Boosting Soup

Ingredients: 1 cup sliced fresh mushrooms (shiitake, maitake, and Reishi), 1 tablespoon dried Astragalus root, 1 tablespoon dried Chaga mushroom powder, 4 cups vegetable broth, 2 minced garlic cloves, 1 chopped onion, 1 tablespoon olive oil, 1 teaspoon thyme, salt, and pepper to taste.
Preparation: Sauté onion and garlic in olive oil until soft. Add the mushrooms, Astragalus root, and Chaga powder, and cook for another 5 minutes. Pour in the vegetable broth and add thyme, salt, and pepper. Simmer for 30 minutes, then strain out the Astragalus root before serving.
Suggested Usage: Enjoy 1-2 bowls weekly to boost immune health and reduce inflammation.
Benefits: Adaptogenic mushrooms like Reishi and Chaga modulate the immune system and reduce inflammation, while Astragalus enhances resilience and protects against illness, making this soup ideal for long-term immune support.

345. Reishi and Turmeric Golden Milk

Ingredients: 1 teaspoon Reishi mushroom powder, 1 teaspoon turmeric powder, 1 cup unsweetened almond milk, 1 teaspoon raw honey, a pinch of black pepper, a pinch of cinnamon.

Preparation: Warm the almond milk over low heat. Stir in Reishi, turmeric, black pepper, and cinnamon until fully dissolved. Remove from heat and add honey. Serve warm.

Suggested Usage: Drink 1 cup before bedtime to reduce inflammation and promote relaxation.

Benefits: Reishi helps calm the nervous system and enhance immune health, while turmeric provides anti-inflammatory support and aids in reducing joint pain and inflammation, making this drink effective for overall well-being.

346. Astragalus and Nettle Nourishing Broth

Ingredients: 1 tablespoon dried Astragalus root, 1 tablespoon dried Nettle leaves, 4 cups vegetable broth, 2 chopped carrots, 2 chopped celery stalks, 1 chopped onion, 2 minced garlic cloves, 1 tablespoon olive oil, salt, and pepper to taste.

Preparation: Sauté onion and garlic in olive oil until soft. Add carrots and celery, cooking for another 5 minutes. Add the broth, Astragalus root, Nettle leaves, salt, and pepper. Simmer for 30 minutes. Strain out the Astragalus root before serving.

Suggested Usage: Enjoy 1 cup daily to support immune health and increase vitality.

Benefits: Astragalus strengthens the immune system, while Nettle provides essential vitamins and minerals, making this broth effective for nourishing the body and boosting overall energy levels.

347. Schisandra and Lemon Balm Nerve Tonic

Ingredients: 1 tablespoon dried Schisandra berries, 1 tablespoon dried Lemon Balm leaves, 3 cups water, 1 teaspoon raw honey.

Preparation: Simmer Schisandra berries in water for 30 minutes. Add Lemon Balm leaves and steep for 10 minutes. Strain and add honey if desired.

Suggested Usage: Drink 1 cup daily to reduce stress and support nervous system health.

Benefits: Schisandra enhances mental clarity and endurance, while Lemon Balm calms the nervous system, making this tonic ideal for reducing stress and supporting emotional well-being.

348. Gotu Kola and Ashwagandha Brain Boost Capsules

Ingredients: ¼ cup dried Gotu Kola powder, ¼ cup dried Ashwagandha root powder, empty vegetable capsules.

Preparation: Mix Gotu Kola and Ashwagandha powders thoroughly. Use a small spoon or capsule machine to fill each capsule. Store in a cool, dry place.

Suggested Usage: Take 1 capsule daily to support cognitive function and reduce stress.

Benefits: Gotu Kola enhances memory and cognitive performance, while Ashwagandha reduces cortisol levels and promotes resilience, making these capsules effective for supporting brain health and managing stress.

349. Cordyceps and Ginger Respiratory Health Tea

Ingredients: 1 tablespoon dried Cordyceps mushroom, 1 tablespoon grated fresh ginger, 2 cups hot water, 1 teaspoon lemon juice.

Preparation: Steep Cordyceps and ginger in hot water for 20 minutes. Strain and add lemon juice.

Suggested Usage: Drink 1 cup up to twice daily to enhance respiratory health and support immune function.

Benefits: Cordyceps improves respiratory function and oxygen utilization, while ginger reduces inflammation and soothes the respiratory tract, making this tea ideal for supporting lung health and enhancing stamina.

350. Maca and Ginseng Energy Capsules

Ingredients: ¼ cup dried Maca root powder, ¼ cup dried Ginseng root powder, empty vegetable capsules.

Preparation: Mix Maca and Ginseng powders thoroughly. Use a small spoon or capsule machine to fill each capsule. Store in a cool, dry place.

Suggested Usage: Take 1-2 capsules daily to boost energy and reduce fatigue.

Benefits: Maca and Ginseng enhance stamina and endurance, improve hormonal balance, and support overall vitality, making these capsules effective for boosting physical and mental energy.

351. Holy Basil and Chamomile Stress Relief Tea

Ingredients: 1 tablespoon dried Holy Basil leaves, 1 tablespoon dried Chamomile flowers, 2 cups hot water, 1 teaspoon raw honey.

Preparation: Steep Holy Basil and Chamomile in hot water for 15 minutes.

Strain and add honey if desired.

Suggested Usage: Drink 1 cup in the evening to reduce anxiety and promote restful sleep.

Benefits: Holy Basil and Chamomile work together to calm the nervous system, reduce cortisol levels, and promote relaxation, making this tea effective for managing stress and supporting emotional health.

352. Astragalus and Reishi Immune Tonic

Ingredients: 1 tablespoon dried Astragalus root, 1 tablespoon dried Reishi mushroom slices, 4 cups water.

Preparation: Simmer Astragalus and Reishi in water for 30-40 minutes. Strain and serve warm.

Suggested Usage: Drink 1 cup daily to support the immune system and enhance energy levels.

Benefits: Astragalus and Reishi are both powerful immune modulators that enhance immune function, reduce inflammation, and promote long-term health, making this tonic ideal for building resilience and protecting against illness.

353. Eleuthero and Rhodiola Adrenal Support Capsules

Ingredients: ¼ cup dried Eleuthero root powder, ¼ cup dried Rhodiola root powder, empty vegetable capsules.

Preparation: Mix Eleuthero and Rhodiola powders thoroughly. Use a small spoon or capsule machine to fill each capsule. Store in a cool, dry place.

Suggested Usage: Take 1 capsule daily to support adrenal health and reduce stress.

Benefits: Eleuthero and Rhodiola enhance adrenal function, reduce fatigue, and improve the body's resilience to stress, making these capsules effective for supporting long-term energy and stress management.

354. Schisandra and Ashwagandha Anti-Stress Tonic

Ingredients: 1 tablespoon dried Schisandra berries, 1 tablespoon dried Ashwagandha root, 3 cups water, 1 teaspoon raw honey.

Preparation: Simmer Schisandra and Ashwagandha in water for 30 minutes. Strain and add honey if desired.

Suggested Usage: Drink 1 cup daily to reduce stress and promote balance.

Benefits: Schisandra and Ashwagandha work synergistically to enhance resilience, support emotional stability, and reduce cortisol levels, making this tonic effective for managing stress and promoting overall health.

355. Adaptogen Berry Smoothie with Schisandra and Goji

Ingredients: 1 teaspoon Schisandra berry powder, 1 tablespoon dried Goji berries (soaked), 1 cup almond milk, ½ cup frozen blueberries, 1 ripe banana, 1 teaspoon raw honey.

Preparation: Blend all ingredients until smooth. Serve immediately.

Suggested Usage: Drink 1 cup in the morning to enhance energy and support cognitive function.

Benefits: Schisandra enhances mental clarity and supports adrenal health, while Goji berries are rich in antioxidants that support immunity and energy, making this smoothie ideal for boosting vitality and overall health.

356. Reishi and Licorice Immune Modulating Tea

Ingredients: 1 tablespoon dried Reishi mushroom slices, 1 tablespoon dried Licorice root, 3 cups hot water, 1 teaspoon raw honey.

Preparation: Simmer Reishi and Licorice root in hot water for 30 minutes. Strain and add honey if desired.

Suggested Usage: Drink 1 cup daily to support immune health and reduce inflammation.

Benefits: Reishi modulates the immune system, while Licorice root soothes mucous membranes and reduces inflammation, making this tea ideal for managing immune health and promoting balance.

357. Tulsi, Lemon Balm, and Chamomile Calming Tea

Ingredients: 1 tablespoon dried Tulsi leaves, 1 tablespoon dried Lemon Balm leaves, 1 tablespoon dried Chamomile flowers, 3 cups hot water.

Preparation: Steep Tulsi, Lemon Balm, and Chamomile in hot water for 15 minutes. Strain and serve warm.

Suggested Usage: Drink 1 cup in the evening to reduce stress and promote restful sleep.

Benefits: Tulsi, Lemon Balm, and Chamomile have calming properties that reduce anxiety, soothe the nervous system, and support emotional health, making this tea ideal for promoting relaxation and reducing stress.

358. Ashwagandha and Cordyceps Performance Elixir

Ingredients: 1 tablespoon Ashwagandha root powder, 1 tablespoon dried Cordyceps mushroom, 3 cups water, 1 teaspoon raw honey.
Preparation: Simmer Ashwagandha and Cordyceps in water for 30 minutes. Strain and add honey if desired.
Suggested Usage: Drink 1 cup before physical activity to enhance energy and stamina.
Benefits: Ashwagandha and Cordyceps increase physical endurance, boost energy levels, and support recovery, making this elixir effective for enhancing athletic performance and overall vitality.

359. Adaptogenic Chai Tea with Reishi and Turmeric

Ingredients: 1 teaspoon Reishi mushroom powder, 1 teaspoon turmeric powder, 1 cup coconut milk, 1 cinnamon stick, 2 whole cloves, 1 teaspoon raw honey, a pinch of black pepper.
Preparation: Heat coconut milk gently and add Reishi, turmeric, cinnamon, cloves, and black pepper. Simmer for 10 minutes, remove from heat, and add honey. Serve warm.
Suggested Usage: Drink 1 cup in the evening to reduce inflammation and promote immune health.
Benefits: Reishi and turmeric reduce inflammation, balance the immune system, and support adrenal health,

making this chai effective for promoting relaxation and overall well-being.

360. Astragalus, Ginger, and Garlic Immunity Broth

Ingredients: 1 tablespoon dried Astragalus root, 2 tablespoons grated fresh ginger, 2 minced garlic cloves, 4 cups vegetable broth, 1 chopped onion, 1 tablespoon olive oil, salt, and pepper to taste.
Preparation: Sauté onion, garlic, and ginger in olive oil until soft. Add the vegetable broth, Astragalus root, salt, and pepper. Simmer for 30 minutes. Strain out the Astragalus root before serving.
Suggested Usage: Enjoy 1-2 cups weekly to boost immunity and support respiratory health.
Benefits: Astragalus enhances immunity and resilience, while ginger and garlic provide anti-inflammatory and antimicrobial support, making this broth effective for preventing illness and promoting overall immune health.

361. Schisandra and Rosehip Antioxidant Tea

Ingredients: 1 tablespoon dried Schisandra berries, 1 tablespoon dried Rosehips, 2 cups hot water, 1 teaspoon raw honey.
Preparation: Steep Schisandra and Rosehips in hot water for 15 minutes. Strain and add honey if desired.
Suggested Usage: Drink 1-2 cups daily to support immune health and increase energy levels.
Benefits: Schisandra and Rosehips are rich in antioxidants that protect against

oxidative stress, support cardiovascular health, and enhance vitality, making this tea effective for long-term health support.

362. Eleuthero and Maca Stamina Capsules

Ingredients: ¼ cup dried Eleuthero root powder, ¼ cup dried Maca root powder, empty vegetable capsules.
Preparation: Mix Eleuthero and Maca powders thoroughly. Use a small spoon or capsule machine to fill each capsule. Store in a cool, dry place.
Suggested Usage: Take 1-2 capsules daily to boost energy and endurance.
Benefits: Eleuthero and Maca increase stamina, reduce fatigue, and support adrenal health, making these capsules ideal for enhancing energy and resilience.

363. Adaptogen Trail Mix with Maca and Schisandra

Ingredients: 1 cup raw almonds, ½ cup dried goji berries, ¼ cup dried Schisandra berries, ¼ cup pumpkin seeds, 1 tablespoon Maca powder, 1 tablespoon shredded coconut.
Preparation: Combine all ingredients in a large bowl and mix thoroughly. Store in an airtight container.
Suggested Usage: Enjoy ¼ cup as a snack to boost energy and support immune health.
Benefits: Schisandra and Maca enhance resilience, energy, and mental clarity, while goji berries and almonds provide additional antioxidant and nutritional support, making this trail mix ideal for boosting vitality.

364. Reishi and Elderberry Immune Elixir

Ingredients: 1 tablespoon dried Reishi mushroom slices, 1 tablespoon dried elderberries, 4 cups water, 1 cup raw honey.
Preparation: Simmer Reishi and elderberries in water for 30 minutes. Strain and return the liquid to the pan. Simmer until reduced by half, then remove from heat and stir in honey. Store in a glass jar.
Suggested Usage: Take 1 tablespoon daily to enhance immune function and reduce inflammation.
Benefits: Reishi and elderberries modulate the immune response, reduce inflammation, and support overall health, making this elixir effective for long-term immune support.

365. Gotu Kola and Ginkgo Biloba Memory Boost Capsules

Ingredients: ¼ cup dried Gotu Kola powder, ¼ cup dried Ginkgo Biloba powder, empty vegetable capsules.
Preparation: Mix Gotu Kola and Ginkgo Biloba powders thoroughly. Use a small spoon or capsule machine to fill each capsule. Store in a cool, dry place.
Suggested Usage: Take 1 capsule daily to support cognitive function and improve memory.
Benefits: Gotu Kola and Ginkgo Biloba enhance circulation to the brain, improve cognitive function, and reduce mental fatigue, making these capsules ideal for supporting brain health and enhancing memory.

366. Holy Basil, Lavender, and Lemon Balm Sleep Tea

Ingredients: 1 tablespoon dried Holy Basil leaves, 1 tablespoon dried Lavender flowers, 1 tablespoon dried Lemon Balm leaves, 2 cups hot water, 1 teaspoon raw honey.
Preparation: Steep Holy Basil, Lavender, and Lemon Balm in hot water for 15 minutes. Strain and add honey if desired.
Suggested Usage: Drink 1 cup in the evening to promote relaxation and restful sleep.
Benefits: Holy Basil helps reduce stress and anxiety, while Lavender and Lemon Balm calm the nervous system and promote restful sleep, making this tea effective for managing insomnia and supporting emotional well-being.

367. Chaga and Ashwagandha Anti-Fatigue Capsules

Ingredients: ¼ cup dried Chaga mushroom powder, ¼ cup dried Ashwagandha root powder, empty vegetable capsules.
Preparation: Mix Chaga and Ashwagandha powders thoroughly. Use a small spoon or capsule machine to fill each capsule. Store in a cool, dry place.
Suggested Usage: Take 1-2 capsules daily to reduce fatigue and enhance energy levels.
Benefits: Chaga boosts immune function and reduces inflammation, while Ashwagandha balances cortisol levels and supports adrenal health, making these capsules ideal for combating chronic fatigue and enhancing resilience.

368. Astragalus, Nettle, and Red Clover Infusion

Ingredients: 1 tablespoon dried Astragalus root, 1 tablespoon dried Nettle leaves, 1 tablespoon dried Red Clover flowers, 4 cups hot water.
Preparation: Combine all herbs in a large jar and pour hot water over them. Seal and let steep for 4-8 hours, then strain.
Suggested Usage: Drink 1-2 cups daily to support immune health and promote vitality.
Benefits: Astragalus enhances immune function, Nettle provides essential vitamins and minerals, and Red Clover supports detoxification, making this infusion effective for nourishing and balancing the body.

369. Cordyceps and Schisandra Exercise Recovery Tea

Ingredients: 1 tablespoon dried Cordyceps mushroom, 1 tablespoon dried Schisandra berries, 2 cups hot water, 1 teaspoon raw honey.
Preparation: Steep Cordyceps and Schisandra in hot water for 20 minutes. Strain and add honey if desired.
Suggested Usage: Drink 1 cup after physical activity to reduce fatigue and support recovery.
Benefits: Cordyceps enhances stamina and improves oxygen utilization, while Schisandra reduces stress and promotes recovery, making this tea ideal for athletes and active individuals.

370. Reishi and Rhodiola Calm Focus Capsules

Ingredients: ¼ cup dried Reishi mushroom powder, ¼ cup dried Rhodiola root powder, empty vegetable capsules.

Preparation: Mix Reishi and Rhodiola powders thoroughly. Use a small spoon or capsule machine to fill each capsule. Store in a cool, dry place.

Suggested Usage: Take 1 capsule daily to promote mental clarity and reduce anxiety.

Benefits: Reishi calms the mind and modulates stress, while Rhodiola enhances focus and mental endurance, making these capsules effective for reducing anxiety and improving cognitive function.

371. Maca and Cordyceps Adaptogen Smoothie

Ingredients: 1 teaspoon Maca powder, 1 teaspoon Cordyceps mushroom powder, 1 cup almond milk, 1 banana, 1 teaspoon raw honey, ¼ teaspoon cinnamon.

Preparation: Blend all ingredients until smooth. Serve immediately.

Suggested Usage: Drink 1 cup in the morning to boost energy and support resilience.

Benefits: Maca and Cordyceps enhance stamina, improve physical performance, and balance hormone levels, making this smoothie ideal for boosting energy and supporting overall vitality.

372. Ashwagandha and Holy Basil Anti-Anxiety Capsules

Ingredients: ¼ cup dried Ashwagandha root powder, ¼ cup dried Holy Basil leaf powder, empty vegetable capsules.

Preparation: Mix Ashwagandha and Holy Basil powders thoroughly. Use a small spoon or capsule machine to fill

each capsule. Store in a cool, dry place.

Suggested Usage: Take 1 capsule daily to reduce anxiety and support adrenal health.

Benefits: Ashwagandha balances cortisol levels and reduces stress, while Holy Basil calms the nervous system and promotes emotional stability, making these capsules effective for managing anxiety and enhancing resilience.

373. Reishi and Turmeric Inflammation Relief Tea

Ingredients: 1 teaspoon Reishi mushroom powder, 1 teaspoon turmeric powder, 1 cup hot water, 1 teaspoon raw honey, a pinch of black pepper.

Preparation: Steep Reishi and turmeric in hot water for 15 minutes. Add black pepper and honey, stirring until dissolved.

Suggested Usage: Drink 1 cup daily to reduce inflammation and support immune health.

Benefits: Reishi modulates the immune response and reduces stress, while turmeric provides strong anti-inflammatory support, making this tea effective for managing chronic inflammation and promoting overall well-being.

374. Eleuthero and Schisandra Hormonal Balance Tonic

Ingredients: 1 tablespoon dried Eleuthero root, 1 tablespoon dried Schisandra berries, 3 cups water, 1 teaspoon raw honey.

Preparation: Simmer Eleuthero and Schisandra in water for 30 minutes. Strain and add honey if desired.

Suggested Usage: Drink 1 cup daily to

support hormonal balance and reduce stress.

Benefits: Eleuthero supports adrenal health and reduces fatigue, while Schisandra balances hormones and enhances resilience, making this tonic ideal for supporting hormonal health and promoting energy.

375. Adaptogen Latte with Ashwagandha and Reishi

Ingredients: 1 teaspoon Ashwagandha powder, 1 teaspoon Reishi mushroom powder, 1 cup unsweetened almond milk, 1 teaspoon raw honey, a pinch of cinnamon.

Preparation: Heat almond milk gently and stir in Ashwagandha, Reishi, and cinnamon until fully dissolved. Add honey and stir until mixed. Serve warm.

Suggested Usage: Drink 1 cup in the evening to reduce stress and promote relaxation.

Benefits: Ashwagandha and Reishi work synergistically to balance the body's stress response, reduce anxiety, and enhance immune health, making this latte ideal for supporting overall well-being.

376. Astragalus and Ginger Immune Boost Tea

Ingredients: 1 tablespoon dried Astragalus root, 1 tablespoon grated fresh ginger, 3 cups hot water, 1 teaspoon raw honey.

Preparation: Simmer Astragalus and ginger in hot water for 30 minutes. Strain and add honey if desired.

Suggested Usage: Drink 1 cup daily to support immune health and reduce inflammation.

Benefits: Astragalus enhances immunity and protects against illness, while ginger provides anti-inflammatory support and soothes the digestive system, making this tea effective for boosting overall health and resilience.

377. Ginseng and Holy Basil Resilience Capsules

Ingredients: ¼ cup dried Ginseng root powder, ¼ cup dried Holy Basil leaf powder, empty vegetable capsules.

Preparation: Mix Ginseng and Holy Basil powders thoroughly. Use a small spoon or capsule machine to fill each capsule. Store in a cool, dry place.

Suggested Usage: Take 1-2 capsules daily to boost resilience and support overall health.

Benefits: Ginseng enhances energy and physical endurance, while Holy Basil reduces stress and supports mental clarity, making these capsules ideal for promoting long-term resilience and vitality.

378. Cordyceps and Eleuthero Performance Tonic

Ingredients: 1 tablespoon dried Cordyceps mushroom, 1 tablespoon dried Eleuthero root, 3 cups water, 1 teaspoon raw honey.

Preparation: Simmer Cordyceps and Eleuthero in water for 30 minutes. Strain and add honey if desired.

Suggested Usage: Drink 1 cup before physical activity to boost stamina and energy.

Benefits: Cordyceps increases oxygen utilization and endurance, while Eleuthero supports adrenal health and reduces fatigue, making this tonic effective for enhancing athletic performance and promoting recovery.

379. Schisandra and Tulsi Adrenal Support Tea

Ingredients: 1 tablespoon dried Schisandra berries, 1 tablespoon dried Tulsi leaves, 2 cups hot water, 1 teaspoon raw honey.
Preparation: Steep Schisandra and Tulsi in hot water for 15 minutes. Strain and add honey if desired.
Suggested Usage: Drink 1 cup in the morning to support adrenal health and reduce stress.
Benefits: Schisandra enhances energy and mental clarity, while Tulsi calms the nervous system and reduces cortisol levels, making this tea effective for balancing adrenal function and managing stress.

380. Adaptogen Energy Bars with Maca and Goji

Ingredients: 1 cup rolled oats, ½ cup chopped almonds, ½ cup dried Goji berries, ¼ cup Maca powder, ¼ cup nut butter, ¼ cup raw honey, 1 teaspoon vanilla extract, a pinch of sea salt.
Preparation: Mix oats, almonds, Goji berries, and Maca powder in a large bowl. In a separate bowl, combine nut butter, honey, vanilla extract, and sea salt. Pour wet ingredients over dry ingredients and mix until combined. Press mixture into a lined baking dish and refrigerate for 2 hours. Cut into bars.
Suggested Usage: Enjoy 1 bar as a snack

to boost energy and support resilience.
Benefits: Maca and Goji berries enhance energy and stamina, while almonds and oats provide sustained fuel, making these bars ideal for promoting long-lasting energy and vitality.

381. Adaptogenic Hot Chocolate with Reishi and Ashwagandha

Ingredients: 1 teaspoon Reishi mushroom powder, 1 teaspoon Ashwagandha powder, 1 tablespoon raw cacao powder, 1 cup unsweetened almond milk, 1 teaspoon raw honey, a pinch of cinnamon.
Preparation: Heat almond milk gently and stir in Reishi, Ashwagandha, and cacao powder until fully dissolved. Remove from heat and add honey and cinnamon. Serve warm.
Suggested Usage: Drink 1 cup in the evening to promote relaxation and support immune health.
Benefits: Reishi and Ashwagandha calm the nervous system and enhance resilience, while raw cacao provides mood-boosting properties, making this hot chocolate ideal for relaxation and overall well-being.

382. Reishi and Nettle Nourishing Tea

Ingredients: 1 tablespoon dried Reishi mushroom slices, 1 tablespoon dried Nettle leaves, 3 cups hot water, 1 teaspoon raw honey.
Preparation: Simmer Reishi and Nettle in hot water for 30 minutes. Strain and add honey if desired.
Suggested Usage: Drink 1 cup daily to support immune health and nourish the

body.

Benefits: Reishi modulates the immune system and reduces inflammation, while Nettle is rich in vitamins and minerals, making this tea ideal for promoting overall health and vitality.

383. Schisandra and Lemon Peel Digestive Tea

Ingredients: 1 tablespoon dried Schisandra berries, 1 tablespoon dried Lemon peel, 2 cups hot water, 1 teaspoon raw honey.

Preparation: Steep Schisandra and Lemon peel in hot water for 15 minutes. Strain and add honey if desired.

Suggested Usage: Drink 1-2 cups daily to support digestive health and reduce inflammation.

Benefits: Schisandra supports liver health and improves digestion, while Lemon peel stimulates digestion and reduces bloating, making this tea ideal for promoting digestive balance and overall well-being.

Book 18: Vitamins and Minerals for Immune Function

A strong and resilient immune system requires a solid nutritional foundation, which begins with essential vitamins and minerals. These nutrients play key roles in supporting the immune response, promoting cellular health, and protecting the body against infections. Inadequate intake of essential nutrients can weaken the immune system, leaving the body more vulnerable to illnesses and reducing its ability to recover efficiently. This chapter delves into the vitamins and minerals that are critical for immune function, highlights herbal sources rich in these nutrients, and provides natural supplementation strategies to ensure optimal health and immunity.

Essential Nutrients for Immune Health

Vitamins and minerals are fundamental for immune health, as they support the development and function of immune cells, regulate inflammatory responses, and promote overall well-being. Some of the most important nutrients for a robust immune system include:

Vitamin C: This potent antioxidant is essential for the production of white blood cells, which defend the body against pathogens. It also enhances the function of phagocytes—cells that "eat" harmful invaders—and supports the health of skin, the body's first line of defense. Vitamin C can be found in high amounts in citrus fruits, bell peppers, strawberries, and herbs like **Rosehips** and **Acerola Cherry**.

Vitamin D: Often referred to as the "sunshine vitamin," Vitamin D plays a crucial role in modulating the immune system. It enhances the pathogen-fighting effects of monocytes and macrophages, two types of white blood cells, and reduces inflammation. A deficiency in Vitamin D is associated with increased susceptibility to infection. The best sources include fatty fish, egg yolks, and exposure to sunlight. Herbal sources are limited, but **Nettle** and **Alfalfa** provide small amounts.

Vitamin A: This vitamin is essential for maintaining the integrity of mucous membranes in the respiratory and digestive tracts, which act as barriers against infections. It also plays a role in the development and function of immune cells like T- and B-cells. Vitamin A can be found in carrots, sweet potatoes, and herbs like **Dandelion**, **Burdock**, and **Chickweed**.

Vitamin E: A powerful antioxidant, Vitamin E helps maintain the health of immune cells by protecting them from oxidative damage. It supports the development of T-cells, which are crucial for adaptive immunity. Rich sources include nuts, seeds, and herbs like **Oatstraw** and **Sunflower Seeds**.

Zinc: This trace mineral is vital for immune cell development and communication, and it plays a critical role in inflammatory response. Zinc deficiency can impair immune function and increase susceptibility to infections. Dietary sources include shellfish, meat, and legumes, as well as herbs like **Pumpkin Seeds** and **Fenugreek**.

Selenium: Selenium is a powerful antioxidant that helps lower oxidative stress, thereby reducing inflammation and enhancing immunity. It is necessary for the production of glutathione peroxidase, an enzyme that helps detoxify harmful substances. Selenium is found in Brazil nuts and grains, and in small amounts in herbs like **Garlic** and **Basil**.

Magnesium: Magnesium supports hundreds of enzymatic reactions in the body, including those involved in energy production and immune cell function. It helps regulate the balance of calcium and Vitamin D, both of which are crucial for immune health. Dark leafy greens, nuts, and seeds, along with herbs like **Nettle** and **Dandelion**, are good sources of magnesium.

Iron: Iron is essential for the production of hemoglobin, which transports oxygen in the blood. It also supports the growth and differentiation of immune cells. Low iron levels can impair the body's ability to mount an effective immune response. Iron-rich foods include red meat, beans, and leafy greens, and herbs like **Nettle**, **Yellow Dock**, and **Mullein**.

Herbal Sources of Vitamins and Minerals

Herbs are often overlooked as nutritional powerhouses, yet many of them are rich in vitamins and minerals that support immune health. Incorporating nutrient-dense herbs into daily meals can help boost immunity and fill potential gaps in the diet. Some of the top herbs for supplying essential nutrients include:

Nettle (Urtica dioica) is a highly nutritious herb rich in iron, calcium, magnesium, and vitamins A, C, and K. It is particularly beneficial for supporting energy levels and overall vitality. Nettle can be consumed as a tea, in soups, or as a tincture.

Oatstraw (Avena sativa) is packed with magnesium and calcium, making it a great herb for supporting nerve and immune health. Oatstraw can be enjoyed as a tea or infusion, providing gentle and sustained nourishment.

Rosehips (Rosa canina) are one of the richest herbal sources of Vitamin C, along with bioflavonoids that enhance its absorption. Rosehips can be used in teas, syrups, or even incorporated into jams and sauces.

Alfalfa (Medicago sativa) is a nutrient-dense herb that provides Vitamins A, D, E, and K, as well as calcium, magnesium, and iron. It can be taken as a tea or sprinkled into smoothies and salads.

Dandelion (Taraxacum officinale) is abundant in vitamins A, C, and K, and is also a good source of iron, calcium, and potassium. The leaves can be added to salads, while the roots can be roasted and used as a coffee substitute.

Burdock Root (Arctium lappa) is rich in iron, magnesium, and potassium, making it ideal for supporting detoxification and immune function. Burdock can be taken as a decoction, tincture, or added to soups and stews.

Chickweed (Stellaria media) is a lesser-known herb that provides Vitamins A and C, as well as iron and calcium. It is best consumed fresh in salads or as a tea.

Red Clover (Trifolium pratense) contains Vitamins C and E, as well as calcium and magnesium. It supports respiratory and reproductive health and is often taken as an infusion or tincture.

Yellow Dock (Rumex crispus) is an excellent source of iron and can help boost energy and support liver health. It is often used as a tincture or decoction.

Pumpkin Seeds (Cucurbita pepo) are not only a great source of zinc, but they also contain magnesium and healthy fats that support overall immune function. Pumpkin seeds can be eaten raw, roasted, or incorporated into herbal powders and trail mixes.

Supplementing Naturally for Optimal Immunity

For those who struggle to meet their nutritional needs through diet alone, herbs can be an effective way to supplement vitamins and minerals naturally. Unlike synthetic supplements, herbal sources are often more bioavailable and come with additional benefits, such as antioxidants and phytonutrients that work synergistically to enhance absorption and support overall health. Here are some natural strategies for supplementing vitamins and minerals using herbs:

1. **Herbal Infusions:** Long infusions, made by steeping herbs in hot water for several hours, can extract more vitamins and minerals from herbs. Nettle, Oatstraw, and Red Clover are particularly effective when prepared as infusions. Simply add a handful of the dried herb to a quart-sized jar, cover with hot water, and let steep for 4-8 hours before straining and consuming.

2. **Herbal Powders:** Herbs like Nettle, Alfalfa, and Dandelion can be dried and ground into a fine powder. These powders can be sprinkled into smoothies, soups, or even capsules to provide concentrated nutrients.

3. **Syrups and Tonics:** Herbs rich in Vitamin C, such as Rosehips and Elderberries, can be simmered with honey to create delicious syrups that boost immunity. These can be taken daily, especially during cold and flu season.

4. **Herbal Vinegars:** Infusing herbs like Nettle, Dandelion, and Chickweed in apple cider vinegar helps extract their minerals and creates a nutrient-rich tonic that can be used in salad dressings or taken by the spoonful.

By incorporating these natural supplementation strategies into your daily routine, you can ensure that your body receives the vitamins and minerals it needs for optimal immune function and overall health.

Book 19: Herbal Teas for Immune Support

Herbal teas are an age-old remedy for nurturing the body, providing comfort, and delivering powerful immune-boosting properties in a gentle yet effective form. They are simple to prepare, easy to incorporate into daily routines, and can be customized to target specific health concerns. This chapter explores the science behind immune-supportive herbal teas, the benefits of different herbal combinations, and how the right blends can enhance immune function, alleviate symptoms, and promote overall health.

Recipes for Immune-Boosting Teas

Herbal teas, also known as tisanes, are infusions or decoctions made from various parts of plants, including leaves, flowers, roots, and seeds. When consumed regularly, herbal teas can provide a consistent supply of vitamins, minerals, antioxidants, and other immune-enhancing phytochemicals. They work by nourishing the body's natural defenses, reducing inflammation, and promoting the production of key immune cells.

The herbs used in these teas have been carefully selected for their ability to strengthen the immune system, combat pathogens, and support recovery from illness. For example, herbs like Echinacea and Elderberry are well-known for their immune-boosting properties and have been extensively studied for their ability to reduce the duration and severity of colds and flu. Similarly, adaptogenic herbs like Holy Basil and Astragalus build long-term resilience by modulating the stress response, which is crucial for maintaining a strong immune system. Including these herbs in teas not only enhances immunity but also provides a therapeutic experience that promotes relaxation and emotional well-being.

By combining immune-boosting herbs with soothing and supportive ingredients like Chamomile or Licorice, herbal teas can address a wide range of health issues, from acute infections to chronic inflammation. The following sections will highlight the benefits of different herbal teas and how to choose the right blend to meet individual health needs.

Benefits of Specific Herbal Teas

Each herbal tea offers a unique profile of benefits, depending on the specific herbs used and the method of preparation. Understanding the properties of these herbs can help you select the most effective teas for enhancing immune function, reducing symptoms of illness, and promoting long-term health.

Echinacea and Elderberry Teas for Immune Activation: Echinacea and Elderberry are two of the most popular herbs for immune support. Echinacea has been shown to activate white blood cells and enhance the production of interferons, which are proteins that inhibit viral replication. Elderberry, rich in anthocyanins, is a powerful antiviral that prevents viruses from attaching to cells, reducing the severity and duration of colds and flu. Teas made with these herbs are best used during the early stages of illness to boost immune activity and prevent the spread of infection.

Astragalus and Adaptogenic Teas for Building Resilience: Adaptogenic herbs like Astragalus, Schisandra, and Reishi mushroom are ideal for supporting long-term immune health. Adaptogens work by regulating the hypothalamic-pituitary-adrenal (HPA) axis and balancing cortisol levels, which, in turn, reduces stress-induced immune suppression. Regular consumption of adaptogenic teas can help build resilience, improve energy levels, and support the body's natural ability to cope with stress and illness.

Vitamin C-Rich Teas for Antioxidant Support: Vitamin C is a critical nutrient for immune function, promoting the activity of phagocytes and enhancing skin barrier function. Herbal teas made from Rosehips, Hibiscus, and Lemon Balm are excellent sources of natural Vitamin C and provide antioxidant support that protects immune cells from oxidative stress. These teas are particularly beneficial during cold and flu season, helping to boost immunity and reduce inflammation.

Anti-Inflammatory Teas for Immune Modulation: Chronic inflammation is a significant contributor to immune dysfunction and increased susceptibility to infections. Herbs like Turmeric, Ginger, and Licorice have strong anti-inflammatory properties that modulate the immune response, reduce inflammation, and promote healing. Teas made from these herbs are ideal for individuals dealing with autoimmune conditions, chronic inflammatory diseases, or recurrent infections.

Calming Teas for Stress and Immune Balance: Herbs like Lemon Balm, Chamomile, and Holy Basil are known for their calming effects on the nervous system. Since chronic stress can weaken the immune system, incorporating calming teas into a daily routine can help lower cortisol levels, reduce anxiety, and promote immune balance. These teas are perfect for evening use, supporting restful sleep and emotional well-being.

Respiratory Teas for Colds and Congestion: Respiratory health is closely linked to immune health, as the respiratory tract is a common entry point for pathogens. Teas made from Mullein, Thyme, and Peppermint help clear congestion, soothe irritated mucous membranes, and reduce coughing. Combined with demulcent herbs like Marshmallow Root, these teas provide comprehensive support for the respiratory system, making them effective for managing colds, bronchitis, and other respiratory infections.

The Role of Herbal Teas in Immune Health

Herbal teas can play a central role in maintaining and enhancing immune function. Unlike other forms of herbal medicine, teas are hydrating, gentle, and often consumed over long periods, which allows for consistent and sustained support. The act of drinking warm tea also provides comfort and can be a meditative experience that promotes relaxation and emotional well-being—factors that are crucial for a strong and balanced immune system.

Moreover, herbal teas offer a convenient way to incorporate a variety of immune-supportive herbs into the diet. Blending different herbs together allows for the synergistic effects of multiple constituents, creating a more comprehensive and effective remedy. For instance, combining antimicrobial herbs like Thyme and Oregano with soothing herbs like Licorice and Marshmallow can provide targeted support for respiratory infections, while adaptogenic teas that blend Reishi, Astragalus, and Holy Basil offer powerful immune modulation and stress resilience.

Choosing the Right Herbal Teas for Immune Support

When selecting herbal teas for immune support, consider the specific health goals and individual needs. For acute conditions like colds or flu, choose teas that contain potent antiviral and immune-stimulating herbs such as Elderberry, Echinacea, and Ginger. For chronic immune imbalances or stress-related suppression, opt for adaptogenic teas that include Reishi, Ashwagandha, or Holy Basil. If the goal is to support respiratory health, focus on teas with Mullein, Thyme, and Peppermint.

It's also important to consider taste and personal preference. Some immune-boosting herbs, like Echinacea and Goldenseal, can have strong, bitter flavors that may not appeal to everyone. In these cases, blending with naturally sweet herbs like Licorice or Lemon Balm can improve palatability without compromising effectiveness.

Incorporating immune-boosting teas into your daily routine is a simple yet powerful way to support overall health. Whether used to fend off infections, reduce inflammation, or build resilience, the right blend of herbs can make a significant difference in maintaining a strong and balanced immune system.

Remedies through Herbal Teas

384. Elderberry and Echinacea Immune-Boosting Tea

Ingredients: 1 tablespoon dried elderberries, 1 tablespoon dried Echinacea root, 1 teaspoon dried ginger root, 2 cups hot water, 1 teaspoon raw honey.
Preparation: Simmer elderberries and Echinacea root in hot water for 20 minutes. Remove from heat, add ginger, and steep for another 10 minutes. Strain and add honey if desired.
Suggested Usage: Drink 1-2 cups daily at the onset of cold or flu symptoms to strengthen the immune system and shorten illness duration.
Benefits: Elderberries provide potent antiviral support and boost immunity with high levels of Vitamin C and flavonoids. Echinacea stimulates immune activity, and ginger adds anti-inflammatory and

warming effects, making this tea ideal for combating infections.

385. Astragalus and Ginger Immunity Tonic

Ingredients: 1 tablespoon dried Astragalus root, 1 tablespoon grated fresh ginger, 3 cups hot water, 1 teaspoon lemon juice.

Preparation: Simmer Astragalus and ginger in hot water for 30 minutes. Strain and add lemon juice.

Suggested Usage: Drink 1 cup daily to enhance immune resilience and support long-term vitality.

Benefits: Astragalus is an adaptogenic herb that builds resilience, strengthens the immune system, and protects against stress. Ginger reduces inflammation and promotes healthy digestion, making this tonic effective for maintaining overall health and immunity.

386. Lemon Balm and Elderflower Antiviral Tea

Ingredients: 1 tablespoon dried Lemon Balm leaves, 1 tablespoon dried Elderflowers, 2 cups hot water, 1 teaspoon raw honey.

Preparation: Steep Lemon Balm and Elderflowers in hot water for 15 minutes. Strain and add honey if desired.

Suggested Usage: Drink 1-2 cups daily during viral outbreaks or cold and flu season to prevent infection and reduce symptoms.

Benefits: Lemon Balm has strong antiviral properties, while Elderflower is known for its ability to reduce fever and clear nasal congestion. Together, they provide gentle yet effective immune support, particularly for respiratory infections.

387. Nettle and Rosehip Vitamin C Tea

Ingredients: 1 tablespoon dried Nettle leaves, 1 tablespoon dried Rosehips, 2 cups hot water, 1 teaspoon raw honey.

Preparation: Steep Nettle and Rosehips in hot water for 15 minutes. Strain and add honey if desired.

Suggested Usage: Drink 1-2 cups daily to boost immunity, increase energy, and support overall vitality.

Benefits: Nettle is packed with vitamins and minerals, including iron and calcium, while Rosehips are one of the richest sources of natural Vitamin C, supporting immune health and protecting against oxidative stress.

388. Chamomile and Licorice Root Soothing Tea

Ingredients: 1 tablespoon dried Chamomile flowers, 1 tablespoon dried Licorice root, 2 cups hot water, 1 teaspoon raw honey.

Preparation: Steep Chamomile and Licorice root in hot water for 15 minutes. Strain and add honey if desired.

Suggested Usage: Drink 1 cup in the evening to soothe the throat and promote relaxation.

Benefits: Chamomile calms the nervous system and reduces inflammation, while Licorice root coats mucous membranes and balances immune responses, making this tea effective for managing sore throats and respiratory irritation.

389. Ginger, Lemon, and Honey Immune Support Tea

Ingredients: 1 tablespoon grated fresh ginger, juice of 1 lemon, 1 teaspoon raw honey, 2 cups hot water.

Preparation: Steep ginger in hot water for 10 minutes. Strain and add lemon juice and honey.

Suggested Usage: Drink 1-2 cups daily during cold and flu season or at the first sign of symptoms.

Benefits: Ginger provides anti-inflammatory and warming properties, lemon is rich in Vitamin C, and honey adds antimicrobial effects, making this tea a powerful remedy for boosting immunity and alleviating cold symptoms.

390. Holy Basil and Turmeric Anti-Inflammatory Tea

Ingredients: 1 tablespoon dried Holy Basil leaves, 1 teaspoon turmeric powder, 2 cups hot water, 1 teaspoon raw honey, a pinch of black pepper.

Preparation: Steep Holy Basil and turmeric in hot water for 15 minutes. Add black pepper and honey, stirring until dissolved.

Suggested Usage: Drink 1-2 cups daily to reduce inflammation and support immune balance.

Benefits: Holy Basil is an adaptogen that reduces stress and inflammation, while turmeric is a potent anti-inflammatory herb. Black pepper enhances the bioavailability of curcumin, the active compound in turmeric, making this tea ideal for managing chronic inflammation and promoting immune health.

391. Reishi and Chaga Adaptogen Immunity Tea

Ingredients: 1 teaspoon dried Reishi mushroom powder, 1 teaspoon dried Chaga mushroom powder, 2 cups hot water, 1 teaspoon raw honey.

Preparation: Steep Reishi and Chaga in hot water for 20 minutes. Strain and add honey if desired.

Suggested Usage: Drink 1 cup daily to build resilience and support long-term immune health.

Benefits: Reishi and Chaga are adaptogenic mushrooms that modulate the immune system, reduce inflammation, and promote overall vitality. This tea is effective for enhancing energy, reducing stress, and supporting immune balance.

392. Tulsi and Lemon Balm Calming Tea

Ingredients: 1 tablespoon dried Tulsi leaves, 1 tablespoon dried Lemon Balm leaves, 2 cups hot water, 1 teaspoon raw honey.

Preparation: Steep Tulsi and Lemon Balm in hot water for 15 minutes. Strain and add honey if desired.

Suggested Usage: Drink 1 cup in the evening to reduce stress and promote restful sleep.

Benefits: Tulsi is known as the "Queen of Herbs" for its ability to balance stress and support immune function, while Lemon Balm calms the nervous system and promotes relaxation, making this tea ideal for managing stress and anxiety.

393. Schisandra and Goji Berry Vitality Tonic

Ingredients: 1 tablespoon dried Schisandra berries, 1 tablespoon dried Goji berries, 3 cups water, 1 teaspoon raw honey.
Preparation: Simmer Schisandra and Goji berries in water for 30 minutes. Strain and add honey if desired.
Suggested Usage: Drink 1 cup daily to boost energy and support immune health.
Benefits: Schisandra enhances resilience and mental clarity, while Goji berries are rich in antioxidants and support liver function. This tonic is effective for boosting vitality and promoting overall well-being.

394. Ashwagandha and Licorice Root Stress Relief Tea

Ingredients: 1 tablespoon dried Ashwagandha root, 1 tablespoon dried Licorice root, 3 cups water, 1 teaspoon raw honey.
Preparation: Simmer Ashwagandha and Licorice in water for 30 minutes. Strain and add honey if desired.
Suggested Usage: Drink 1 cup in the evening to reduce stress and support adrenal health.
Benefits: Ashwagandha is a powerful adaptogen that reduces cortisol levels and promotes emotional balance, while Licorice supports adrenal health and soothes mucous membranes, making this tea effective for managing chronic stress and promoting resilience.

395. Peppermint and Thyme Respiratory Support Tea

Ingredients: 1 tablespoon dried Peppermint leaves, 1 tablespoon dried Thyme, 2 cups hot water, 1 teaspoon raw honey.
Preparation: Steep Peppermint and Thyme in hot water for 15 minutes. Strain and add honey if desired.
Suggested Usage: Drink 1-2 cups daily to support respiratory health and reduce congestion.
Benefits: Peppermint opens up the respiratory passages and reduces inflammation, while Thyme provides strong antimicrobial and expectorant properties, making this tea effective for relieving congestion and supporting respiratory health.

396. Elderflower and Yarrow Fever-Reducing Tea

Ingredients: 1 tablespoon dried Elderflowers, 1 tablespoon dried Yarrow flowers, 2 cups hot water, 1 teaspoon raw honey.
Preparation: Steep Elderflowers and Yarrow in hot water for 15 minutes. Strain and add honey if desired.
Suggested Usage: Drink 1 cup up to 3 times daily during fevers to reduce temperature and support immune function.
Benefits: Elderflower and Yarrow promote sweating and help the body regulate temperature, making this tea ideal for managing fevers and reducing the severity of cold and flu symptoms.

397. Ginger, Turmeric, and Cinnamon Warming Tea

Ingredients: 1 tablespoon grated fresh ginger, 1 teaspoon turmeric powder, 1 cinnamon stick, 2 cups hot water, 1 teaspoon raw honey.
Preparation: Simmer ginger, turmeric, and cinnamon in hot water for 15 minutes. Strain and add honey.
Suggested Usage: Drink 1-2 cups daily during cold weather or at the onset of illness to boost immunity and warm the body.
Benefits: Ginger, turmeric, and cinnamon provide anti-inflammatory, antimicrobial, and warming properties that help stimulate circulation, reduce inflammation, and support the immune system.

398. Sage and Lemon Throat Soother

Ingredients: 1 tablespoon dried Sage leaves, juice of 1 lemon, 2 cups hot water, 1 teaspoon raw honey.
Preparation: Steep Sage in hot water for 10 minutes. Strain and add lemon juice and honey.
Suggested Usage: Drink 1 cup up to 3 times daily to relieve sore throat and reduce inflammation.
Benefits: Sage is a powerful antimicrobial herb that helps soothe sore throats and reduce inflammation, while lemon provides Vitamin C and honey coats the throat, making this tea effective for managing throat irritation.

399. Holy Basil and Chamomile Bedtime Tea

Ingredients: 1 tablespoon dried Holy Basil leaves, 1 tablespoon dried Chamomile flowers, 2 cups hot water, 1 teaspoon raw honey.
Preparation: Steep Holy Basil and Chamomile in hot water for 15 minutes. Strain and add honey if desired.
Suggested Usage: Drink 1 cup in the evening to promote relaxation and support restful sleep.
Benefits: Holy Basil calms the mind and reduces cortisol levels, while Chamomile relaxes the nervous system and promotes sleep, making this tea ideal for managing stress and improving sleep quality.

400. Hibiscus and Lemon Peel Antioxidant Tea

Ingredients: 1 tablespoon dried Hibiscus flowers, 1 tablespoon dried Lemon peel, 2 cups hot water, 1 teaspoon raw honey.
Preparation: Steep Hibiscus and Lemon peel in hot water for 15 minutes. Strain and add honey if desired.
Suggested Usage: Drink 1-2 cups daily to support cardiovascular health and boost immunity.
Benefits: Hibiscus is rich in antioxidants and supports heart health, while Lemon peel enhances Vitamin C absorption and adds digestive support, making this tea effective for overall vitality and immune health.

401. Eucalyptus and Peppermint Respiratory Tea

Ingredients: 1 tablespoon dried Eucalyptus leaves, 1 tablespoon dried Peppermint leaves, 2 cups hot water.
Preparation: Steep Eucalyptus and

The Complete Collection of Barbara O'Neill   Jacqueline Bridge

Peppermint in hot water for 15 minutes. Strain and serve.

Suggested Usage: Drink 1 cup up to 3 times daily to clear congestion and support respiratory health.

Benefits: Eucalyptus helps open up the airways and reduce congestion, while Peppermint soothes the respiratory tract and reduces inflammation, making this tea effective for managing colds, bronchitis, and other respiratory issues.

402. Astragalus, Reishi, and Schisandra Immune Tonic

Ingredients: 1 tablespoon dried Astragalus root, 1 tablespoon dried Reishi mushroom, 1 tablespoon dried Schisandra berries, 4 cups water.

Preparation: Simmer Astragalus, Reishi, and Schisandra in water for 40 minutes. Strain and serve warm.

Suggested Usage: Drink 1 cup daily to support immune function and reduce the impact of stress.

Benefits: Astragalus strengthens the immune system, Reishi modulates immune response and reduces inflammation, and Schisandra enhances resilience, making this tonic ideal for long-term immune support.

403. Marshmallow Root and Slippery Elm Soothing Tea

Ingredients: 1 tablespoon dried Marshmallow root, 1 tablespoon dried Slippery Elm bark, 2 cups hot water, 1 teaspoon raw honey.

Preparation: Steep Marshmallow root and Slippery Elm in hot water for 20 minutes. Strain and add honey if desired.

Suggested Usage: Drink 1-2 cups daily to soothe sore throats and calm digestive irritation.

Benefits: Marshmallow root and Slippery Elm provide mucilaginous properties that coat mucous membranes, reduce inflammation, and promote healing, making this tea effective for managing sore throats, coughs, and digestive discomfort.

404. Rosemary and Ginger Circulation Tea

Ingredients: 1 tablespoon dried Rosemary leaves, 1 tablespoon grated fresh ginger, 2 cups hot water, 1 teaspoon raw honey.

Preparation: Steep Rosemary and ginger in hot water for 15 minutes. Strain and add honey if desired.

Suggested Usage: Drink 1-2 cups daily to improve circulation and support cognitive function.

Benefits: Rosemary stimulates circulation and enhances memory, while ginger warms the body and reduces inflammation, making this tea ideal for promoting healthy blood flow and cognitive health.

405. Elderberry, Rosehip, and Hibiscus Vitamin C Tea

Ingredients: 1 tablespoon dried Elderberries, 1 tablespoon dried Rosehips, 1 tablespoon dried Hibiscus flowers, 2 cups hot water, 1 teaspoon raw honey.

Preparation: Simmer Elderberries and Rosehips in hot water for 20 minutes. Remove from heat, add Hibiscus, and steep for 10 minutes. Strain and add honey if desired.

164

Suggested Usage: Drink 1-2 cups daily to support immune function and increase antioxidant intake.

Benefits: Elderberries, Rosehips, and Hibiscus are all rich in Vitamin C and antioxidants, making this tea effective for boosting immunity, reducing inflammation, and promoting overall health.

406. Mullein and Licorice Root Cough Relief Tea

Ingredients: 1 tablespoon dried Mullein leaves, 1 tablespoon dried Licorice root, 2 cups hot water, 1 teaspoon raw honey.

Preparation: Steep Mullein and Licorice in hot water for 20 minutes. Strain and add honey if desired.

Suggested Usage: Drink 1 cup up to 3 times daily to relieve coughs and soothe irritated airways.

Benefits: Mullein soothes the respiratory tract and acts as an expectorant, while Licorice root coats mucous membranes and reduces inflammation, making this tea ideal for managing coughs and respiratory discomfort.

407. Goldenseal and Ginger Sinus Clearing Tea

Ingredients: 1 teaspoon dried Goldenseal root, 1 tablespoon grated fresh ginger, 2 cups hot water, 1 teaspoon lemon juice.

Preparation: Steep Goldenseal and ginger in hot water for 20 minutes. Strain and add lemon juice.

Suggested Usage: Drink 1 cup up to twice daily to reduce sinus congestion and support immune function.

Benefits: Goldenseal has antimicrobial properties that help fight infections, while ginger reduces inflammation and promotes sinus drainage, making this tea effective for relieving sinus congestion.

408. Oregano and Thyme Antimicrobial Tea

Ingredients: 1 tablespoon dried Oregano leaves, 1 tablespoon dried Thyme leaves, 2 cups hot water, 1 teaspoon raw honey.

Preparation: Steep Oregano and Thyme in hot water for 15 minutes. Strain and add honey if desired.

Suggested Usage: Drink 1 cup up to twice daily to combat infections and support respiratory health.

Benefits: Oregano and Thyme are both strong antimicrobial herbs that help fight bacterial and viral infections, making this tea ideal for supporting respiratory health and immune defense.

409. Garlic and Lemon Immune Support Tea

Ingredients: 1 garlic clove (crushed), juice of 1 lemon, 2 cups hot water, 1 teaspoon raw honey.

Preparation: Steep crushed garlic in hot water for 10 minutes. Strain and add lemon juice and honey.

Suggested Usage: Drink 1 cup daily to boost immunity and fight off infections.

Benefits: Garlic has potent antibacterial and antiviral properties, while lemon provides Vitamin C and antioxidants, making this tea effective for supporting the immune system and preventing illness.

410. Calendula and Red Clover Lymphatic Tea

Ingredients: 1 tablespoon dried Calendula flowers, 1 tablespoon dried Red Clover flowers, 2 cups hot water.
Preparation: Steep Calendula and Red Clover in hot water for 15 minutes. Strain and serve warm.
Suggested Usage: Drink 1 cup up to twice daily to support lymphatic drainage and detoxification.
Benefits: Calendula and Red Clover promote lymphatic health, reduce inflammation, and support detoxification, making this tea ideal for enhancing the body's natural cleansing processes.

411. Lemon Balm and Passionflower Stress Relief Tea

Ingredients: 1 tablespoon dried Lemon Balm leaves, 1 tablespoon dried Passionflower, 2 cups hot water, 1 teaspoon raw honey.
Preparation: Steep Lemon Balm and Passionflower in hot water for 15 minutes. Strain and add honey if desired.
Suggested Usage: Drink 1 cup in the evening to reduce anxiety and promote relaxation.
Benefits: Lemon Balm calms the nervous system and supports emotional balance, while Passionflower reduces anxiety and promotes restful sleep, making this tea effective for managing stress and improving sleep quality.

412. Dandelion and Burdock Root Liver Support Tea

Ingredients: 1 tablespoon dried Dandelion root, 1 tablespoon dried Burdock root, 3 cups water.
Preparation: Simmer Dandelion and Burdock root in water for 30 minutes. Strain and serve warm.
Suggested Usage: Drink 1 cup up to twice daily to support liver health and detoxification.
Benefits: Dandelion and Burdock root stimulate liver function, support detoxification, and promote healthy digestion, making this tea ideal for cleansing the liver and supporting overall vitality.

413. Ginseng and Holy Basil Adaptogen Tea

Ingredients: 1 tablespoon dried Ginseng root slices, 1 tablespoon dried Holy Basil leaves, 3 cups water, 1 teaspoon raw honey.
Preparation: Simmer Ginseng in water for 20 minutes. Remove from heat, add Holy Basil, and steep for another 15 minutes. Strain and add honey if desired.
Suggested Usage: Drink 1 cup daily to reduce stress and support energy levels.
Benefits: Ginseng enhances energy and cognitive function, while Holy Basil reduces cortisol levels and balances the nervous system, making this tea effective for promoting resilience and managing stress.

414. Cinnamon and Clove Antiviral Tea

Ingredients: 1 cinnamon stick, 4 whole cloves, 2 cups hot water, 1 teaspoon raw honey.

Preparation: Simmer cinnamon and cloves in hot water for 15 minutes. Strain and add honey if desired.
Suggested Usage: Drink 1-2 cups daily during cold and flu season to reduce the risk of infection.
Benefits: Cinnamon and cloves have strong antiviral and antimicrobial properties, making this tea effective for protecting against infections and supporting immune health.

415. Linden and Chamomile Calming Immune Tea

Ingredients: 1 tablespoon dried Linden flowers, 1 tablespoon dried Chamomile flowers, 2 cups hot water, 1 teaspoon raw honey.
Preparation: Steep Linden and Chamomile in hot water for 15 minutes. Strain and add honey if desired.
Suggested Usage: Drink 1 cup in the evening to promote relaxation and support immune health.
Benefits: Linden and Chamomile calm the nervous system, reduce inflammation, and support restful sleep, making this tea ideal for managing stress and promoting overall immune balance.

416. Sage, Rosemary, and Thyme Immune Support Tea

Ingredients: 1 tablespoon dried Sage leaves, 1 tablespoon dried Rosemary leaves, 1 tablespoon dried Thyme leaves, 2 cups hot water.
Preparation: Steep Sage, Rosemary, and Thyme in hot water for 15 minutes. Strain and serve warm.
Suggested Usage: Drink 1 cup daily to enhance immunity and support respiratory health.
Benefits: Sage, Rosemary, and Thyme are rich in antioxidants and have strong antimicrobial properties, making this tea effective for supporting immune function and reducing the risk of infections.

417. Cat's Claw and Licorice Root Antiviral Tea

Ingredients: 1 tablespoon dried Cat's Claw bark, 1 tablespoon dried Licorice root, 3 cups water.
Preparation: Simmer Cat's Claw and Licorice root in water for 30 minutes. Strain and serve warm.
Suggested Usage: Drink 1 cup up to twice daily to reduce inflammation and support immune health.
Benefits: Cat's Claw has strong antiviral and anti-inflammatory properties, while Licorice root helps modulate immune response and soothe mucous membranes, making this tea ideal for managing viral infections and supporting respiratory health.

418. Fenugreek and Ginger Respiratory Relief Tea

Ingredients: 1 tablespoon dried Fenugreek seeds, 1 tablespoon grated fresh ginger, 2 cups hot water, 1 teaspoon lemon juice.
Preparation: Simmer Fenugreek and ginger in hot water for 15 minutes. Strain and add lemon juice.
Suggested Usage: Drink 1-2 cups daily to reduce mucus and support respiratory health.
Benefits: Fenugreek helps clear excess

mucus from the respiratory tract, while ginger provides warming and anti-inflammatory effects, making this tea effective for relieving congestion and supporting respiratory function.

419. Tulsi, Lemon, and Ginger Digestion Tea

Ingredients: 1 tablespoon dried Tulsi leaves, 1 tablespoon grated fresh ginger, juice of ½ lemon, 2 cups hot water.
Preparation: Steep Tulsi and ginger in hot water for 15 minutes. Strain and add lemon juice.
Suggested Usage: Drink 1 cup after meals to support digestion and reduce bloating.
Benefits: Tulsi balances digestion and reduces stress, while ginger and lemon stimulate digestive enzymes, making this tea ideal for promoting healthy digestion and reducing gastrointestinal discomfort.

420. Maca and Cacao Adaptogen Mood-Boosting Tea

Ingredients: 1 teaspoon Maca powder, 1 teaspoon raw cacao powder, 1 cup hot almond milk, 1 teaspoon raw honey, a pinch of cinnamon.
Preparation: Stir Maca, cacao, and cinnamon into hot almond milk until fully dissolved. Add honey and serve warm.
Suggested Usage: Drink 1 cup in the morning to enhance mood and support energy.
Benefits: Maca and cacao work synergistically to boost mood, balance hormones, and enhance energy levels, making this tea effective for promoting emotional well-being and overall vitality.

421. Lavender, Lemon Balm, and Valerian Relaxation Tea

Ingredients: 1 tablespoon dried Lavender flowers, 1 tablespoon dried Lemon Balm leaves, 1 teaspoon dried Valerian root, 2 cups hot water.
Preparation: Steep Lavender, Lemon Balm, and Valerian in hot water for 15 minutes. Strain and serve warm.
Suggested Usage: Drink 1 cup before bedtime to promote restful sleep and reduce anxiety.
Benefits: Lavender and Lemon Balm calm the nervous system, while Valerian promotes deep, restful sleep, making this tea effective for managing insomnia and supporting emotional health.

422. Elderberry and Ginger Immune Syrup Tea

Ingredients: 1 tablespoon dried Elderberries, 1 tablespoon grated fresh ginger, 2 cups hot water, 1 teaspoon raw honey.
Preparation: Simmer Elderberries and ginger in hot water for 20 minutes. Strain and add honey if desired.
Suggested Usage: Drink 1 cup daily during cold and flu season to boost immunity.
Benefits: Elderberries are rich in immune-boosting flavonoids, while ginger provides anti-inflammatory and warming effects, making this tea effective for preventing illness and supporting overall immune health.

423. Licorice Root and Peppermint Antiviral Tea

Ingredients: 1 tablespoon dried Licorice root, 1 tablespoon dried Peppermint leaves, 2 cups hot water.

Preparation: Steep Licorice root and Peppermint in hot water for 15 minutes. Strain and serve warm.

Suggested Usage: Drink 1 cup up to twice daily to reduce inflammation and support respiratory health.

Benefits: Licorice root helps soothe mucous membranes and provides antiviral support, while Peppermint opens the airways and reduces inflammation, making this tea ideal for managing colds, coughs, and other respiratory issues.

424. Chamomile and Lemon Peel Immune-Calming Tea

Ingredients: 1 tablespoon dried Chamomile flowers, 1 tablespoon dried Lemon peel, 2 cups hot water, 1 teaspoon raw honey.

Preparation: Steep Chamomile and Lemon peel in hot water for 15 minutes. Strain and add honey if desired.

Suggested Usage: Drink 1 cup in the evening to reduce stress and support immune health.

Benefits: Chamomile calms the nervous system and reduces inflammation, while Lemon peel provides Vitamin C and supports digestion, making this tea ideal for promoting relaxation and overall immune health.

425. Holy Basil and Ashwagandha Adaptogen Tonic Tea

Ingredients: 1 tablespoon dried Holy Basil leaves, 1 tablespoon dried Ashwagandha root, 3 cups hot water.

Preparation: Simmer Holy Basil and Ashwagandha in hot water for 30 minutes. Strain and serve warm.

Suggested Usage: Drink 1 cup daily to reduce stress and support resilience.

Benefits: Holy Basil balances cortisol levels and reduces anxiety, while Ashwagandha supports adrenal health and enhances energy, making this tea effective for promoting resilience and managing chronic stress.

426. Ginger, Clove, and Cayenne Warming Immune Tea

Ingredients: 1 tablespoon grated fresh ginger, ½ teaspoon ground cloves, a pinch of cayenne, 2 cups hot water, 1 teaspoon raw honey.

Preparation: Steep ginger, cloves, and cayenne in hot water for 15 minutes. Strain and add honey.

Suggested Usage: Drink 1 cup up to twice daily during cold weather or at the onset of cold symptoms.

Benefits: Ginger, clove, and cayenne stimulate circulation, clear congestion, and boost immunity, making this tea effective for warming the body and preventing illness.

427. Fennel and Mint Digestive Immune Tea

Ingredients: 1 tablespoon dried Fennel seeds, 1 tablespoon dried Mint leaves, 2 cups hot water.

Preparation: Steep Fennel and Mint in hot water for 15 minutes. Strain and serve warm.

Suggested Usage: Drink 1 cup after meals to support digestion and boost immunity.

Benefits: Fennel reduces bloating and supports digestive function, while Mint calms the digestive tract and enhances nutrient absorption, making this tea ideal for promoting digestive health and immune balance.

428. Astragalus, Elderberry, and Ginger Resilience Tea

Ingredients: 1 tablespoon dried Astragalus root, 1 tablespoon dried Elderberries, 1 tablespoon grated fresh ginger, 4 cups water.
Preparation: Simmer Astragalus, Elderberries, and ginger in water for 30 minutes. Strain and serve warm.
Suggested Usage: Drink 1 cup daily to enhance immune resilience and support overall vitality.
Benefits: Astragalus is a powerful adaptogen that boosts immune function, while Elderberries provide potent antiviral support. Ginger adds anti-inflammatory properties, making this tea ideal for building long-term resilience and protecting against illness.

429. Thyme, Oregano, and Garlic Antibacterial Tea

Ingredients: 1 tablespoon dried Thyme leaves, 1 tablespoon dried Oregano leaves, 2 minced garlic cloves, 2 cups hot water, 1 teaspoon raw honey.
Preparation: Steep Thyme, Oregano, and garlic in hot water for 20 minutes. Strain and add honey if desired.
Suggested Usage: Drink 1 cup up to twice daily to fight bacterial infections and support respiratory health.
Benefits: Thyme and Oregano are strong antimicrobial herbs that help combat bacterial and viral infections, while garlic enhances immune function and provides additional antibacterial properties, making this tea effective for supporting immune health.

430. Eleuthero and Reishi Immunity Boost Tea

Ingredients: 1 tablespoon dried Eleuthero root, 1 tablespoon dried Reishi mushroom slices, 3 cups water.
Preparation: Simmer Eleuthero and Reishi in water for 30 minutes. Strain and serve warm.
Suggested Usage: Drink 1 cup daily to reduce stress and support immune health.
Benefits: Eleuthero boosts energy and reduces fatigue, while Reishi modulates immune function and calms the nervous system, making this tea ideal for supporting long-term immune resilience and managing stress.

431. Burdock Root and Dandelion Blood Cleanse Tea

Ingredients: 1 tablespoon dried Burdock root, 1 tablespoon dried Dandelion root, 4 cups water.
Preparation: Simmer Burdock and Dandelion root in water for 30 minutes. Strain and serve warm.
Suggested Usage: Drink 1 cup up to twice daily to support detoxification and cleanse the blood.

Benefits: Burdock and Dandelion roots are renowned for their ability to cleanse the blood, support liver function, and promote healthy skin, making this tea effective for enhancing detoxification and promoting overall vitality.

432. Schisandra and Lemon Peel Liver Support Tea

Ingredients: 1 tablespoon dried Schisandra berries, 1 tablespoon dried Lemon peel, 3 cups hot water, 1 teaspoon raw honey.
Preparation: Steep Schisandra and Lemon peel in hot water for 20 minutes. Strain and add honey if desired.
Suggested Usage: Drink 1 cup daily to support liver health and enhance detoxification.
Benefits: Schisandra berries support liver function, enhance resilience, and reduce stress, while Lemon peel aids in digestion and provides antioxidant support, making this tea ideal for promoting liver health and overall well-being.

433. Gotu Kola and Rosemary Brain Boost Tea

Ingredients: 1 tablespoon dried Gotu Kola leaves, 1 tablespoon dried Rosemary leaves, 2 cups hot water, 1 teaspoon raw honey.
Preparation: Steep Gotu Kola and Rosemary in hot water for 15 minutes. Strain and add honey if desired.
Suggested Usage: Drink 1 cup daily to enhance cognitive function and support memory.
Benefits: Gotu Kola improves circulation to the brain and enhances cognitive performance, while Rosemary stimulates memory and focus, making this tea effective for supporting brain health and promoting mental clarity.

Book 20: Lifestyle Practices to Enhance Immunity

A strong and resilient immune system is built through a holistic approach that integrates not only herbal remedies but also lifestyle choices that nourish the body, mind, and spirit. Herbs are incredibly powerful tools for supporting immunity, but they are most effective when combined with a healthy lifestyle that includes a balanced diet, regular exercise, adequate sleep, and stress management. This chapter explores how to create a lifestyle that enhances immune health naturally and sustainably, focusing on holistic practices, the integration of herbs with physical activity, and strategies for managing stress to keep the immune system robust and balanced.

Holistic Lifestyle Tips for Immune Health

The immune system is influenced by every aspect of our lifestyle, from the food we eat to the amount of rest we get. To support optimal immune health, it's essential to adopt habits that nourish the entire body. A balanced diet rich in whole foods, regular physical activity, and sufficient hydration are the cornerstones of immune health. Here are some key lifestyle changes that can have a profound impact on the immune system:

Prioritize a Nutrient-Dense Diet: A diet rich in fruits, vegetables, whole grains, lean proteins, and healthy fats provides the vitamins and minerals needed to support immune cell function. Nutrients like Vitamin C, zinc, and selenium are particularly important for immunity, while antioxidants from colorful fruits and vegetables help protect immune cells from oxidative damage. Incorporating herbs like Nettle, Oatstraw, and Rosehips, which are high in essential nutrients, can further enrich the diet and support overall immune health.

Maintain Gut Health: The gut is home to a significant portion of the immune system, and a healthy microbiome is crucial for proper immune function. Consuming fermented foods like yogurt, kefir, and sauerkraut, as well as prebiotic-rich foods like garlic, onions, and asparagus, helps maintain a healthy balance of gut flora. Adding digestive-supportive herbs like Peppermint, Chamomile, and Fennel to daily meals can promote gut health and improve nutrient absorption.

Get Adequate Sleep: Sleep is essential for immune regulation and recovery. During sleep, the body produces and releases cytokines, proteins that are necessary for fighting infection and inflammation. Poor sleep quality or insufficient sleep can weaken the immune response and increase susceptibility to illness. Establishing a regular sleep schedule and incorporating calming herbal teas, such as Chamomile, Lemon Balm, or Valerian, can promote restful sleep and support overall immunity.

Stay Hydrated: Proper hydration is key for maintaining mucous membranes, which act as a barrier to pathogens, and for supporting lymphatic flow, which helps remove toxins and waste from the body. Drinking plenty of water throughout the day, along with hydrating herbal teas like Nettle, Hibiscus, or Dandelion leaf, helps keep the body well-hydrated and supports immune function.

Engage in Regular Physical Activity: Exercise has a profound impact on immune health, enhancing circulation, reducing inflammation, and promoting the efficient movement of immune cells throughout the body. Moderate exercise, such as walking, yoga, or swimming, is particularly beneficial. High-intensity workouts should be balanced with adequate recovery to avoid overtraining, which can suppress immune function. Including adaptogenic herbs like Ashwagandha and Rhodiola can support energy and recovery, making exercise more effective and sustainable.

Minimize Exposure to Environmental Toxins: Environmental toxins, such as pollutants, chemicals, and heavy metals, can weaken the immune system and increase oxidative stress. Limiting exposure to these toxins and supporting detoxification pathways through herbs like Milk Thistle, Dandelion root, and Burdock root can help protect the body and promote a healthier immune response.

Combining Herbs with Physical Activity

The benefits of regular physical activity extend far beyond physical fitness—it's also one of the most effective ways to strengthen the immune system. Exercise enhances circulation, increases the activity of natural killer cells, and helps reduce inflammation, all of which are crucial for a healthy immune response. When combined with herbal remedies, the effects of exercise can be amplified, leading to greater resilience and overall health.

Pre-Workout Herbal Boosters: Adaptogenic herbs like Rhodiola, Eleuthero, and Cordyceps are ideal for supporting energy and endurance during physical activity. They help the body adapt to stress, improve stamina, and reduce fatigue, making exercise more effective. Taking these herbs in the form of a tea, tincture, or capsule 30 minutes before exercise can provide a natural boost.

Post-Workout Recovery with Anti-Inflammatory Herbs: After exercise, the body enters a recovery phase where inflammation and muscle repair occur. Anti-inflammatory herbs like Turmeric, Ginger, and Holy Basil can help reduce post-exercise inflammation and support faster recovery. Incorporating these herbs into post-workout smoothies, teas, or broths can promote muscle healing and enhance the benefits of exercise.

Herbal Teas for Hydration and Detoxification: Staying hydrated during and after exercise is crucial for maintaining electrolyte balance and supporting detoxification. Herbs like Hibiscus, Lemon Balm, and Peppermint can be added to homemade electrolyte drinks or consumed as teas to support hydration. These herbs not only help replenish fluids but also provide antioxidants and anti-inflammatory properties, making them ideal for supporting overall immune health.

Yoga and Mindfulness with Calming Herbs: Combining exercise with mindfulness practices like yoga or meditation can reduce stress and promote immune balance. Calming herbs such as Chamomile, Lemon Balm, and Lavender can be taken as a tea or in aromatherapy form to deepen relaxation and enhance the mind-body connection during these activities.

Stress Management for a Stronger Immune System

Chronic stress is one of the biggest threats to immune health. High levels of stress hormones like cortisol suppress the immune system, increase inflammation, and make the body more susceptible to infections and chronic illnesses. Managing stress through lifestyle practices, herbs, and relaxation techniques is essential for maintaining a strong and resilient immune system.

Herbs for Stress Reduction: Adaptogenic herbs like Ashwagandha, Holy Basil, and Reishi mushroom are known for their ability to modulate the body's response to stress. These herbs help balance cortisol levels, reduce anxiety, and enhance overall resilience. Taking these herbs as part of a daily tea blend or in capsule form can provide long-term support for managing stress and promoting immune health.

Mindfulness and Meditation: Practices like mindfulness, deep breathing, and meditation help calm the nervous system, lower cortisol levels, and promote relaxation. Regular meditation has been shown to enhance immune function by increasing the activity of natural killer cells and reducing inflammation. Combining these practices with calming herbs like Lemon Balm, Chamomile, or Passionflower can deepen the relaxation response and provide greater stress relief.

Breathing Exercises for Immune Health: Deep breathing exercises, such as diaphragmatic breathing or alternate nostril breathing, increase oxygen flow, reduce stress, and enhance lymphatic circulation. Practicing these techniques for just a few minutes each day can have a significant impact on reducing stress and supporting immune function.

Creating a Calming Environment: Environmental factors can also influence stress levels. Incorporating calming scents like Lavender, Rose, or Sandalwood through aromatherapy can promote relaxation and reduce anxiety. Using herbal-infused oils or diffusers in the home environment can help create a sense of calm and support mental and emotional well-being.

Establishing a Routine for Balance: Having a regular routine that includes time for self-care, exercise, and relaxation can help reduce the impact of stress on the immune system. Setting aside time for herbal teas, meditation, and gentle movement each day creates a structured environment that supports overall health and well-being.

By integrating these holistic lifestyle practices with herbal remedies, it's possible to create a comprehensive plan that supports the immune system, enhances resilience, and promotes long-term health. Combining diet, exercise, stress management, and herbal support provides a multifaceted approach to immune health that is both sustainable and effective.

Section III: Digestive Health

Book 21: Natural Remedies for Indigestion

Indigestion is a common digestive issue characterized by discomfort in the upper abdomen, often accompanied by symptoms such as bloating, gas, heartburn, and nausea. While occasional indigestion may be triggered by overeating or consuming certain foods, chronic digestive discomfort can be indicative of underlying digestive imbalances. This chapter explores how to alleviate these symptoms through the use of herbs that calm and support the digestive system, and it emphasizes the importance of addressing the root causes of indigestion through dietary and lifestyle adjustments.

Herbs to Soothe Digestive Discomfort

Herbs have been used for centuries to treat digestive disorders, and many are known for their carminative, anti-inflammatory, and soothing properties. By using herbs that target the underlying causes of indigestion, such as excess gas, inflammation, or sluggish digestion, it's possible to achieve both immediate relief and long-term digestive balance.

One of the most effective categories of herbs for managing indigestion is **carminative herbs**, which work by relaxing the smooth muscles of the digestive tract, reducing the formation of gas, and relieving bloating. Examples include **Peppermint**, **Fennel**, and **Ginger**. These herbs are often used in combination, as they complement each other and enhance overall digestive function. Peppermint, for instance, helps alleviate spasms in the gastrointestinal tract, while Fennel seeds reduce gas and promote the expulsion of trapped air.

Anti-inflammatory herbs, such as **Chamomile** and **Licorice Root**, play a crucial role in reducing irritation and inflammation in the stomach and intestines. Chamomile not only soothes the digestive system but also calms the nervous system, making it an excellent choice for individuals whose digestive discomfort is triggered by stress. Licorice root, particularly in its deglycyrrhizinated form (DGL), helps coat and protect the mucous membranes, reducing acid reflux and promoting healing of the esophagus.

For individuals experiencing **heartburn** or **acid reflux**, demulcent herbs like **Slippery Elm** and **Marshmallow Root** are highly beneficial. These herbs are rich in mucilage, a gel-like substance that coats the lining of the digestive tract, providing a protective barrier against stomach acid and soothing irritation. They are also effective for managing conditions such as gastritis and peptic ulcers, as they reduce inflammation and promote tissue repair.

In cases of **indigestion caused by poor liver function or sluggish bile flow**, bitter herbs such as **Dandelion Root** and **Artichoke Leaf** are recommended. Bitters stimulate the production of digestive enzymes and bile, improving the breakdown and absorption of nutrients while reducing bloating and heaviness after meals. Regular use of bitter herbs can also enhance overall liver health, promoting detoxification and reducing the burden on the digestive system.

Recipes for Digestive Teas and Tinctures

In addition to identifying the right herbs for specific digestive concerns, it's essential to choose the appropriate form of delivery. Herbal teas and tinctures are two of the most popular methods for supporting digestive health. Teas are gentle, hydrating, and comforting, making them ideal for calming acute symptoms like nausea or bloating. Tinctures, on the other hand, are more concentrated and can deliver potent doses of active compounds quickly and effectively.

When preparing digestive teas, consider combining herbs that provide complementary actions. For example, a soothing tea for **bloating** might include **Fennel** (to reduce gas), **Peppermint** (to relieve spasms), and **Ginger** (to stimulate digestion). A tea for **acid reflux** might feature **Chamomile** (to reduce inflammation), **Licorice Root** (to coat and protect the mucous membranes), and **Marshmallow Root** (to provide additional mucilage).

Tinctures can be particularly useful for **stimulating digestion before meals**. A small dose of **Dandelion Root** and **Gentian** tincture taken 10-15 minutes before eating can help prime the digestive system, promoting the secretion of digestive juices and bile. Tinctures are also effective for managing more **chronic digestive issues** like **IBS**, as they can deliver therapeutic doses of herbs over an extended period.

When using herbal remedies for indigestion, it's important to remember that everyone's digestive system is unique. Some individuals may find relief with warming herbs like **Ginger** and **Cinnamon**, while others may benefit more from cooling and calming herbs like **Peppermint** and **Chamomile**. Taking note of which herbs and formulations work best for your body can help create a personalized approach to digestive health.

Finally, it's essential to consider lifestyle factors that contribute to indigestion. Eating slowly, chewing food thoroughly, and avoiding large meals late at night can all help reduce the burden on the digestive system. Combining these habits with the regular use of digestive-supportive herbs can lead to lasting improvements in digestive function and overall well-being.

Book 22: Herbal Solutions for Irritable Bowel Syndrome (IBS)

Irritable Bowel Syndrome (IBS) is a common gastrointestinal disorder characterized by a combination of symptoms, including abdominal pain, bloating, gas, and altered bowel habits such as diarrhea, constipation, or a mixture of both. It is a functional disorder, meaning that while the structure of the digestive system is normal, its function is impaired, leading to significant discomfort and disruption in daily life. Managing IBS requires a multifaceted approach that addresses not only the symptoms but also the underlying triggers, which may include stress, food sensitivities, and imbalances in gut flora. Herbs can play a powerful role in alleviating IBS symptoms and promoting overall gut health by calming the digestive tract, modulating inflammation, and supporting a balanced gut environment.

Managing IBS Symptoms Naturally

The unpredictable nature of IBS symptoms can make it challenging to find effective treatments, as triggers and symptoms vary widely from person to person. However, certain herbs have shown promise in managing specific IBS symptoms, providing a natural way to reduce discomfort and improve quality of life.

For Abdominal Pain and Cramping: Abdominal pain is a hallmark symptom of IBS, often caused by spasms in the muscles of the gastrointestinal tract. Antispasmodic herbs like **Peppermint** and **Fennel** are highly effective for relieving these spasms and calming intestinal contractions. Peppermint oil, in particular, has been widely studied for its ability to reduce pain and discomfort in individuals with IBS. The menthol in peppermint helps relax smooth muscle tissue, alleviating cramping and reducing the sensation of pain. Fennel works similarly, reducing spasms and promoting the expulsion of gas, which can relieve the sensation of bloating and fullness.

For Gas and Bloating: Carminative herbs, which promote the expulsion of gas and soothe the digestive tract, are ideal for managing bloating and gas. **Chamomile**, **Ginger**, and **Lemon Balm** are gentle carminatives that also have calming effects on the nervous system, making them particularly useful for individuals whose symptoms are worsened by stress or anxiety. These herbs help relax the digestive tract, reduce the formation of gas, and promote smooth digestion, alleviating the discomfort of bloating.

For Diarrhea-Predominant IBS: Individuals with diarrhea-predominant IBS (IBS-D) often experience urgent bowel movements, loose stools, and frequent trips to the bathroom. Astringent herbs like **Slippery Elm** and **Marshmallow Root** are beneficial for managing diarrhea, as they form a soothing, gel-like coating over the mucous membranes of the intestines, reducing irritation and slowing down transit time. **Chamomile** is another effective herb for IBS-D, as it reduces inflammation and spasm, helping to normalize bowel movements.

For Constipation-Predominant IBS: In constipation-predominant IBS (IBS-C), sluggish bowel movements can lead to discomfort, bloating, and abdominal pain. Gentle laxative herbs like **Aloe Vera** and **Psyllium Husk** help promote regularity without causing harsh cramping. **Dandelion Root** and **Ginger** are also effective for stimulating digestion and promoting healthy bile flow, which can help ease constipation. It's important to choose herbs that do not cause dependency and to support overall gut motility rather than relying on stimulant laxatives.

For Stress and Anxiety: Stress and anxiety are major triggers for IBS, as the gut and brain are closely connected through the gut-brain axis. Adaptogenic and calming herbs like **Ashwagandha**, **Holy Basil**, and **Lemon Balm** can help regulate the body's response to stress and reduce anxiety-related digestive symptoms. These herbs help balance cortisol levels, promote a sense of calm, and reduce the frequency and severity of stress-induced IBS flare-ups.

For Balancing Gut Flora: Dysbiosis, or an imbalance of gut bacteria, is often a contributing factor in IBS. Herbs like **Garlic**, **Oregano**, and **Thyme** have natural antimicrobial properties that help reduce harmful bacteria and support a balanced gut microbiome. **Chamomile** and **Licorice Root** are also beneficial for promoting a healthy gut environment, as they reduce inflammation and soothe the gut lining, creating a more favorable environment for beneficial bacteria.

Herbal Blends for Gut Health

Creating specific herbal blends that address the unique needs of individuals with IBS can be a powerful way to support gut health and alleviate symptoms. By combining herbs that work synergistically to calm the digestive tract, balance gut flora, and promote regularity, it's possible to create effective formulations tailored to different IBS presentations.

Calming Blend for Abdominal Pain and Spasms: A blend of **Peppermint**, **Fennel**, and **Chamomile** can be used to soothe abdominal pain and reduce cramping. This combination works by relaxing smooth muscle tissue, reducing inflammation, and promoting the expulsion of trapped gas. Taking this blend as a tea before or after meals can provide immediate relief from discomfort.

Gut Healing Blend for Inflammation and Irritation: Individuals with IBS often have an inflamed and irritated gut lining, which can contribute to symptoms like pain and diarrhea. A blend of **Slippery Elm**, **Marshmallow Root**, and **Licorice Root** helps coat and soothe the mucous membranes, promoting healing and reducing inflammation. This blend can be taken as a tea or in powdered form, mixed into water or a smoothie.

Digestive Motility Blend for Constipation: For those with constipation-predominant IBS, a combination of **Dandelion Root**, **Ginger**, and **Aloe Vera** can help stimulate digestion and promote healthy bowel movements. This blend supports liver function, increases bile flow, and gently encourages regularity without causing harsh cramping. Taking this blend in tea or tincture form 20 minutes before meals can help ease constipation and promote digestive comfort.

Stress Relief Blend for Anxiety-Triggered IBS: For individuals whose IBS symptoms are closely linked to stress, a calming blend of **Lemon Balm**, **Holy Basil**, and **Ashwagandha** can help reduce anxiety and support a balanced nervous system. These herbs work together to lower cortisol levels, promote relaxation, and reduce the severity of stress-related digestive symptoms. This blend can be taken as a tea in the evening or as a tincture during times of high stress.

Microbiome Balance Blend for Gut Flora Health: A blend of **Garlic**, **Oregano**, and **Thyme** can be used to reduce harmful bacteria and promote a healthy balance of gut flora. This antimicrobial blend can be taken as a tincture or in capsule form and should be combined with a probiotic regimen to support overall gut health. Including anti-inflammatory herbs like **Chamomile** and **Licorice Root** in the blend can further support a healthy gut environment and reduce irritation.

By addressing the unique symptoms and underlying causes of IBS with targeted herbal blends, it's possible to create a comprehensive approach to managing this complex condition. Alongside dietary adjustments, stress management techniques, and lifestyle changes, herbal remedies offer a natural and effective way to alleviate symptoms, promote gut health, and improve quality of life for individuals living with IBS.

Remedies for IBS

434. Peppermint and Fennel Bloating Relief Tea

Ingredients: 1 tablespoon dried Peppermint leaves, 1 teaspoon Fennel seeds, 2 cups hot water.
Preparation: Steep Peppermint leaves and Fennel seeds in hot water for 15 minutes. Strain and serve warm.
Suggested Usage: Drink 1 cup after meals to reduce bloating and ease digestive discomfort.
Benefits: Peppermint relaxes the smooth muscles of the digestive tract, while Fennel helps expel trapped gas, making this tea highly effective for relieving bloating and abdominal discomfort.

435. Chamomile and Ginger Anti-Spasm Tea

Ingredients: 1 tablespoon dried Chamomile flowers, 1 teaspoon grated fresh Ginger, 2 cups hot water, 1 teaspoon raw honey.
Preparation: Steep Chamomile and Ginger in hot water for 10-15 minutes. Strain and add honey if desired.

Suggested Usage: Drink 1 cup before or after meals to alleviate cramping and reduce spasms.

Benefits: Chamomile's antispasmodic properties help relax the muscles of the digestive tract, while Ginger reduces inflammation and stimulates digestion, making this tea ideal for calming abdominal spasms and pain.

436. Slippery Elm and Marshmallow Gut-Soothing Powder

Ingredients: 1 tablespoon Slippery Elm powder, 1 tablespoon Marshmallow Root powder, 1 cup warm water.

Preparation: Mix Slippery Elm and Marshmallow Root powder into warm water, stirring until fully dissolved.

Suggested Usage: Take 1 tablespoon of the mixture up to twice daily to coat and soothe the digestive tract.

Benefits: Both Slippery Elm and Marshmallow Root are rich in mucilage, which forms a protective layer over the mucous membranes, reducing inflammation and promoting healing, making this blend effective for managing gastritis, acid reflux, and other inflammatory gut conditions.

437. Licorice Root and Aloe Vera Heartburn Relief Syrup

Ingredients: 1 tablespoon dried Licorice Root, 1 tablespoon Aloe Vera gel, 2 cups water, 1 teaspoon raw honey.

Preparation: Simmer Licorice Root in water for 20 minutes. Remove from heat, cool, and add Aloe Vera gel and honey. Stir until well combined.

Suggested Usage: Take 1 tablespoon before meals to soothe acid reflux and prevent heartburn.

Benefits: Licorice Root helps protect the stomach lining and reduces acid production, while Aloe Vera soothes irritation and promotes healing, making this syrup effective for relieving heartburn and acid reflux symptoms.

438. Lemon Balm and Peppermint Gas Relief Tea

Ingredients: 1 tablespoon dried Lemon Balm leaves, 1 tablespoon dried Peppermint leaves, 2 cups hot water.

Preparation: Steep Lemon Balm and Peppermint in hot water for 10-15 minutes. Strain and serve warm.

Suggested Usage: Drink 1-2 cups daily to reduce gas and soothe the digestive system.

Benefits: Lemon Balm calms the nervous system and reduces digestive upset, while Peppermint relaxes the muscles of the gastrointestinal tract, making this tea effective for relieving gas, bloating, and digestive spasms.

439. Fennel and Anise Seed Carminative Tea

Ingredients: 1 tablespoon Fennel seeds, 1 teaspoon Anise seeds, 2 cups hot water.

Preparation: Steep Fennel and Anise seeds in hot water for 15 minutes. Strain and serve warm.

Suggested Usage: Drink 1 cup before or after meals to prevent gas and bloating.

Benefits: Fennel and Anise seeds are powerful carminatives that help expel gas from the digestive tract, reduce bloating, and promote smooth digestion, making this tea ideal for managing post-meal discomfort.

440. Holy Basil and Ashwagandha Stress Relief Tonic

Ingredients: 1 tablespoon dried Holy Basil leaves, 1 teaspoon dried Ashwagandha root, 3 cups water.
Preparation: Simmer Holy Basil and Ashwagandha in water for 20 minutes. Strain and serve warm.
Suggested Usage: Drink 1 cup in the evening to reduce stress and support adrenal health.
Benefits: Holy Basil and Ashwagandha are adaptogenic herbs that help regulate cortisol levels, reduce stress, and promote resilience, making this tonic effective for managing stress-related IBS symptoms and enhancing overall well-being.

441. Dandelion Root and Burdock Liver Support Decoction

Ingredients: 1 tablespoon dried Dandelion Root, 1 tablespoon dried Burdock Root, 4 cups water.
Preparation: Simmer Dandelion and Burdock Root in water for 30 minutes. Strain and serve warm.
Suggested Usage: Drink 1 cup daily to support liver health and promote digestion.
Benefits: Dandelion and Burdock Root are both powerful liver tonics that stimulate bile production, support detoxification, and enhance overall digestive function, making this decoction effective for reducing bloating and supporting liver health.

442. Psyllium Husk and Aloe Vera Constipation Relief Drink

Ingredients: 1 tablespoon Psyllium Husk, 1 tablespoon Aloe Vera gel, 1 cup warm water.
Preparation: Mix Psyllium Husk and Aloe Vera gel into warm water, stirring until fully dissolved.
Suggested Usage: Drink 1 cup in the morning to promote regular bowel movements.
Benefits: Psyllium Husk is a bulk-forming fiber that promotes bowel regularity, while Aloe Vera soothes the digestive tract and supports smooth bowel movements, making this drink ideal for relieving constipation without causing cramping.

443. Ginger and Turmeric Digestive Fire Tea

Ingredients: 1 tablespoon grated fresh Ginger, 1 teaspoon Turmeric powder, 1 teaspoon lemon juice, 2 cups hot water.
Preparation: Simmer Ginger and Turmeric in hot water for 10 minutes. Strain, add lemon juice, and serve warm.
Suggested Usage: Drink 1 cup before meals to stimulate digestion and reduce bloating.
Benefits: Ginger and Turmeric stimulate the production of digestive enzymes and reduce inflammation, making this tea effective for enhancing digestion, promoting healthy bile flow, and reducing post-meal discomfort.

444. Peppermint Oil Capsules for Cramping

Ingredients: 2-3 drops Peppermint essential oil, empty gel capsules.
Preparation: Add 2-3 drops of Peppermint essential oil into an empty gel capsule. Seal tightly.
Suggested Usage: Take 1 capsule up to twice daily to alleviate cramping and spasms.
Benefits: Peppermint oil helps relax the smooth muscles of the digestive tract and reduces cramping, making it highly effective for managing IBS-related abdominal pain and discomfort.

445. Artichoke Leaf and Gentian Digestive Bitters

Ingredients: 1 tablespoon dried Artichoke Leaf, 1 teaspoon dried Gentian Root, 1 cup vodka or brandy (for tincture base).
Preparation: Place Artichoke Leaf and Gentian Root in a glass jar and cover with vodka or brandy. Seal tightly and let steep for 2-4 weeks, shaking occasionally. Strain and store in a dark glass bottle.
Suggested Usage: Take ½ teaspoon in a small amount of water 15-20 minutes before meals to stimulate digestion.
Benefits: Artichoke Leaf and Gentian are bitter herbs that enhance the secretion of digestive juices, improve bile flow, and reduce bloating, making this blend effective for promoting healthy digestion and preventing indigestion.

446. Chamomile and Licorice Root Anti-Inflammatory Tea

Ingredients: 1 tablespoon dried Chamomile flowers, 1 teaspoon dried Licorice Root, 2 cups hot water.
Preparation: Steep Chamomile and Licorice Root in hot water for 15 minutes. Strain and serve warm.
Suggested Usage: Drink 1 cup up to twice daily to reduce inflammation and soothe the digestive tract.
Benefits: Chamomile calms the digestive system and reduces inflammation, while Licorice Root protects the mucous membranes and promotes healing, making this tea ideal for managing inflammatory digestive conditions like gastritis and acid reflux.

447. Lemon Balm and Lavender Relaxation Tea

Ingredients: 1 tablespoon dried Lemon Balm leaves, 1 tablespoon dried Lavender flowers, 2 cups hot water, 1 teaspoon raw honey.
Preparation: Steep Lemon Balm and Lavender in hot water for 10-15 minutes. Strain and add honey if desired.
Suggested Usage: Drink 1 cup in the evening to promote relaxation and alleviate stress-related digestive issues.
Benefits: Lemon Balm and Lavender calm the nervous system, reduce anxiety, and support restful sleep, making this tea effective for managing stress-induced digestive symptoms and promoting emotional well-being.

448. Aloe Vera and Slippery Elm Gut-Healing Gel

Ingredients: 1 tablespoon Aloe Vera gel, 1 teaspoon Slippery Elm powder, 1 cup water.
Preparation: Mix Aloe Vera gel and Slippery Elm powder into water, stirring until fully combined.

Suggested Usage: Take 1 tablespoon before meals to coat and protect the digestive tract.

Benefits: Aloe Vera soothes irritation and promotes healing, while Slippery Elm coats the mucous membranes, forming a protective barrier that reduces inflammation and promotes tissue repair, making this gel ideal for managing acid reflux, ulcers, and other inflammatory gut conditions.

449. Ashwagandha and Rhodiola Cortisol-Balancing Capsules

Ingredients: 1 tablespoon Ashwagandha powder, 1 tablespoon Rhodiola powder, empty gel capsules.

Preparation: Mix Ashwagandha and Rhodiola powders thoroughly. Fill the empty gel capsules with the powder mixture and seal.

Suggested Usage: Take 1 capsule in the morning and 1 in the evening to balance cortisol levels and reduce stress.

Benefits: Ashwagandha and Rhodiola are adaptogenic herbs that help regulate cortisol production, reduce anxiety, and promote resilience, making these capsules effective for managing stress-related IBS symptoms and improving overall energy levels.

450. Cinnamon and Cardamom Warming Digestive Tea

Ingredients: 1 cinnamon stick, 3 whole Cardamom pods, 2 cups hot water, 1 teaspoon raw honey.

Preparation: Simmer Cinnamon and Cardamom in hot water for 15 minutes. Strain and add honey if desired.

Suggested Usage: Drink 1 cup after meals to stimulate digestion and reduce bloating.

Benefits: Cinnamon and Cardamom are warming spices that enhance circulation, stimulate digestion, and reduce gas, making this tea effective for promoting healthy digestion and relieving post-meal discomfort.

451. Oregano and Garlic Antimicrobial Tincture

Ingredients: 1 tablespoon dried Oregano leaves, 1 tablespoon minced fresh Garlic, 1 cup vodka or brandy.

Preparation: Place Oregano and Garlic in a glass jar and cover with vodka or brandy. Seal tightly and let steep for 2-4 weeks, shaking occasionally. Strain and store in a dark glass bottle.

Suggested Usage: Take ½ teaspoon up to twice daily in a small amount of water to reduce harmful bacteria and support gut health.

Benefits: Oregano and Garlic have strong antimicrobial properties that help eliminate pathogenic bacteria and support a healthy balance of gut flora, making this tincture effective for managing dysbiosis and improving overall digestive health.

452. Thyme and Ginger Gut Microbiome Balance Tea

Ingredients: 1 tablespoon dried Thyme leaves, 1 tablespoon grated fresh Ginger, 2 cups hot water.

Preparation: Steep Thyme and Ginger in hot water for 15 minutes. Strain and serve warm.

Suggested Usage: Drink 1-2 cups daily to support gut health and reduce

inflammation.

Benefits: Thyme and Ginger help reduce harmful bacteria and support a balanced gut microbiome, while also promoting digestion and reducing inflammation, making this tea effective for improving overall gut health.

453. Caraway and Coriander Seed Digestive Ease Tea

Ingredients: 1 tablespoon Caraway seeds, 1 tablespoon Coriander seeds, 2 cups hot water.

Preparation: Steep Caraway and Coriander seeds in hot water for 15 minutes. Strain and serve warm.

Suggested Usage: Drink 1 cup after meals to alleviate gas and bloating.

Benefits: Caraway and Coriander seeds are carminative herbs that reduce gas, promote digestion, and soothe the digestive tract, making this tea effective for relieving bloating and post-meal discomfort.

454. Peppermint and Chamomile IBS-Calming Tea

Ingredients: 1 tablespoon dried Peppermint leaves, 1 tablespoon dried Chamomile flowers, 2 cups hot water.

Preparation: Steep Peppermint and Chamomile in hot water for 10-15 minutes. Strain and serve warm.

Suggested Usage: Drink 1-2 cups daily to calm the digestive tract and reduce spasms.

Benefits: Peppermint relaxes the muscles of the digestive tract, while Chamomile reduces inflammation and promotes relaxation, making this tea effective for

managing IBS symptoms like cramping, gas, and bloating.

455. Valerian and Passionflower Sleep Support Tea

Ingredients: 1 tablespoon dried Valerian root, 1 tablespoon dried Passionflower, 2 cups hot water, 1 teaspoon raw honey.

Preparation: Steep Valerian and Passionflower in hot water for 15 minutes. Strain and add honey if desired.

Suggested Usage: Drink 1 cup in the evening to promote restful sleep and reduce stress-related digestive symptoms.

Benefits: Valerian and Passionflower are calming herbs that support relaxation and promote deep, restful sleep, making this tea effective for managing stress and improving sleep quality, which are essential for reducing IBS flare-ups.

456. Skullcap and Lemon Balm Nerve-Soothing Tincture

Ingredients: 1 tablespoon dried Skullcap, 1 tablespoon dried Lemon Balm, 1 cup vodka or brandy (for tincture base).

Preparation: Place Skullcap and Lemon Balm in a glass jar and cover with vodka or brandy. Seal tightly and let steep for 4-6 weeks, shaking occasionally. Strain and store in a dark glass bottle.

Suggested Usage: Take ½ teaspoon up to twice daily to calm the nervous system and reduce anxiety-related digestive symptoms.

Benefits: Skullcap and Lemon Balm are nervine herbs that help calm the mind, reduce anxiety, and promote relaxation, making this tincture ideal for managing stress-induced IBS symptoms.

457. Cinnamon, Fennel, and Clove Bloating Relief Tea

Ingredients: 1 cinnamon stick, 1 teaspoon Fennel seeds, 3 whole Cloves, 2 cups hot water.
Preparation: Simmer Cinnamon, Fennel, and Cloves in hot water for 15 minutes. Strain and serve warm.
Suggested Usage: Drink 1 cup after meals to reduce bloating and relieve gas.
Benefits: Cinnamon warms the digestive system and reduces inflammation, while Fennel and Clove work as carminative herbs to expel trapped gas and relieve bloating, making this tea effective for post-meal digestive discomfort.

458. Dandelion Root and Yellow Dock Detox Tea

Ingredients: 1 tablespoon dried Dandelion Root, 1 tablespoon dried Yellow Dock Root, 3 cups water.
Preparation: Simmer Dandelion and Yellow Dock Root in water for 30 minutes. Strain and serve warm.
Suggested Usage: Drink 1 cup up to twice daily to support detoxification and enhance liver health.
Benefits: Dandelion and Yellow Dock Roots are powerful liver-supportive herbs that stimulate bile production and promote detoxification, making this tea effective for cleansing the liver and reducing digestive sluggishness.

459. Licorice Root and Marshmallow Soothing Gut Tea

Ingredients: 1 tablespoon dried Licorice Root, 1 tablespoon dried Marshmallow Root, 2 cups hot water.
Preparation: Steep Licorice Root and Marshmallow Root in hot water for 20 minutes. Strain and serve warm.
Suggested Usage: Drink 1-2 cups daily to coat the digestive tract and reduce irritation.
Benefits: Licorice Root and Marshmallow Root are demulcent herbs that form a protective coating over the mucous membranes, reducing inflammation and soothing irritated tissues, making this tea effective for managing gastritis, acid reflux, and other inflammatory digestive conditions.

460. Ginger and Artichoke Leaf Appetite Stimulation Tonic

Ingredients: 1 tablespoon grated fresh Ginger, 1 tablespoon dried Artichoke Leaf, 2 cups water.
Preparation: Simmer Ginger and Artichoke Leaf in water for 15 minutes. Strain and serve warm.
Suggested Usage: Drink ½ cup 20 minutes before meals to stimulate appetite and enhance digestion.
Benefits: Ginger stimulates the production of digestive enzymes and bile, while Artichoke Leaf promotes healthy liver function and appetite, making this tonic effective for enhancing digestive health and supporting those with poor appetite.

461. Lemon Balm, Fennel, and Ginger Spasm Relief Tea

Ingredients: 1 tablespoon dried Lemon Balm leaves, 1 teaspoon Fennel seeds, 1 teaspoon grated fresh Ginger, 2 cups hot water.

Preparation: Steep Lemon Balm, Fennel, and Ginger in hot water for 15 minutes. Strain and serve warm.

Suggested Usage: Drink 1 cup as needed to reduce digestive spasms and alleviate discomfort.

Benefits: Lemon Balm calms the nervous system, while Fennel and Ginger work as antispasmodics to reduce cramping and promote smooth digestion, making this tea effective for managing IBS-related abdominal pain and spasms.

462. Marshmallow Root and Plantain Gut-Healing Syrup

Ingredients: 1 tablespoon dried Marshmallow Root, 1 tablespoon dried Plantain Leaf, 2 cups water, 1 cup raw honey.

Preparation: Simmer Marshmallow Root and Plantain in water for 20 minutes. Strain and add honey, stirring until fully dissolved. Store in a glass jar.

Suggested Usage: Take 1 tablespoon up to twice daily to soothe the digestive tract and promote healing.

Benefits: Marshmallow and Plantain are rich in mucilage, which soothes and protects the mucous membranes, reduces inflammation, and promotes tissue repair, making this syrup ideal for managing ulcers, acid reflux, and other inflammatory gut conditions.

463. Ginger, Peppermint, and Anise Nausea Relief Tea

Ingredients: 1 tablespoon grated fresh Ginger, 1 tablespoon dried Peppermint leaves, 1 teaspoon Anise seeds, 2 cups hot water.

Preparation: Steep Ginger, Peppermint, and Anise in hot water for 15 minutes. Strain and serve warm.

Suggested Usage: Drink 1 cup as needed to reduce nausea and settle the stomach.

Benefits: Ginger and Peppermint are well-known for their anti-nausea properties, while Anise reduces gas and bloating, making this tea effective for relieving nausea and calming the digestive system.

464. Slippery Elm and Chamomile Esophageal Soother

Ingredients: 1 tablespoon Slippery Elm powder, 1 tablespoon dried Chamomile flowers, 2 cups hot water.

Preparation: Steep Chamomile in hot water for 10 minutes, then stir in Slippery Elm powder until dissolved.

Suggested Usage: Drink 1 cup before meals to coat and protect the esophagus.

Benefits: Slippery Elm and Chamomile form a soothing, protective coating over the mucous membranes, reducing inflammation and irritation, making this tea ideal for managing acid reflux and esophageal discomfort.

465. Psyllium Husk, Flaxseed, and Aloe Bowel Regularity Drink

Ingredients: 1 tablespoon Psyllium Husk, 1 tablespoon ground Flaxseed, 1 tablespoon Aloe Vera gel, 1 cup warm water.

Preparation: Mix Psyllium, Flaxseed, and Aloe Vera into warm water, stirring until fully combined.

Suggested Usage: Drink 1 cup in the

morning to promote regular bowel movements.

Benefits: Psyllium and Flaxseed provide soluble fiber that promotes bowel regularity, while Aloe Vera soothes the digestive tract, making this drink effective for relieving constipation and supporting gut health.

466. Nettle and Peppermint Antioxidant Support Tea

Ingredients: 1 tablespoon dried Nettle leaves, 1 tablespoon dried Peppermint leaves, 2 cups hot water.
Preparation: Steep Nettle and Peppermint in hot water for 15 minutes. Strain and serve warm.
Suggested Usage: Drink 1-2 cups daily to support antioxidant levels and promote overall vitality.
Benefits: Nettle is rich in vitamins and minerals, while Peppermint enhances digestion and reduces inflammation, making this tea ideal for boosting overall health and supporting immune function.

467. Turmeric and Licorice Gut Healing Capsules

Ingredients: 1 tablespoon Turmeric powder, 1 tablespoon Licorice Root powder, empty gel capsules.
Preparation: Mix Turmeric and Licorice Root powders thoroughly. Fill the empty gel capsules with the powder mixture and seal.
Suggested Usage: Take 1 capsule up to twice daily to reduce inflammation and promote gut healing.
Benefits: Turmeric has strong anti-inflammatory and antioxidant properties,

while Licorice Root soothes mucous membranes and supports tissue repair, making these capsules effective for managing inflammatory digestive conditions and promoting gut health.

468. Oatstraw and Holy Basil Stress Relief Tea

Ingredients: 1 tablespoon dried Oatstraw, 1 tablespoon dried Holy Basil leaves, 2 cups hot water, 1 teaspoon raw honey.
Preparation: Steep Oatstraw and Holy Basil in hot water for 15 minutes. Strain and add honey if desired.
Suggested Usage: Drink 1 cup in the evening to reduce stress and support nervous system health.
Benefits: Oatstraw nourishes and calms the nervous system, while Holy Basil acts as an adaptogen to reduce stress and promote resilience, making this tea ideal for managing stress-induced digestive symptoms and supporting overall emotional well-being.

469. Dandelion and Milk Thistle Liver Cleansing Capsules

Ingredients: 1 tablespoon Dandelion Root powder, 1 tablespoon Milk Thistle seed powder, empty gel capsules.
Preparation: Mix Dandelion Root and Milk Thistle powders thoroughly. Fill the empty gel capsules with the powder mixture and seal.
Suggested Usage: Take 1 capsule daily to support liver health and promote detoxification.
Benefits: Dandelion Root and Milk Thistle both enhance liver function and promote detoxification, making these

capsules effective for supporting digestion and reducing digestive sluggishness.

470. Valerian and Hops Deep Relaxation Tea

Ingredients: 1 tablespoon dried Valerian Root, 1 tablespoon dried Hops flowers, 2 cups hot water.
Preparation: Steep Valerian and Hops in hot water for 15 minutes. Strain and serve warm.
Suggested Usage: Drink 1 cup before bedtime to promote deep relaxation and restful sleep.
Benefits: Valerian and Hops are calming nervine herbs that promote deep relaxation and reduce anxiety, making this tea effective for improving sleep quality and reducing stress-related digestive issues.

471. Lemon Balm and Skullcap Anxiety Soother

Ingredients: 1 tablespoon dried Lemon Balm leaves, 1 tablespoon dried Skullcap, 2 cups hot water, 1 teaspoon raw honey.
Preparation: Steep Lemon Balm and Skullcap in hot water for 15 minutes. Strain and add honey if desired.
Suggested Usage: Drink 1 cup in the evening to reduce anxiety and promote relaxation.
Benefits: Lemon Balm calms the nervous system and reduces anxiety, while Skullcap acts as a nervine to relieve tension and promote a sense of calm, making this tea effective for managing stress and anxiety-induced digestive symptoms.

472. Ginger and Cinnamon Digestive Motility Tea

Ingredients: 1 tablespoon grated fresh Ginger, 1 cinnamon stick, 2 cups hot water, 1 teaspoon raw honey.
Preparation: Simmer Ginger and Cinnamon in hot water for 15 minutes. Strain and add honey if desired.
Suggested Usage: Drink 1 cup before meals to stimulate digestion and promote healthy bowel movements.
Benefits: Ginger and Cinnamon both enhance digestive motility, reduce inflammation, and stimulate the production of digestive enzymes, making this tea effective for improving digestion and relieving constipation.

473. Psyllium and Ginger Gut Mobility Capsules

Ingredients: 1 tablespoon Psyllium Husk powder, 1 tablespoon Ginger powder, empty gel capsules.
Preparation: Mix Psyllium Husk and Ginger powders thoroughly. Fill the empty gel capsules with the powder mixture and seal.
Suggested Usage: Take 1 capsule in the morning with a full glass of water to promote regularity and gut motility.
Benefits: Psyllium Husk is a bulk-forming fiber that supports bowel regularity, while Ginger stimulates digestion and reduces inflammation, making these capsules effective for relieving constipation and promoting gut health.

474. Chamomile and Fennel Anti-Bloat Tea

Ingredients: 1 tablespoon dried Chamomile flowers, 1 teaspoon Fennel seeds, 2 cups hot water.
Preparation: Steep Chamomile and Fennel in hot water for 15 minutes. Strain and serve warm.
Suggested Usage: Drink 1 cup after meals to reduce bloating and promote smooth digestion.
Benefits: Chamomile calms the digestive tract and reduces inflammation, while Fennel helps expel trapped gas and relieve bloating, making this tea ideal for managing post-meal discomfort.

475. Peppermint and Caraway Gas Relief Tea

Ingredients: 1 tablespoon dried Peppermint leaves, 1 tablespoon Caraway seeds, 2 cups hot water.
Preparation: Steep Peppermint and Caraway seeds in hot water for 15 minutes. Strain and serve warm.
Suggested Usage: Drink 1 cup as needed to reduce gas and alleviate bloating.
Benefits: Peppermint relaxes the muscles of the digestive tract, while Caraway reduces gas production and promotes digestion, making this tea effective for relieving gas, bloating, and abdominal discomfort.

476. Slippery Elm and Marshmallow Root Acid Reflux Relief Tea

Ingredients: 1 tablespoon Slippery Elm powder, 1 tablespoon dried Marshmallow Root, 2 cups hot water.
Preparation: Steep Marshmallow Root in hot water for 20 minutes. Stir in Slippery Elm powder until fully dissolved.
Suggested Usage: Drink 1 cup before meals to coat and protect the digestive tract.
Benefits: Slippery Elm and Marshmallow Root form a protective coating over the mucous membranes, reducing irritation and promoting healing, making this tea ideal for managing acid reflux and esophageal discomfort.

477. Licorice Root and Cinnamon Gut-Healing Tonic

Ingredients: 1 tablespoon dried Licorice Root, 1 cinnamon stick, 2 cups water.
Preparation: Simmer Licorice Root and Cinnamon in water for 20 minutes. Strain and serve warm.
Suggested Usage: Drink 1 cup up to twice daily to soothe and heal the digestive tract.
Benefits: Licorice Root soothes mucous membranes and reduces inflammation, while Cinnamon stimulates digestion and reduces gas, making this tonic effective for promoting gut healing and supporting healthy digestion.

478. Ginger, Turmeric, and Fennel Digestion-Enhancing Tea

Ingredients: 1 tablespoon grated fresh Ginger, 1 teaspoon Turmeric powder, 1 teaspoon Fennel seeds, 2 cups hot water, 1 teaspoon raw honey.
Preparation: Simmer Ginger, Turmeric, and Fennel in hot water for 15 minutes. Strain and add honey if desired.
Suggested Usage: Drink 1 cup before meals to stimulate digestion and reduce post-meal discomfort.
Benefits: Ginger and Turmeric both

enhance the production of digestive enzymes and reduce inflammation, while Fennel expels trapped gas and soothes the digestive tract, making this tea ideal for promoting smooth digestion and reducing bloating.

479. Valerian and Lemon Balm Nighttime Calming Tea

Ingredients: 1 tablespoon dried Valerian Root, 1 tablespoon dried Lemon Balm leaves, 2 cups hot water, 1 teaspoon raw honey.
Preparation: Steep Valerian and Lemon Balm in hot water for 15 minutes. Strain and add honey if desired.
Suggested Usage: Drink 1 cup 30 minutes before bedtime to promote restful sleep and reduce nighttime digestive discomfort.
Benefits: Valerian promotes deep relaxation and restful sleep, while Lemon Balm calms the nervous system and supports emotional balance, making this tea effective for managing stress and improving sleep quality, which in turn supports digestive health.

480. Skullcap and Chamomile Stress-Reducing Tea

Ingredients: 1 tablespoon dried Skullcap, 1 tablespoon dried Chamomile flowers, 2 cups hot water.
Preparation: Steep Skullcap and Chamomile in hot water for 15 minutes. Strain and serve warm.
Suggested Usage: Drink 1 cup in the evening to calm the mind and reduce anxiety-induced digestive issues.
Benefits: Skullcap is a nervine herb that helps alleviate tension and reduce stress,

while Chamomile soothes the digestive tract and promotes relaxation, making this tea effective for reducing stress-related IBS symptoms.

481. Peppermint, Fennel, and Ginger Cramps Relief Tea

Ingredients: 1 tablespoon dried Peppermint leaves, 1 teaspoon Fennel seeds, 1 tablespoon grated fresh Ginger, 2 cups hot water.
Preparation: Steep Peppermint, Fennel, and Ginger in hot water for 15 minutes. Strain and serve warm.
Suggested Usage: Drink 1 cup after meals to relieve cramping and reduce bloating.
Benefits: Peppermint relaxes the muscles of the digestive tract, Fennel reduces gas, and Ginger stimulates digestion, making this tea effective for relieving abdominal cramps, bloating, and other IBS-related symptoms.

482. Milk Thistle and Dandelion Root Digestive Tonic

Ingredients: 1 tablespoon Milk Thistle seed powder, 1 tablespoon dried Dandelion Root, 3 cups water.
Preparation: Simmer Milk Thistle and Dandelion Root in water for 20 minutes. Strain and serve warm.
Suggested Usage: Drink 1 cup daily to support liver function and promote healthy digestion.
Benefits: Milk Thistle and Dandelion Root are powerful liver-supportive herbs that enhance bile production, promote detoxification, and support overall digestive health, making this tonic ideal

for improving digestion and reducing bloating.

483. Artichoke Leaf and Gentian Digestive Support Capsules

Ingredients: 1 tablespoon dried Artichoke Leaf powder, 1 tablespoon Gentian Root powder, empty gel capsules.

Preparation: Mix Artichoke Leaf and Gentian powders thoroughly. Fill empty gel capsules with the powder mixture and seal.

Suggested Usage: Take 1 capsule 15-20 minutes before meals to stimulate digestion and prevent indigestion.

Benefits: Artichoke Leaf and Gentian are bitter herbs that stimulate the secretion of digestive enzymes and bile, enhancing digestion and preventing bloating and gas, making these capsules effective for managing indigestion and promoting healthy appetite.

484. Holy Basil and Lemon Balm Cortisol Balancing Capsules

Ingredients: 1 tablespoon Holy Basil powder, 1 tablespoon Lemon Balm powder, empty gel capsules.

Preparation: Mix Holy Basil and Lemon Balm powders thoroughly. Fill empty gel capsules with the powder mixture and seal.

Suggested Usage: Take 1 capsule in the morning and 1 in the evening to reduce stress and balance cortisol levels.

Benefits: Holy Basil and Lemon Balm are adaptogenic and nervine herbs that help regulate the body's response to stress, promote a sense of calm, and reduce cortisol levels, making these capsules effective for managing stress-related digestive issues and supporting overall emotional well-being.

Book 23: Detoxifying the Digestive System

The digestive system plays a crucial role in overall health and wellness, as it is responsible for breaking down food, absorbing nutrients, and eliminating waste and toxins from the body. However, over time, the accumulation of toxins from processed foods, environmental pollutants, and stress can overwhelm the digestive system, leading to sluggishness, discomfort, and a host of other health issues. Detoxifying the digestive system through the use of specific herbs and natural cleansing protocols can help restore balance, support optimal organ function, and improve overall vitality. This chapter explores the use of herbs that support liver and kidney health, comprehensive detox strategies, and recipes for internal cleansing.

Herbs for Liver and Kidney Support

The liver and kidneys are two of the body's primary detoxification organs, filtering toxins, waste products, and harmful substances from the blood and excreting them through urine and bile. Supporting these organs with the right herbs can enhance their function, promote the efficient elimination of toxins, and prevent the buildup of harmful substances that can lead to chronic health issues. Here are some of the most effective herbs for supporting liver and kidney health:

Milk Thistle (Silybum marianum): Milk Thistle is one of the most well-known liver-supportive herbs. It contains silymarin, a powerful antioxidant compound that protects liver cells from damage, stimulates the regeneration of liver tissue, and enhances the detoxification of harmful substances. Regular use of Milk Thistle can help prevent liver damage from toxins, alcohol, and heavy metals, making it an essential herb for liver health.

Dandelion Root (Taraxacum officinale): Dandelion Root is a gentle but effective liver tonic that stimulates bile production and improves digestion. It also acts as a mild diuretic, promoting the elimination of toxins through the kidneys. Dandelion Root is particularly useful for individuals experiencing digestive sluggishness, bloating, or water retention, as it helps support both liver and kidney function.

Burdock Root (Arctium lappa): Burdock Root is a powerful blood cleanser that enhances liver and kidney function by promoting the elimination of waste products and toxins. It is rich in antioxidants and has anti-inflammatory properties, making it beneficial for detoxifying the body and supporting overall digestive health. Burdock Root also has a mild diuretic effect, which helps flush toxins out through the urinary system.

Artichoke Leaf (Cynara scolymus): Artichoke Leaf is a bitter herb that stimulates bile production and supports liver detoxification. It enhances the digestion of fats, reduces cholesterol levels, and promotes liver health. Artichoke Leaf can be particularly beneficial for individuals with gallbladder issues or sluggish bile flow, as it helps optimize the liver's ability to process and eliminate toxins.

Nettle Leaf (Urtica dioica): Nettle Leaf is a nutrient-rich herb that supports kidney health by promoting urine flow and reducing the accumulation of toxins. It is high in vitamins and minerals, including iron, calcium, and magnesium, which support overall health and vitality. Nettle Leaf is often used in combination with other herbs in detox blends to enhance kidney function and promote the elimination of metabolic waste.

Yellow Dock Root (Rumex crispus): Yellow Dock Root is a mild laxative and liver tonic that helps cleanse the digestive tract and support liver function. It promotes bile flow, enhances digestion, and encourages the elimination of toxins through the intestines. Yellow Dock is also known for its ability to reduce skin conditions like eczema and acne, which can be linked to poor liver function.

Parsley (Petroselinum crispum): Parsley is a gentle diuretic and kidney-supportive herb that promotes the elimination of toxins through increased urine production. It also helps reduce water retention and supports the kidneys in filtering waste products from the blood. Parsley can be used in teas, smoothies, and tinctures as part of a comprehensive detox program.

Corn Silk (Zea mays): Corn Silk is a soothing herb that supports kidney health by reducing inflammation and promoting urine flow. It is often used to relieve urinary tract discomfort and prevent the formation of kidney stones. Corn Silk can be used in combination with other kidney-supportive herbs to promote healthy kidney function and eliminate toxins.

Natural Detox Protocols

Effective detoxification involves more than just targeting specific organs—it requires a holistic approach that addresses diet, hydration, and lifestyle factors. The following are comprehensive detox protocols that utilize herbal remedies to cleanse the digestive system, support liver and kidney health, and promote overall detoxification:

Liver and Gallbladder Flush:
This protocol focuses on enhancing liver and gallbladder function, stimulating bile flow, and eliminating toxins from the liver. It typically involves a short period of fasting, the consumption of liver-supportive teas (such as Milk Thistle, Dandelion, and Burdock Root), and the use of lemon juice and olive oil to stimulate the expulsion of bile and gallstones. It's recommended to perform this flush under the guidance of a healthcare practitioner, as it can be intense for those with existing liver or gallbladder issues.

Kidney Cleanse Program:
A kidney cleanse focuses on promoting healthy urine flow, reducing inflammation in the urinary tract, and preventing the buildup of toxins in the kidneys. This program typically includes diuretic herbs like Nettle Leaf, Parsley, and Corn Silk, as well as hydrating beverages such as herbal teas and infused waters. Adequate hydration is crucial during a kidney cleanse to ensure that toxins are efficiently flushed out of the body.

Digestive System Reset:
This protocol is designed to cleanse the entire digestive system, support gut health, and eliminate waste buildup. It involves the use of fiber-rich herbs like Psyllium Husk and Flaxseed to promote bowel regularity, combined with soothing demulcent herbs like Slippery Elm and Marshmallow Root to protect and heal the digestive lining. Liver-supportive herbs like Artichoke and Milk Thistle are also included to enhance detoxification and improve bile flow.

Daily Detox Routine:
A gentle daily detox routine involves incorporating detoxifying herbs and foods into everyday meals. This can include starting the day with a warm cup of Lemon and Ginger tea, adding detoxifying greens like Dandelion and Nettle to smoothies, and sipping on herbal teas like Peppermint and Burdock throughout the day. Maintaining a diet rich in whole foods, avoiding processed foods, and staying well-hydrated are essential components of a daily detox routine.

Recipes for Internal Cleansing

The following are examples of herbal recipes that support internal cleansing and promote optimal digestive health:

Liver-Supportive Tea: Combine equal parts of Milk Thistle, Dandelion Root, and Burdock Root. Steep 1 tablespoon of the blend in 2 cups of hot water for 20 minutes. Drink 1 cup daily to support liver function and promote detoxification.

Kidney-Cleansing Juice: Blend 1 cucumber, 1 handful of Parsley, 1 green apple, and 1 lemon (juiced) with 2 cups of water. Drink this juice in the morning to support kidney health and flush out toxins.

Digestive Detox Tonic: Combine 1 tablespoon of Yellow Dock Root and 1 tablespoon of Ginger Root in 2 cups of water. Simmer for 15 minutes, strain, and drink 1 cup before meals to stimulate digestion and promote elimination.

By incorporating these herbs and protocols into a comprehensive detox strategy, it's possible to cleanse the digestive system, support organ health, and promote overall vitality and well-being.

Book 24: Natural Constipation and Diarrhea Remedies

Herbs to Regulate Bowel Movements

The balance of bowel movements is a critical aspect of digestive health, reflecting the overall function of the gastrointestinal system. Any disruption in this balance—manifested as either constipation or diarrhea—signals that something in the digestive process is amiss. Herbs have been used for centuries to support healthy digestion and can play an essential role in normalizing bowel movements. By using gentle yet effective natural remedies, it is possible to address the root causes of these issues, restore regularity, and promote digestive comfort.

For constipation, which is characterized by infrequent, hard, or painful bowel movements, herbal laxatives and bulk-forming agents can be highly effective. Psyllium Husk, for example, is one of the most reliable natural remedies for constipation. A soluble fiber that absorbs water and forms a gel-like mass, Psyllium helps to soften the stool and promote smooth passage through the intestines. It works without irritating the bowel, making it suitable for long-term use. Another gentle yet powerful option is Flaxseed. When ground, Flaxseed provides both soluble and insoluble fiber, which adds bulk to the stool and helps stimulate peristalsis, the wave-like muscle contractions that move food through the digestive tract.

For individuals who need a stronger effect, stimulant laxative herbs like Senna and Cascara Sagrada can be used cautiously. These herbs directly stimulate the muscles of the intestines, prompting bowel movements within a few hours. However, because of their potency, they should only be used for short-term relief and not as a daily remedy, as overuse can lead to dependency and weaken the natural function of the bowels.

Dandelion Root and Artichoke Leaf are two additional herbs that can help relieve constipation by enhancing bile production. Bile, produced by the liver, acts as a natural lubricant in the intestines and helps break down fats. An increase in bile flow can promote smoother digestion and alleviate sluggish bowels, making these herbs particularly beneficial for individuals with digestive complaints linked to poor liver function.

In contrast, diarrhea is often the result of inflammation, irritation, or a loss of control in the digestive system, leading to frequent, loose stools. Astringent herbs such as Blackberry Leaf and Agrimony are effective for firming up stools and reducing excess fluid in the intestines. Blackberry Leaf is especially rich in tannins, which have a strong astringent effect on the digestive tract, helping to restore normal stool consistency and reduce the urgency of bowel movements. Agrimony, another traditional astringent herb, works similarly, toning the tissues of the gut and helping to alleviate symptoms of acute diarrhea.

Demulcent herbs, which coat and soothe the mucous membranes of the intestines, are also beneficial for managing diarrhea. Slippery Elm and Marshmallow Root are two of the best-known demulcent herbs. Both are rich in mucilage, a gel-like substance that forms a protective barrier over the lining of the intestines, reducing irritation and promoting healing. This makes them ideal for managing diarrhea caused by inflammatory conditions such as irritable bowel syndrome (IBS) or gastroenteritis. When combined with anti-inflammatory herbs like Chamomile, which calms spasms and reduces gut inflammation, these herbs can quickly restore balance to an overactive bowel.

By using the right combination of herbs, it's possible to support healthy bowel function, reduce discomfort, and promote a balanced digestive system. Understanding how each herb works, and selecting those that address the specific symptoms and root causes of digestive imbalances, is key to creating effective natural remedies for bowel regulation.

Balancing Digestive Function Naturally

Achieving digestive balance involves more than just treating symptoms when they arise. It requires a holistic approach that considers diet, hydration, stress management, and lifestyle practices to promote long-term digestive health. A balanced digestive system not only supports healthy bowel movements but also enhances nutrient absorption, boosts immunity, and contributes to overall well-being. The following strategies, when combined with herbal remedies, can help maintain digestive health and prevent recurring issues like constipation or diarrhea.

One of the most critical components of digestive health is diet. A diet rich in whole foods, including plenty of fruits, vegetables, whole grains, and legumes, provides the fiber needed to maintain regular bowel movements. For constipation, increasing the intake of fiber is often the first step. However, it's important to introduce fiber slowly and balance it with adequate hydration. Fiber absorbs water as it moves through the intestines, so without sufficient fluid intake, it can worsen constipation. Hydrating herbal teas, such as those made with Peppermint, Ginger, or Chamomile, can support hydration and soothe the digestive tract.

Individuals with diarrhea, on the other hand, may need to reduce their intake of certain fibers, particularly insoluble fibers found in foods like raw vegetables and whole grains, which can further irritate the gut. Instead, soluble fiber from sources like oats, apples, and bananas is recommended, as it absorbs excess water in the intestines and helps firm up stools. Probiotic-rich foods such as yogurt, kefir, and fermented vegetables can also help restore a healthy balance of gut bacteria, which is often disrupted during episodes of diarrhea.

In addition to diet, regular physical activity is essential for maintaining digestive health. Exercise helps stimulate peristalsis, the natural contractions of the digestive muscles that move food through the intestines. Gentle activities like walking, yoga, and stretching are particularly effective for relieving constipation and promoting overall gut health. For individuals with diarrhea, moderate exercise can help reduce stress, which is often a contributing factor to digestive imbalances.

Managing stress is another crucial aspect of maintaining digestive health. The gut and brain are connected through the gut-brain axis, meaning that psychological stress can have a direct impact on bowel function. Chronic stress can either slow down the bowels, leading to constipation, or speed them up, resulting in diarrhea. Incorporating relaxation techniques such as deep breathing, meditation, or progressive muscle relaxation can help regulate the body's response to stress and reduce its impact on the digestive system. Adaptogenic herbs like Ashwagandha, Holy Basil, and Lemon Balm can further support the body's stress response, promoting emotional balance and reducing the frequency and severity of stress-induced digestive symptoms.

Hydration is another key component of digestive balance. Drinking enough water is crucial for both preventing constipation and managing diarrhea. In the case of constipation, staying well-hydrated ensures that the stool remains soft and easy to pass. For diarrhea, which leads to rapid fluid loss, rehydration is essential to prevent dehydration and restore electrolyte balance. Herbal teas, such as Nettle or Peppermint, can support hydration while also providing soothing benefits to the digestive system.

By integrating these strategies into daily routines and using herbal remedies to support specific needs, it's possible to achieve lasting digestive health and maintain regular bowel function. This holistic approach not only alleviates acute symptoms but also strengthens the digestive system over time, ensuring resilience and balance.

Remedies for Constipation and Diarrhea

485. Psyllium Husk and Flaxseed Constipation Relief Drink

Ingredients: 1 tablespoon Psyllium Husk, 1 tablespoon ground Flaxseed, 1 cup warm water.
Preparation: Mix Psyllium Husk and Flaxseed into the warm water, stirring until fully dissolved.
Suggested Usage: Drink once daily, preferably in the morning, followed by an additional glass of water to support bowel regularity.
Benefits: Psyllium and Flaxseed provide a balanced mix of soluble and insoluble fiber, which absorbs water and forms a gel-like consistency, adding bulk to the stool and promoting smooth, regular bowel movements.

486. Slippery Elm and Marshmallow Root Soothing Tea for Diarrhea

Ingredients: 1 tablespoon Slippery Elm powder, 1 tablespoon dried Marshmallow Root, 2 cups hot water.
Preparation: Steep Marshmallow Root in hot water for 20 minutes, then stir in Slippery Elm powder until fully dissolved.
Suggested Usage: Drink 1 cup up to twice daily to reduce irritation and promote healing of the digestive tract.
Benefits: Slippery Elm and Marshmallow Root are rich in mucilage, which coats and soothes the lining of the intestines, making this tea highly effective for managing diarrhea and protecting the mucous membranes.

487. Chamomile and Peppermint Anti-Spasm Tea for IBS Symptoms

Ingredients: 1 tablespoon dried Chamomile flowers, 1 tablespoon dried Peppermint leaves, 2 cups hot water.
Preparation: Steep Chamomile and Peppermint in hot water for 10-15 minutes. Strain and serve warm.
Suggested Usage: Drink 1-2 cups daily to relieve spasms and calm the digestive system.
Benefits: Chamomile and Peppermint are well-known antispasmodic herbs that relax the smooth muscles of the digestive tract, reduce cramping, and alleviate discomfort, making this tea ideal for individuals with IBS.

488. Dandelion Root and Aloe Vera Gut-Stimulating Tonic

Ingredients: 1 tablespoon dried Dandelion Root, 1 tablespoon Aloe Vera gel, 2 cups water.
Preparation: Simmer Dandelion Root in water for 15 minutes. Remove from heat, cool, and add Aloe Vera gel. Stir well.
Suggested Usage: Take ½ cup before meals to stimulate digestion and relieve constipation.
Benefits: Dandelion Root enhances bile production, promoting smoother digestion, while Aloe Vera soothes the digestive tract and gently stimulates bowel movements.

489. Senna and Ginger Quick-Relief Laxative Tea

Ingredients: 1 teaspoon dried Senna leaves, 1 tablespoon grated fresh Ginger, 2 cups hot water.
Preparation: Steep Senna and Ginger in hot water for 10 minutes. Strain and serve warm.
Suggested Usage: Drink 1 cup as needed for quick constipation relief. Use sparingly to avoid dependency.
Benefits: Senna is a potent herbal laxative that stimulates intestinal muscles, while Ginger reduces the cramping often associated with stimulant laxatives, providing a balanced approach to quick constipation relief.

490. Blackberry Leaf and Agrimony Astringent Tea for Diarrhea

Ingredients: 1 tablespoon dried Blackberry Leaf, 1 tablespoon dried Agrimony, 2 cups hot water.
Preparation: Steep Blackberry Leaf and Agrimony in hot water for 15 minutes. Strain and serve warm.
Suggested Usage: Drink 1 cup up to twice daily to firm up stools and reduce fluid

loss.

Benefits: Blackberry Leaf and Agrimony are strong astringent herbs that help tone the digestive tract, reduce excess fluid in the intestines, and alleviate diarrhea.

491. Licorice Root and Cinnamon Gut-Healing Capsules for Constipation

Ingredients: 1 tablespoon Licorice Root powder, 1 tablespoon Cinnamon powder, empty gel capsules.
Preparation: Mix Licorice Root and Cinnamon powders thoroughly. Fill the empty gel capsules with the mixture and seal.
Suggested Usage: Take 1 capsule up to twice daily to soothe the digestive tract and support regular bowel movements.
Benefits: Licorice Root soothes and protects the mucous membranes, while Cinnamon stimulates digestion and reduces inflammation, making these capsules effective for managing constipation associated with inflammatory digestive conditions.

492. Fennel and Anise Seed Gas-Reducing Tea

Ingredients: 1 tablespoon Fennel seeds, 1 teaspoon Anise seeds, 2 cups hot water.
Preparation: Steep Fennel and Anise seeds in hot water for 15 minutes. Strain and serve warm.
Suggested Usage: Drink 1 cup after meals to reduce gas and bloating.
Benefits: Fennel and Anise are carminative herbs that promote the expulsion of gas, reduce bloating, and soothe the digestive tract, making this tea

highly effective for managing post-meal discomfort.

493. Peppermint and Ginger Bloating Relief Tea

Ingredients: 1 tablespoon dried Peppermint leaves, 1 tablespoon grated fresh Ginger, 2 cups hot water.
Preparation: Steep Peppermint and Ginger in hot water for 10-15 minutes. Strain and serve warm.
Suggested Usage: Drink 1-2 cups daily to relieve bloating and support digestion.
Benefits: Peppermint relaxes the digestive tract, while Ginger stimulates the production of digestive enzymes and bile, making this tea ideal for reducing bloating and promoting healthy digestion.

494. Aloe Vera and Psyllium Husk Constipation Drink

Ingredients: 1 tablespoon Aloe Vera gel, 1 tablespoon Psyllium Husk, 1 cup warm water.
Preparation: Mix Aloe Vera gel and Psyllium Husk into warm water, stirring until fully dissolved.
Suggested Usage: Drink 1 cup in the morning, followed by a full glass of water, to promote regularity.
Benefits: Aloe Vera gently stimulates the bowels, while Psyllium Husk adds bulk and moisture to the stool, making this drink effective for relieving constipation and promoting smooth bowel movements.

495. Chamomile and Lemon Balm Relaxation Tea for Stress-Related Digestive Issues

Ingredients: 1 tablespoon dried Chamomile flowers, 1 tablespoon dried Lemon Balm leaves, 2 cups hot water.

Preparation: Steep Chamomile and Lemon Balm in hot water for 15 minutes. Strain and serve warm.

Suggested Usage: Drink 1 cup in the evening to promote relaxation and reduce stress-related digestive symptoms.

Benefits: Chamomile and Lemon Balm calm the nervous system and reduce anxiety, making this tea effective for managing digestive symptoms triggered by stress or emotional tension.

496. Yellow Dock and Burdock Root Liver Support Decoction

Ingredients: 1 tablespoon dried Yellow Dock Root, 1 tablespoon dried Burdock Root, 4 cups water.

Preparation: Simmer Yellow Dock and Burdock Root in water for 30 minutes. Strain and serve warm.

Suggested Usage: Drink 1 cup daily to support liver function and promote detoxification.

Benefits: Yellow Dock and Burdock Root are powerful liver-supportive herbs that enhance bile production, support detoxification, and promote overall digestive health, making this decoction ideal for individuals with sluggish digestion or liver congestion.

497. Marshmallow Root and Plantain Demulcent Syrup

Ingredients: 1 tablespoon dried Marshmallow Root, 1 tablespoon dried Plantain Leaf, 2 cups water, 1 cup raw honey.

Preparation: Simmer Marshmallow Root and Plantain Leaf in water for 20 minutes. Strain and add honey, stirring until fully dissolved. Store in a glass jar.

Suggested Usage: Take 1 tablespoon up to twice daily to soothe the digestive tract and reduce inflammation.

Benefits: Marshmallow and Plantain are rich in mucilage, forming a soothing layer over the digestive mucous membranes, making this syrup highly effective for managing inflammatory conditions like gastritis and acid reflux.

498. Artichoke Leaf and Gentian Digestive Bitters Capsules

Ingredients: 1 tablespoon dried Artichoke Leaf powder, 1 tablespoon Gentian Root powder, empty gel capsules.

Preparation: Mix Artichoke Leaf and Gentian powders thoroughly. Fill the empty gel capsules with the powder mixture and seal.

Suggested Usage: Take 1 capsule 15-20 minutes before meals to stimulate digestive secretions and prevent bloating.

Benefits: Artichoke Leaf and Gentian are powerful bitter herbs that promote the production of digestive enzymes and bile, supporting healthy digestion and preventing symptoms of indigestion.

499. Ginger, Fennel, and Cinnamon Digestive Fire Tea

Ingredients: 1 tablespoon grated fresh Ginger, 1 teaspoon Fennel seeds, 1 cinnamon stick, 2 cups hot water, 1 teaspoon raw honey.

Preparation: Simmer Ginger, Fennel, and Cinnamon in hot water for 15 minutes.

Strain and add honey if desired.

Suggested Usage: Drink 1 cup before meals to enhance digestive fire and reduce post-meal discomfort.

Benefits: Ginger and Cinnamon stimulate digestion, while Fennel reduces gas and bloating, making this tea ideal for promoting healthy digestion and reducing post-meal heaviness.

500. Agrimony and Raspberry Leaf Diarrhea Control Tea

Ingredients: 1 tablespoon dried Agrimony, 1 tablespoon dried Raspberry Leaf, 2 cups hot water.

Preparation: Steep Agrimony and Raspberry Leaf in hot water for 15 minutes. Strain and serve warm.

Suggested Usage: Drink 1-2 cups daily to firm up stools and reduce diarrhea.

Benefits: Agrimony and Raspberry Leaf are astringent herbs that tone the digestive tract and reduce excess fluid in the intestines, making this tea highly effective for managing acute diarrhea.

501. Ashwagandha and Holy Basil Stress-Relief Capsules for Gut Health

Ingredients: 1 tablespoon Ashwagandha Root powder, 1 tablespoon Holy Basil powder, empty gel capsules.

Preparation: Mix Ashwagandha and Holy Basil powders thoroughly. Fill the empty gel capsules with the powder mixture and seal.

Suggested Usage: Take 1 capsule in the morning and 1 in the evening to reduce stress and promote emotional balance.

Benefits: Ashwagandha and Holy Basil are adaptogenic herbs that help regulate cortisol levels, reduce anxiety, and support overall resilience, making these capsules ideal for managing stress-induced digestive symptoms.

502. Blackberry Leaf and Chamomile Anti-Diarrheal Tea

Ingredients: 1 tablespoon dried Blackberry Leaf, 1 tablespoon dried Chamomile flowers, 2 cups hot water.

Preparation: Steep Blackberry Leaf and Chamomile in hot water for 15 minutes. Strain and serve warm.

Suggested Usage: Drink 1 cup up to twice daily to reduce diarrhea and soothe the digestive system.

Benefits: Blackberry Leaf's strong astringent properties help firm up stools, while Chamomile reduces inflammation and calms the digestive tract, making this tea highly effective for managing both acute and chronic diarrhea.

503. Ginger, Peppermint, and Lemon Bloating Relief Tea

Ingredients: 1 tablespoon grated fresh Ginger, 1 tablespoon dried Peppermint leaves, 1 teaspoon lemon juice, 2 cups hot water.

Preparation: Steep Ginger and Peppermint in hot water for 15 minutes. Strain, add lemon juice, and serve warm.

Suggested Usage: Drink 1 cup after meals to relieve bloating and support healthy digestion.

Benefits: Ginger stimulates digestion and reduces inflammation, while Peppermint relaxes the digestive tract and lemon enhances bile flow, making this tea ideal for reducing gas, bloating, and digestive discomfort.

504. Milk Thistle and Dandelion Liver-Detox Capsules

Ingredients: 1 tablespoon Milk Thistle seed powder, 1 tablespoon Dandelion Root powder, empty gel capsules.
Preparation: Mix Milk Thistle and Dandelion powders thoroughly. Fill the empty gel capsules with the powder mixture and seal.
Suggested Usage: Take 1 capsule daily to support liver health and promote detoxification.
Benefits: Milk Thistle protects liver cells and stimulates regeneration, while Dandelion enhances bile flow and promotes detoxification, making these capsules ideal for supporting liver function and overall digestive health.

505. Senna and Licorice Overnight Laxative Tea

Ingredients: 1 teaspoon dried Senna leaves, 1 teaspoon dried Licorice Root, 2 cups hot water.
Preparation: Steep Senna and Licorice in hot water for 10 minutes. Strain and serve warm.
Suggested Usage: Drink 1 cup in the evening for overnight constipation relief. Use sparingly to prevent dependency.
Benefits: Senna is a potent stimulant laxative that promotes bowel movements, while Licorice Root soothes and protects the digestive tract, making this tea a balanced remedy for occasional constipation.

506. Chamomile, Fennel, and Caraway Gas and Bloat-Reducing Tea

Ingredients: 1 tablespoon dried Chamomile flowers, 1 teaspoon Fennel seeds, 1 teaspoon Caraway seeds, 2 cups hot water.
Preparation: Steep Chamomile, Fennel, and Caraway in hot water for 15 minutes. Strain and serve warm.
Suggested Usage: Drink 1 cup after meals to reduce gas and prevent bloating.
Benefits: Chamomile calms the digestive tract, Fennel reduces gas, and Caraway stimulates digestion, making this tea ideal for reducing bloating and promoting digestive comfort.

507. Lemon Balm and Lavender Anti-Spasm Tea

Ingredients: 1 tablespoon dried Lemon Balm leaves, 1 tablespoon dried Lavender flowers, 2 cups hot water.
Preparation: Steep Lemon Balm and Lavender in hot water for 15 minutes. Strain and serve warm.
Suggested Usage: Drink 1 cup in the evening to reduce digestive spasms and promote relaxation.
Benefits: Lemon Balm and Lavender are gentle antispasmodic herbs that help calm the digestive tract and reduce tension, making this tea effective for managing cramping and stress-related digestive symptoms.

508. Ginger, Turmeric, and Cinnamon Bowel Regularity Capsules

Ingredients: 1 tablespoon Ginger powder, 1 tablespoon Turmeric powder, 1 tablespoon Cinnamon powder, empty gel capsules.

Preparation: Mix Ginger, Turmeric, and Cinnamon powders thoroughly. Fill empty gel capsules with the powder mixture and seal.

Suggested Usage: Take 1 capsule up to twice daily to promote regular bowel movements and reduce inflammation.

Benefits: Ginger and Turmeric stimulate digestive motility and reduce inflammation, while Cinnamon supports healthy digestion, making these capsules effective for maintaining bowel regularity.

509. Marshmallow Root and Licorice Acid Reflux Relief Tea

Ingredients: 1 tablespoon dried Marshmallow Root, 1 tablespoon dried Licorice Root, 2 cups hot water.

Preparation: Steep Marshmallow and Licorice Roots in hot water for 15 minutes. Strain and serve warm.

Suggested Usage: Drink 1 cup before meals to soothe the digestive tract and reduce acid reflux.

Benefits: Marshmallow Root and Licorice Root form a protective coating over the mucous membranes, reducing irritation and promoting healing, making this tea highly effective for managing acid reflux and other inflammatory digestive conditions.

510. Nettle and Peppermint Soothing Tea for Gut Health

Ingredients: 1 tablespoon dried Nettle leaves, 1 tablespoon dried Peppermint leaves, 2 cups hot water.

Preparation: Steep Nettle and Peppermint in hot water for 15 minutes. Strain and serve warm.

Suggested Usage: Drink 1 cup up to twice daily to support digestive health and reduce inflammation.

Benefits: Nettle is rich in nutrients and supports overall vitality, while Peppermint calms the digestive tract, making this tea ideal for managing digestive discomfort and promoting overall gut health.

511. Psyllium Husk and Oat Bran Daily Constipation Support Drink

Ingredients: 1 tablespoon Psyllium Husk, 1 tablespoon Oat Bran, 1 cup warm water.

Preparation: Mix Psyllium Husk and Oat Bran into the warm water, stirring until fully dissolved.

Suggested Usage: Drink once daily in the morning to promote regularity and support digestive health.

Benefits: Psyllium and Oat Bran are rich in soluble fiber, which absorbs water and adds bulk to the stool, making this drink effective for promoting regular bowel movements and preventing constipation.

512. Black Walnut and Wormwood Parasite Cleanse Tincture

Ingredients: 1 tablespoon dried Black Walnut Hulls, 1 tablespoon dried Wormwood, 1 cup vodka or brandy.

Preparation: Place Black Walnut Hulls and Wormwood in a glass jar and cover with vodka or brandy. Seal tightly and let steep for 4-6 weeks, shaking occasionally. Strain and store in a dark glass bottle.

Suggested Usage: Take ½ teaspoon up to twice daily for 2 weeks to eliminate parasites.

Benefits: Black Walnut and Wormwood are powerful antiparasitic herbs that help eliminate intestinal parasites and support overall gut health, making this tincture effective for cleansing the digestive system.

513. Lemon Balm and Skullcap Stress-Reducing Capsules

Ingredients: 1 tablespoon Lemon Balm powder, 1 tablespoon Skullcap powder, empty gel capsules.

Preparation: Mix Lemon Balm and Skullcap powders thoroughly. Fill empty gel capsules with the powder mixture and seal.

Suggested Usage: Take 1 capsule in the evening to reduce stress and promote relaxation.

Benefits: Lemon Balm and Skullcap are calming nervine herbs that help reduce anxiety, alleviate tension, and promote restful sleep, making these capsules ideal for managing stress-related digestive symptoms.

514. Aloe Vera and Ginger Gut-Healing Gel

Ingredients: 1 tablespoon Aloe Vera gel, 1 teaspoon grated fresh Ginger, 1 cup water.

Preparation: Blend Aloe Vera gel and Ginger with water until smooth. Store in a glass jar.

Suggested Usage: Take 1 tablespoon before meals to soothe the digestive tract and promote healing.

Benefits: Aloe Vera and Ginger soothe inflammation, stimulate digestion, and promote tissue repair, making this gel highly effective for managing gut inflammation and supporting overall digestive health.

515. Agrimony and Yarrow Intestinal Health Tea

Ingredients: 1 tablespoon dried Agrimony, 1 tablespoon dried Yarrow, 2 cups hot water.

Preparation: Steep Agrimony and Yarrow in hot water for 15 minutes. Strain and serve warm.

Suggested Usage: Drink 1 cup up to twice daily to support intestinal health and relieve diarrhea.

Benefits: Agrimony and Yarrow are astringent herbs that help tone the digestive tract and reduce excess fluid in the intestines, making this tea effective for managing diarrhea and promoting gut health.

516. Fenugreek and Ginger IBS Support Tea

Ingredients: 1 tablespoon Fenugreek seeds, 1 tablespoon grated fresh Ginger, 2 cups hot water.

Preparation: Simmer Fenugreek seeds and Ginger in hot water for 15 minutes. Strain and serve warm.

Suggested Usage: Drink 1 cup before meals to reduce cramping and support digestion.

Benefits: Fenugreek and Ginger reduce inflammation, enhance digestion, and support healthy bowel movements, making this tea ideal for managing IBS symptoms.

517. Licorice Root and Marshmallow Root Gut-Healing Powder

Ingredients: 1 tablespoon Licorice Root powder, 1 tablespoon Marshmallow Root powder.
Preparation: Mix Licorice and Marshmallow powders thoroughly. Store in a glass jar.
Suggested Usage: Take ½ teaspoon mixed in warm water before meals to soothe and heal the digestive tract.
Benefits: Licorice and Marshmallow Root are demulcent herbs that coat and protect the digestive lining, reduce inflammation, and promote healing, making this powder effective for managing acid reflux and other inflammatory conditions.

518. Dandelion Root and Artichoke Leaf Digestive Stimulation Capsules

Ingredients: 1 tablespoon Dandelion Root powder, 1 tablespoon Artichoke Leaf powder, empty gel capsules.
Preparation: Mix Dandelion Root and Artichoke powders thoroughly. Fill empty gel capsules with the mixture and seal.
Suggested Usage: Take 1 capsule before meals to stimulate digestion and prevent bloating.
Benefits: Dandelion Root and Artichoke Leaf promote bile flow and enhance digestion, making these capsules effective for supporting liver health and reducing symptoms of indigestion.

519. Peppermint and Chamomile Relaxation Tea for Cramps

Ingredients: 1 tablespoon dried Peppermint leaves, 1 tablespoon dried Chamomile flowers, 2 cups hot water.
Preparation: Steep Peppermint and Chamomile in hot water for 15 minutes. Strain and serve warm.
Suggested Usage: Drink 1 cup after meals to relieve cramping and reduce bloating.
Benefits: Peppermint relaxes the digestive tract, while Chamomile reduces inflammation and calms spasms, making this tea ideal for managing cramps and promoting digestive comfort.

520. Yellow Dock and Gentian Root Bitter Capsules

Ingredients: 1 tablespoon Yellow Dock Root powder, 1 tablespoon Gentian Root powder, empty gel capsules.
Preparation: Mix Yellow Dock and Gentian powders thoroughly. Fill empty gel capsules with the mixture and seal.
Suggested Usage: Take 1 capsule 15-20 minutes before meals to stimulate digestive secretions and enhance digestion.
Benefits: Yellow Dock and Gentian are powerful bitter herbs that promote the secretion of digestive enzymes and bile, making these capsules effective for preventing indigestion and promoting appetite.

525. Agrimony and Black Walnut Astringent Tea for Diarrhea

Ingredients: 1 tablespoon dried Agrimony, 1 tablespoon dried Black Walnut Leaf, 2 cups hot water.
Preparation: Steep Agrimony and Black Walnut Leaf in hot water for 15 minutes. Strain and serve warm.
Suggested Usage: Drink 1 cup up to twice daily to reduce diarrhea and firm up stools.
Benefits: Agrimony and Black Walnut have strong astringent properties that tone the mucous membranes of the digestive tract, helping to reduce excess fluid and control diarrhea effectively.

526. Milk Thistle and Artichoke Leaf Liver-Cleansing Capsules

Ingredients: 1 tablespoon Milk Thistle seed powder, 1 tablespoon Artichoke Leaf powder, empty gel capsules.
Preparation: Mix Milk Thistle and Artichoke powders thoroughly. Fill empty gel capsules with the mixture and seal.
Suggested Usage: Take 1 capsule daily to support liver function and promote detoxification.
Benefits: Milk Thistle protects and regenerates liver cells, while Artichoke Leaf enhances bile flow and supports digestion, making these capsules effective for promoting liver health and detoxification.

527. Lemon Balm and Peppermint IBS-Soothing Tea

Ingredients: 1 tablespoon dried Lemon Balm leaves, 1 tablespoon dried Peppermint leaves, 2 cups hot water.
Preparation: Steep Lemon Balm and Peppermint in hot water for 15 minutes.

Strain and serve warm.
Suggested Usage: Drink 1-2 cups daily to soothe IBS symptoms and calm the digestive system.
Benefits: Lemon Balm and Peppermint are gentle antispasmodics that relax the smooth muscles of the digestive tract, reduce cramping, and alleviate discomfort, making this tea ideal for managing IBS-related symptoms.

528. Aloe Vera and Flaxseed Constipation Drink

Ingredients: 1 tablespoon Aloe Vera gel, 1 tablespoon ground Flaxseed, 1 cup warm water.
Preparation: Mix Aloe Vera gel and Flaxseed into the warm water, stirring until fully combined.
Suggested Usage: Drink once daily, preferably in the morning, followed by an additional glass of water to support regular bowel movements.
Benefits: Aloe Vera gently stimulates the bowels, while Flaxseed adds bulk and moisture to the stool, making this drink highly effective for relieving constipation and promoting smooth bowel movements.

529. Valerian and Passionflower Calming Tea for Stress-Induced Digestive Upset

Ingredients: 1 tablespoon dried Valerian Root, 1 tablespoon dried Passionflower, 2 cups hot water.
Preparation: Steep Valerian and Passionflower in hot water for 15 minutes. Strain and serve warm.
Suggested Usage: Drink 1 cup in the evening to promote relaxation and reduce

stress-related digestive issues.

Benefits: Valerian and Passionflower are calming nervine herbs that reduce anxiety and promote restful sleep, making this tea effective for managing stress-induced digestive symptoms such as cramping or indigestion.

530. Cinnamon and Licorice Root Bowel-Soothing Capsules

Ingredients: 1 tablespoon Cinnamon powder, 1 tablespoon Licorice Root powder, empty gel capsules.
Preparation: Mix Cinnamon and Licorice powders thoroughly. Fill empty gel capsules with the mixture and seal.
Suggested Usage: Take 1 capsule up to twice daily to soothe the digestive tract and promote healthy digestion.
Benefits: Cinnamon and Licorice Root reduce inflammation, protect mucous membranes, and support healthy digestion, making these capsules ideal for managing inflammatory bowel conditions.

531. Black Walnut and Garlic Parasite Cleanse Capsules

Ingredients: 1 tablespoon Black Walnut Hull powder, 1 tablespoon Garlic powder, empty gel capsules.
Preparation: Mix Black Walnut and Garlic powders thoroughly. Fill empty gel capsules with the mixture and seal.
Suggested Usage: Take 1 capsule up to twice daily for 2 weeks to eliminate parasites.
Benefits: Black Walnut and Garlic are powerful antiparasitic herbs that support the elimination of intestinal parasites,

making these capsules effective for cleansing the digestive system.

532. Ginger, Fennel, and Peppermint Nausea Relief Tea

Ingredients: 1 tablespoon grated fresh Ginger, 1 tablespoon Fennel seeds, 1 tablespoon dried Peppermint leaves, 2 cups hot water.
Preparation: Steep Ginger, Fennel, and Peppermint in hot water for 15 minutes. Strain and serve warm.
Suggested Usage: Drink 1 cup as needed to reduce nausea and settle the stomach.
Benefits: Ginger and Peppermint are well-known for their anti-nausea properties, while Fennel reduces bloating and gas, making this tea ideal for relieving nausea and calming the digestive system.

533. Slippery Elm and Chamomile Mucilage-Forming Gut Tea

Ingredients: 1 tablespoon Slippery Elm powder, 1 tablespoon dried Chamomile flowers, 2 cups hot water.
Preparation: Steep Chamomile in hot water for 10 minutes, then stir in Slippery Elm powder until fully dissolved.
Suggested Usage: Drink 1 cup before meals to coat and protect the digestive tract.
Benefits: Slippery Elm and Chamomile form a protective coating over the mucous membranes, reducing irritation and promoting healing, making this tea ideal for managing acid reflux and esophageal discomfort.

534. Dandelion and Yellow Dock Liver Support Capsules

Ingredients: 1 tablespoon Dandelion Root powder, 1 tablespoon Yellow Dock Root powder, empty gel capsules.
Preparation: Mix Dandelion Root and Yellow Dock powders thoroughly. Fill empty gel capsules with the mixture and seal.
Suggested Usage: Take 1 capsule daily to support liver function and promote detoxification.
Benefits: Dandelion and Yellow Dock both enhance liver function and promote bile flow, making these capsules ideal for supporting healthy digestion and detoxification.

535. Lemon Balm, Skullcap, and Lavender Calming Tea for Digestive Health

Ingredients: 1 tablespoon dried Lemon Balm leaves, 1 tablespoon dried Skullcap, 1 tablespoon dried Lavender flowers, 2 cups hot water.
Preparation: Steep Lemon Balm, Skullcap, and Lavender in hot water for 15 minutes. Strain and serve warm.
Suggested Usage: Drink 1 cup in the evening to reduce stress and support digestive health.
Benefits: Lemon Balm, Skullcap, and Lavender are calming nervine herbs that help reduce anxiety and tension, making this tea effective for managing stress-related digestive symptoms.

536. Fennel and Peppermint IBS-Calming Tea

Ingredients: 1 tablespoon Fennel seeds, 1 tablespoon dried Peppermint leaves, 2 cups hot water.
Preparation: Steep Fennel and Peppermint in hot water for 15 minutes. Strain and serve warm.
Suggested Usage: Drink 1 cup up to twice daily to reduce IBS symptoms and promote digestive comfort.
Benefits: Fennel reduces gas and bloating, while Peppermint relaxes the digestive tract, making this tea ideal for managing IBS-related discomfort.

537. Marshmallow Root and Slippery Elm Intestinal Healing Gel

Ingredients: 1 tablespoon Marshmallow Root powder, 1 tablespoon Slippery Elm powder, 1 cup water.
Preparation: Mix Marshmallow Root and Slippery Elm powders into the water, stirring until a gel-like consistency forms.
Suggested Usage: Take 1 tablespoon up to twice daily to soothe the digestive tract and promote healing.
Benefits: Marshmallow and Slippery Elm are rich in mucilage, which coats and protects the intestinal lining, making this gel ideal for managing inflammatory conditions and promoting gut healing.

538. Valerian and Skullcap Anti-Anxiety Capsules for Gut Health

Ingredients: 1 tablespoon Valerian Root powder, 1 tablespoon Skullcap powder, empty gel capsules.
Preparation: Mix Valerian and Skullcap

powders thoroughly. Fill empty gel capsules with the mixture and seal.

Suggested Usage: Take 1 capsule in the evening to reduce anxiety and support gut health.

Benefits: Valerian and Skullcap calm the nervous system and reduce stress, making these capsules effective for managing stress-related digestive symptoms.

539. Psyllium Husk and Oat Straw Constipation Relief Capsules

Ingredients: 1 tablespoon Psyllium Husk powder, 1 tablespoon Oat Straw powder, empty gel capsules.

Preparation: Mix Psyllium Husk and Oat Straw powders thoroughly. Fill empty gel capsules with the mixture and seal.

Suggested Usage: Take 1 capsule up to twice daily with a full glass of water to promote bowel regularity.

Benefits: Psyllium Husk and Oat Straw add bulk to the stool and promote smooth bowel movements, making these capsules effective for relieving constipation.

540. Dandelion and Milk Thistle Liver Support Elixir

Ingredients: 1 tablespoon dried Dandelion Root, 1 tablespoon Milk Thistle seeds, 1 cup vodka or brandy (for tincture base).

Preparation: Place Dandelion and Milk Thistle in a glass jar and cover with vodka or brandy. Seal tightly and let steep for 4-6 weeks, shaking occasionally. Strain and store in a dark glass bottle.

Suggested Usage: Take ½ teaspoon up to twice daily to support liver function and promote detoxification.

Benefits: Dandelion and Milk Thistle enhance liver function and support the detoxification process, making this elixir ideal for promoting overall digestive health and vitality.

Book 25: Healing the Gut with Herbs

A healthy gut is central to overall wellness, influencing not only digestion but also immune function, mental health, and even the body's ability to ward off chronic diseases. The gut is often referred to as the "second brain" due to its intricate connection with the central nervous system and its role in producing neurotransmitters that affect mood and cognition. This delicate and complex system relies heavily on the balance of gut flora—beneficial bacteria that reside in the intestines and support various bodily functions. Disruptions to this balance, whether due to poor diet, stress, antibiotic use, or other factors, can lead to an array of digestive issues, such as bloating, constipation, diarrhea, and inflammatory bowel conditions. To promote a healthy gut environment and restore balance, herbs can play a significant role. Herbal remedies, when used correctly, offer gentle, natural ways to heal the gut, reduce inflammation, and foster a thriving microbiome.

Promoting Gut Health and Microbiome Balance

The gut microbiome consists of trillions of bacteria, fungi, and other microorganisms that live symbiotically in the intestines. A diverse and balanced microbiome is essential for maintaining gut health, as it aids in the digestion of food, synthesizes vitamins, and plays a critical role in modulating the immune system. When the balance of gut bacteria is disrupted, a state known as dysbiosis occurs, leading to inflammation, impaired nutrient absorption, and increased susceptibility to digestive disorders such as irritable bowel syndrome (IBS) and inflammatory bowel disease (IBD).

Herbs can support the microbiome by promoting the growth of beneficial bacteria, reducing harmful pathogens, and soothing inflammation in the gut lining. Some herbs, such as Marshmallow Root and Licorice Root, are known for their ability to form a protective mucilaginous layer over the gut lining, which can help reduce irritation and support the regeneration of healthy tissues. This soothing action is especially beneficial for conditions like leaky gut syndrome, where the integrity of the gut lining is compromised, allowing undigested food particles and toxins to enter the bloodstream.

Herbs like Slippery Elm, rich in mucilage, not only protect the gut lining but also provide nourishment for beneficial bacteria, acting as a prebiotic. Prebiotics are non-digestible fibers that serve as food for probiotics, the beneficial bacteria in the gut. By incorporating prebiotic herbs into the diet, it's possible to create a more hospitable environment for these beneficial bacteria to thrive. Other herbs, such as Fennel and Peppermint, are carminative, meaning they help relax the digestive tract and reduce gas, bloating, and cramping, all of which can disrupt the balance of the gut flora.

Anti-inflammatory herbs such as Chamomile and Turmeric also play a vital role in promoting gut health. Inflammation in the gut is a common symptom of many digestive disorders, and reducing this inflammation can significantly improve gut function and overall health. Chamomile, with its gentle anti-inflammatory and antispasmodic properties, helps calm the digestive tract and alleviate discomfort, while Turmeric's active compound, curcumin, has been extensively studied for its powerful anti-inflammatory and antioxidant effects.

In addition to these supportive herbs, it's crucial to include a diet rich in diverse fibers, vitamins, and minerals to maintain a balanced gut microbiome. Consuming a wide variety of colorful fruits, vegetables, and whole grains provides essential nutrients that feed both the gut lining and its microbial inhabitants. Pairing these foods with gut-supportive herbs can enhance their effects and create a foundation for long-term gut health.

Herbal Probiotics and Prebiotics

Probiotics and prebiotics are key players in maintaining a healthy gut microbiome. Probiotics are live beneficial bacteria that help replenish the gut flora, while prebiotics are types of dietary fibers that nourish these bacteria, allowing them to thrive. While most people are familiar with probiotic foods like yogurt, kefir, and sauerkraut, certain herbs also contain probiotic and prebiotic properties, making them valuable additions to a gut-healing protocol.

Herbs such as Dandelion Root, Burdock Root, and Chicory Root are rich in inulin, a type of prebiotic fiber that feeds beneficial bacteria in the colon, particularly Bifidobacteria. Inulin helps increase the population of these friendly bacteria, improving digestion, enhancing nutrient absorption, and supporting the body's natural detoxification processes. Dandelion Root, in particular, is known for its ability to stimulate bile production, supporting liver function and aiding in the breakdown of fats, which further enhances its role in promoting a healthy digestive environment.

Marshmallow Root and Slippery Elm, in addition to their soothing properties, also act as prebiotics. Their high mucilage content provides a protective layer over the gut lining, which not only reduces inflammation but also serves as a food source for beneficial bacteria. By incorporating these herbs into teas, powders, or tinctures, individuals can support the growth of a healthy microbiome and reduce the risk of dysbiosis.

Herbs like Fermented Ginger and Garlic offer natural probiotic benefits. Fermentation is a process that encourages the growth of beneficial bacteria, transforming these herbs into potent probiotic sources that help repopulate the gut with healthy microbes. Fermented Ginger is particularly useful for supporting digestive health, as it not only replenishes the gut flora but also reduces nausea and improves overall digestion. Similarly, Fermented Garlic is a strong antimicrobial herb that targets harmful bacteria while promoting the growth of beneficial strains, making it ideal for balancing the microbiome.

Another herb to consider is Triphala, a traditional Ayurvedic blend of three fruits: Amalaki (Emblica officinalis), Haritaki (Terminalia chebula), and Bibhitaki (Terminalia bellirica). Triphala has long been used to support digestive health and regularity. It acts as both a gentle laxative and a prebiotic, providing nourishment for the beneficial bacteria in the gut. Its unique combination of antioxidant and anti-inflammatory properties makes it a versatile herb for promoting gut health and maintaining a balanced microbiome.

To incorporate herbal probiotics and prebiotics into the diet, consider the following strategies:

1. Prebiotic-Rich Teas and Tinctures: Brew teas using Dandelion Root, Burdock Root, or Chicory Root, and consume them daily to increase prebiotic intake. Alternatively, use these herbs in tincture form for a more concentrated dose.
2. Fermented Herbal Preparations: Prepare fermented herbal blends using Ginger, Garlic, or other herbs known for their antimicrobial and gut-supportive properties. These can be taken as daily supplements to maintain gut flora balance.
3. Triphala Powder: Add Triphala powder to smoothies or teas to support digestion and provide prebiotic benefits. This blend not only enhances gut health but also supports regular bowel movements and detoxification.
4. Herbal Infusions with Marshmallow Root or Slippery Elm: Create herbal infusions using mucilaginous herbs like Marshmallow Root and Slippery Elm. These can be consumed as teas or mixed into smoothies to soothe the gut lining and promote the growth of beneficial bacteria.

By understanding the role of herbal probiotics and prebiotics and incorporating them into daily routines, it's possible to create a balanced and healthy gut environment that supports overall health and vitality.

Remedies for Gut Healing

541. Slippery Elm and Marshmallow Root Gut-Healing Tea

Ingredients: 1 tablespoon dried Slippery Elm Bark, 1 tablespoon dried Marshmallow Root, 2 cups hot water.
Preparation: Steep Slippery Elm and Marshmallow Root in hot water for 15 minutes. Strain and serve warm.
Suggested Usage: Drink 1 cup up to twice daily to soothe and protect the digestive tract.
Benefits: Slippery Elm and Marshmallow Root form a mucilaginous layer over the gut lining, reducing inflammation and promoting healing, making this tea ideal for managing conditions like leaky gut and gastritis.

542. Licorice Root and Aloe Vera Acid Reflux Relief Drink

Ingredients: 1 tablespoon Licorice Root powder, 1 tablespoon Aloe Vera gel, 1 cup warm water.

Preparation: Mix Licorice Root powder and Aloe Vera gel into warm water, stirring until fully dissolved.

Suggested Usage: Drink 1 cup before meals to reduce acid reflux and soothe the digestive tract.

Benefits: Licorice Root and Aloe Vera coat and protect the esophagus, reduce acidity, and promote healing of the mucous membranes, making this drink highly effective for managing acid reflux.

543. Chamomile and Lemon Balm Anti-Spasm Tea

Ingredients: 1 tablespoon dried Chamomile flowers, 1 tablespoon dried Lemon Balm leaves, 2 cups hot water.

Preparation: Steep Chamomile and Lemon Balm in hot water for 15 minutes. Strain and serve warm.

Suggested Usage: Drink 1 cup up to twice daily to relieve spasms and calm the digestive system.

Benefits: Chamomile and Lemon Balm are gentle antispasmodic herbs that relax the smooth muscles of the digestive tract, making this tea effective for reducing cramping, gas, and bloating.

544. Dandelion Root and Burdock Liver Support Tea

Ingredients: 1 tablespoon dried Dandelion Root, 1 tablespoon dried Burdock Root, 4 cups water.

Preparation: Simmer Dandelion Root and Burdock Root in water for 30 minutes. Strain and serve warm.

Suggested Usage: Drink 1 cup daily to support liver function and promote detoxification.

Benefits: Dandelion and Burdock Roots are powerful liver-supportive herbs that enhance bile production, improve digestion, and support the body's natural detoxification processes.

545. Peppermint and Ginger Bloating Relief Tea

Ingredients: 1 tablespoon dried Peppermint leaves, 1 tablespoon grated fresh Ginger, 2 cups hot water.

Preparation: Steep Peppermint and Ginger in hot water for 15 minutes. Strain and serve warm.

Suggested Usage: Drink 1-2 cups daily to relieve bloating and support digestion.

Benefits: Peppermint relaxes the digestive tract, while Ginger stimulates the production of digestive enzymes and bile, making this tea effective for reducing bloating and promoting digestive health.

546. Nettle and Peppermint Soothing Tea for Gut Health

Ingredients: 1 tablespoon dried Nettle leaves, 1 tablespoon dried Peppermint leaves, 2 cups hot water.

Preparation: Steep Nettle and Peppermint in hot water for 15 minutes. Strain and serve warm.

Suggested Usage: Drink 1 cup up to twice daily to soothe the digestive system and reduce inflammation.

Benefits: Nettle is rich in nutrients that support overall health, while Peppermint calms the digestive tract, making this tea ideal for managing digestive discomfort and promoting gut health.

547. Turmeric and Ginger Anti-Inflammatory Tonic

Ingredients: 1 tablespoon grated fresh Ginger, 1 teaspoon Turmeric powder, 1 teaspoon raw honey, 1 cup hot water.
Preparation: Steep Ginger and Turmeric in hot water for 10 minutes. Strain and add honey if desired.
Suggested Usage: Drink 1 cup daily to reduce inflammation and support gut health.
Benefits: Turmeric's active compound, curcumin, has strong anti-inflammatory properties, while Ginger enhances digestion, making this tonic highly effective for reducing inflammation in the digestive tract.

548. Psyllium Husk and Flaxseed Constipation Relief Drink

Ingredients: 1 tablespoon Psyllium Husk, 1 tablespoon ground Flaxseed, 1 cup warm water.
Preparation: Mix Psyllium Husk and Flaxseed into warm water, stirring until fully dissolved.
Suggested Usage: Drink once daily, followed by an additional glass of water, to promote bowel regularity.
Benefits: Psyllium and Flaxseed provide a balanced mix of soluble and insoluble fiber, which absorbs water, adds bulk to the stool, and promotes smooth, regular bowel movements.

549. Fenugreek and Ginger Gut-Calming Tea

Ingredients: 1 tablespoon Fenugreek seeds, 1 tablespoon grated fresh Ginger, 2 cups hot water.
Preparation: Simmer Fenugreek seeds and Ginger in hot water for 15 minutes. Strain and serve warm.
Suggested Usage: Drink 1 cup before meals to reduce inflammation and support digestion.
Benefits: Fenugreek and Ginger reduce gut inflammation, promote healthy digestion, and alleviate symptoms of IBS, making this tea ideal for calming an irritated digestive system.

550. Fennel and Anise Seed Carminative Tea

Ingredients: 1 tablespoon Fennel seeds, 1 teaspoon Anise seeds, 2 cups hot water.
Preparation: Steep Fennel and Anise seeds in hot water for 15 minutes. Strain and serve warm.
Suggested Usage: Drink 1 cup after meals to reduce gas and bloating.
Benefits: Fennel and Anise are carminative herbs that promote the expulsion of gas, reduce bloating, and soothe the digestive tract, making this tea highly effective for managing post-meal discomfort.

551. Licorice Root and Cinnamon Gut-Healing Capsules

Ingredients: 1 tablespoon Licorice Root powder, 1 tablespoon Cinnamon powder, empty gel capsules.
Preparation: Mix Licorice Root and Cinnamon powders thoroughly. Fill the empty gel capsules with the mixture and seal.

Suggested Usage: Take 1 capsule up to twice daily to soothe the digestive tract and reduce inflammation.
Benefits: Licorice Root soothes and protects the mucous membranes, while Cinnamon stimulates digestion and reduces inflammation, making these capsules effective for managing inflammatory digestive conditions.

552. Artichoke Leaf and Gentian Digestive Support Tea

Ingredients: 1 tablespoon dried Artichoke Leaf, 1 teaspoon dried Gentian Root, 2 cups hot water.
Preparation: Steep Artichoke Leaf and Gentian in hot water for 15 minutes. Strain and serve warm.
Suggested Usage: Drink 1 cup before meals to enhance digestive function and prevent bloating.
Benefits: Artichoke Leaf and Gentian are powerful bitter herbs that stimulate the production of digestive enzymes and bile, making this tea effective for enhancing digestion and relieving symptoms of indigestion.

553. Milk Thistle and Dandelion Liver-Detox Capsules

Ingredients: 1 tablespoon Milk Thistle seed powder, 1 tablespoon Dandelion Root powder, empty gel capsules.
Preparation: Mix Milk Thistle and Dandelion powders thoroughly. Fill the empty gel capsules with the powder mixture and seal.
Suggested Usage: Take 1 capsule daily to support liver function and promote detoxification.

Benefits: Milk Thistle protects liver cells and stimulates regencration, while Dandelion enhances bile flow and promotes detoxification, making these capsules effective for supporting liver function and overall digestive health.

554. Calendula and Chamomile Gut-Soothing Tea

Ingredients: 1 tablespoon dried Calendula flowers, 1 tablespoon dried Chamomile flowers, 2 cups hot water.
Preparation: Steep Calendula and Chamomile in hot water for 15 minutes. Strain and serve warm.
Suggested Usage: Drink 1 cup up to twice daily to soothe the digestive system and reduce inflammation.
Benefits: Calendula and Chamomile are gentle anti-inflammatory herbs that reduce irritation, promote healing, and calm the digestive system, making this tea ideal for managing inflammatory digestive conditions.

555. Ginger, Fennel, and Peppermint Nausea Relief Tea

Ingredients: 1 tablespoon grated fresh Ginger, 1 tablespoon Fennel seeds, 1 tablespoon dried Peppermint leaves, 2 cups hot water.
Preparation: Steep Ginger, Fennel, and Peppermint in hot water for 15 minutes. Strain and serve warm.
Suggested Usage: Drink 1 cup as needed to reduce nausea and settle the stomach.
Benefits: Ginger and Peppermint are well-known for their anti-nausea properties, while Fennel reduces bloating and gas,

making this tea ideal for relieving nausea and calming the digestive system.

556. Lemon Balm and Skullcap Stress-Relief Tea

Ingredients: 1 tablespoon dried Lemon Balm leaves, 1 tablespoon dried Skullcap, 2 cups hot water.
Preparation: Steep Lemon Balm and Skullcap in hot water for 15 minutes. Strain and serve warm.
Suggested Usage: Drink 1 cup in the evening to reduce stress and promote relaxation.
Benefits: Lemon Balm and Skullcap are calming nervine herbs that help reduce anxiety, alleviate tension, and promote restful sleep, making this tea effective for managing stress-related digestive symptoms.

557. Triphala Gut-Toning Tincture

Ingredients: 1 tablespoon Triphala powder, 1 cup vodka or brandy (for tincture base).
Preparation: Combine Triphala powder and alcohol in a glass jar. Seal tightly and let steep for 4-6 weeks, shaking occasionally. Strain and store in a dark glass bottle.
Suggested Usage: Take ½ teaspoon up to twice daily to support digestion and bowel regularity.
Benefits: Triphala is a traditional Ayurvedic blend that gently supports gut health, promotes regular bowel movements, and nourishes the intestinal tract, making it ideal for maintaining overall digestive health.

558. Aloe Vera and Ginger Gut-Healing Gel

Ingredients: 1 tablespoon Aloe Vera gel, 1 tablespoon grated fresh Ginger, 1 cup water.
Preparation: Blend Aloe Vera gel and Ginger with water until smooth. Store in a glass jar.
Suggested Usage: Take 1 tablespoon before meals to soothe the digestive tract and reduce inflammation.
Benefits: Aloe Vera and Ginger are both anti-inflammatory and soothing, making this gel effective for managing gut inflammation, calming irritation, and promoting overall digestive health.

559. Agrimony and Raspberry Leaf Astringent Tea for Diarrhea

Ingredients: 1 tablespoon dried Agrimony, 1 tablespoon dried Raspberry Leaf, 2 cups hot water.
Preparation: Steep Agrimony and Raspberry Leaf in hot water for 15 minutes. Strain and serve warm.
Suggested Usage: Drink 1-2 cups daily to firm up stools and reduce diarrhea.
Benefits: Agrimony and Raspberry Leaf are strong astringent herbs that tone the digestive tract and reduce excess fluid in the intestines, making this tea highly effective for managing diarrhea.

560. Holy Basil and Ashwagandha Stress-Balancing Capsules

Ingredients: 1 tablespoon Holy Basil powder, 1 tablespoon Ashwagandha Root

powder, empty gel capsules.

Preparation: Mix Holy Basil and Ashwagandha powders thoroughly. Fill empty gel capsules with the mixture and seal.

Suggested Usage: Take 1 capsule up to twice daily to reduce stress and promote emotional balance.

Benefits: Holy Basil and Ashwagandha are adaptogenic herbs that help regulate cortisol levels, support emotional resilience, and reduce the impact of stress on the digestive system.

561. Chamomile and Licorice Root Anti-Inflammatory Tea

Ingredients: 1 tablespoon dried Chamomile flowers, 1 tablespoon dried Licorice Root, 2 cups hot water.

Preparation: Steep Chamomile and Licorice in hot water for 15 minutes. Strain and serve warm.

Suggested Usage: Drink 1 cup up to twice daily to reduce inflammation and support digestive healing.

Benefits: Chamomile and Licorice Root reduce inflammation, calm the digestive tract, and promote healing, making this tea ideal for managing inflammatory conditions like gastritis or IBD.

562. Marshmallow Root and Licorice Throat and Gut-Coating Syrup

Ingredients: 1 tablespoon dried Marshmallow Root, 1 tablespoon Licorice Root, 2 cups water, 1 cup raw honey.

Preparation: Simmer Marshmallow Root and Licorice Root in water for 20 minutes. Strain and add honey, stirring until fully dissolved. Store in a glass jar.

Suggested Usage: Take 1 tablespoon up to twice daily to coat and protect the digestive and esophageal linings.

Benefits: Marshmallow Root and Licorice Root create a soothing gel that coats mucous membranes, providing relief from irritation and promoting healing of inflamed or damaged tissue.

563. Yellow Dock and Burdock Digestive Detox Capsules

Ingredients: 1 tablespoon Yellow Dock powder, 1 tablespoon Burdock Root powder, empty gel capsules.

Preparation: Mix Yellow Dock and Burdock powders thoroughly. Fill empty gel capsules with the mixture and seal.

Suggested Usage: Take 1 capsule daily to support liver function and promote detoxification.

Benefits: Yellow Dock and Burdock are powerful liver-supportive herbs that enhance bile production, promote detoxification, and support overall digestive health.

564. Peppermint and Chamomile Relaxation Tea for IBS

Ingredients: 1 tablespoon dried Peppermint leaves, 1 tablespoon dried Chamomile flowers, 2 cups hot water.

Preparation: Steep Peppermint and Chamomile in hot water for 15 minutes. Strain and serve warm.

Suggested Usage: Drink 1-2 cups daily to soothe IBS symptoms and calm the digestive system.

Benefits: Peppermint and Chamomile are gentle antispasmodic herbs that relax the digestive tract, reduce cramping, and alleviate discomfort, making this tea ideal for managing IBS-related symptoms.

565. Lemon Balm and Peppermint Anti-Spasm Capsules

Ingredients: 1 tablespoon Lemon Balm powder, 1 tablespoon Peppermint powder, empty gel capsules.
Preparation: Mix Lemon Balm and Peppermint powders thoroughly. Fill empty gel capsules with the mixture and seal.
Suggested Usage: Take 1 capsule up to twice daily to relieve digestive spasms and reduce gas.
Benefits: Lemon Balm and Peppermint are effective at calming the smooth muscles of the digestive tract, making these capsules highly effective for reducing cramping, gas, and bloating.

566. Psyllium and Aloe Vera Daily Gut Cleanse Drink

Ingredients: 1 tablespoon Psyllium Husk, 1 tablespoon Aloe Vera gel, 1 cup warm water.
Preparation: Mix Psyllium and Aloe Vera into the warm water, stirring until fully dissolved.
Suggested Usage: Drink once daily in the morning to promote regularity and support gut health.
Benefits: Psyllium and Aloe Vera gently cleanse the digestive tract, add bulk to the stool, and promote smooth bowel movements, making this drink ideal for maintaining regularity.

567. Black Walnut and Wormwood Parasite Cleanse Capsules

Ingredients: 1 tablespoon Black Walnut Hull powder, 1 tablespoon Wormwood powder, empty gel capsules.
Preparation: Mix Black Walnut and Wormwood powders thoroughly. Fill empty gel capsules with the mixture and seal.
Suggested Usage: Take 1 capsule up to twice daily for 2 weeks to eliminate parasites.
Benefits: Black Walnut and Wormwood are powerful antiparasitic herbs that support the elimination of intestinal parasites, making these capsules effective for cleansing the digestive system.

568. Licorice Root and Marshmallow Gut-Soothing Powder

Ingredients: 1 tablespoon Licorice Root powder, 1 tablespoon Marshmallow Root powder.
Preparation: Mix Licorice and Marshmallow powders thoroughly. Store in a glass jar.
Suggested Usage: Take ½ teaspoon mixed in warm water before meals to coat and protect the digestive tract.
Benefits: Licorice and Marshmallow are demulcent herbs that coat and protect the gut lining, reduce inflammation, and promote healing, making this powder ideal for managing acid reflux and other inflammatory conditions.

569. Chamomile, Lavender, and Lemon Balm Relaxation Tea

Ingredients: 1 tablespoon dried Chamomile flowers, 1 tablespoon dried Lavender flowers, 1 tablespoon dried Lemon Balm leaves, 2 cups hot water.

Preparation: Steep Chamomile, Lavender, and Lemon Balm in hot water for 15 minutes. Strain and serve warm.

Suggested Usage: Drink 1 cup in the evening to promote relaxation and reduce stress-related digestive issues.

Benefits: Chamomile, Lavender, and Lemon Balm calm the nervous system and reduce anxiety, making this tea effective for managing stress-induced digestive symptoms.

570. Dandelion Root and Artichoke Leaf Digestive Bitters Capsules

Ingredients: 1 tablespoon Dandelion Root powder, 1 tablespoon Artichoke Leaf powder, empty gel capsules.

Preparation: Mix Dandelion Root and Artichoke powders thoroughly. Fill empty gel capsules with the mixture and seal.

Suggested Usage: Take 1 capsule before meals to stimulate digestive secretions and prevent bloating.

Benefits: Dandelion Root and Artichoke Leaf are powerful bitter herbs that stimulate bile production and digestive enzyme release, making these capsules highly effective for enhancing digestion and preventing symptoms of indigestion.

571. Slippery Elm and Plantain Gut-Healing Powder

Ingredients: 1 tablespoon Slippery Elm powder, 1 tablespoon Plantain Leaf powder.

Preparation: Mix Slippery Elm and Plantain powders thoroughly. Store in a glass jar.

Suggested Usage: Take ½ teaspoon mixed in warm water before meals to coat and protect the gut lining.

Benefits: Slippery Elm and Plantain provide a soothing layer of mucilage that protects the mucous membranes of the digestive tract, making this powder effective for managing inflammatory bowel conditions and promoting gut healing.

572. Peppermint and Ginger Anti-Nausea Capsules

Ingredients: 1 tablespoon Peppermint powder, 1 tablespoon Ginger powder, empty gel capsules.

Preparation: Mix Peppermint and Ginger powders thoroughly. Fill empty gel capsules with the mixture and seal.

Suggested Usage: Take 1 capsule up to twice daily to relieve nausea and promote digestion.

Benefits: Peppermint and Ginger are well-known anti-nausea herbs that calm the digestive tract, reduce inflammation, and alleviate discomfort, making these capsules ideal for managing nausea and digestive upset.

573. Valerian and Skullcap Stress-Reducing Capsules

Ingredients: 1 tablespoon Valerian Root powder, 1 tablespoon Skullcap powder, empty gel capsules.

Preparation: Mix Valerian and Skullcap powders thoroughly. Fill empty gel capsules with the mixture and seal.

Suggested Usage: Take 1 capsule in the evening to reduce anxiety and promote restful sleep.

Benefits: Valerian and Skullcap are calming nervine herbs that help relax the nervous system, reduce anxiety, and support deep, restorative sleep, making these capsules effective for managing stress-related digestive issues.

574. Triphala and Ginger Digestive Support Capsules

Ingredients: 1 tablespoon Triphala powder, 1 tablespoon Ginger powder, empty gel capsules.

Preparation: Mix Triphala and Ginger powders thoroughly. Fill empty gel capsules with the mixture and seal.

Suggested Usage: Take 1 capsule up to twice daily to support digestion and maintain bowel regularity.

Benefits: Triphala tones and cleanses the digestive tract, while Ginger enhances digestion and reduces inflammation, making these capsules ideal for supporting gut health and regularity.

575. Calendula and Slippery Elm Mucilage-Forming Tea

Ingredients: 1 tablespoon dried Calendula flowers, 1 tablespoon Slippery Elm powder, 2 cups hot water.

Preparation: Steep Calendula in hot water for 10 minutes, then stir in Slippery Elm powder until fully dissolved.

Suggested Usage: Drink 1 cup up to twice daily to coat and protect the digestive tract.

Benefits: Calendula and Slippery Elm reduce irritation, promote healing, and form a protective mucilaginous layer over the gut lining, making this tea ideal for managing conditions like leaky gut and acid reflux.

576. Fennel, Ginger, and Cardamom Digestive Comfort Tea

Ingredients: 1 tablespoon Fennel seeds, 1 tablespoon grated fresh Ginger, 1 teaspoon Cardamom pods, 2 cups hot water.

Preparation: Steep Fennel, Ginger, and Cardamom in hot water for 15 minutes. Strain and serve warm.

Suggested Usage: Drink 1 cup after meals to support digestion and reduce bloating.

Benefits: Fennel, Ginger, and Cardamom are warming digestive herbs that stimulate digestion, reduce gas, and alleviate discomfort, making this tea highly effective for promoting healthy digestion.

577. Yellow Dock and Gentian Bitter Capsules

Ingredients: 1 tablespoon Yellow Dock Root powder, 1 tablespoon Gentian Root powder, empty gel capsules.

Preparation: Mix Yellow Dock and Gentian powders thoroughly. Fill empty gel capsules with the mixture and seal.

Suggested Usage: Take 1 capsule 15-20 minutes before meals to stimulate digestive secretions and improve digestion.

Benefits: Yellow Dock and Gentian are powerful bitter herbs that enhance bile flow and stimulate the production of digestive enzymes, making these capsules ideal for improving digestion and preventing indigestion.

578. Ginger, Lemon, and Honey Bloating Relief Tea

Ingredients: 1 tablespoon grated fresh Ginger, 1 teaspoon lemon juice, 1 teaspoon raw honey, 2 cups hot water.
Preparation: Steep Ginger in hot water for 10 minutes. Strain, add lemon juice and honey, and serve warm.
Suggested Usage: Drink 1 cup after meals to reduce bloating and promote digestion.
Benefits: Ginger and lemon enhance digestion and reduce bloating, while honey soothes the digestive tract, making this tea effective for relieving post-meal discomfort.

579. Aloe Vera and Chamomile Gut-Healing Tincture

Ingredients: 1 tablespoon Aloe Vera gel, 1 tablespoon dried Chamomile flowers, 1 cup vodka or brandy (for tincture base).
Preparation: Combine Aloe Vera gel, Chamomile flowers, and alcohol in a glass jar. Seal tightly and let steep for 4-6 weeks, shaking occasionally. Strain and store in a dark glass bottle.
Suggested Usage: Take ½ teaspoon up to twice daily to soothe the gut lining and reduce inflammation.
Benefits: Aloe Vera and Chamomile reduce inflammation, promote healing, and soothe the gut lining, making this tincture highly effective for managing inflammatory digestive conditions.

580. Lemon Balm and Peppermint IBS-Support Tea

Ingredients: 1 tablespoon dried Lemon Balm leaves, 1 tablespoon dried Peppermint leaves, 2 cups hot water.
Preparation: Steep Lemon Balm and Peppermint in hot water for 15 minutes. Strain and serve warm.
Suggested Usage: Drink 1-2 cups daily to soothe IBS symptoms and calm the digestive system.
Benefits: Lemon Balm and Peppermint are gentle antispasmodic herbs that relax the smooth muscles of the digestive tract, reduce cramping, and alleviate discomfort, making this tea ideal for managing IBS-related symptoms.

581. Milk Thistle and Dandelion Liver-Support Capsules

Ingredients: 1 tablespoon Milk Thistle seed powder, 1 tablespoon Dandelion Root powder, empty gel capsules.
Preparation: Mix Milk Thistle and Dandelion powders thoroughly. Fill empty gel capsules with the mixture and seal.
Suggested Usage: Take 1 capsule daily to support liver function and promote detoxification.
Benefits: Milk Thistle protects liver cells and stimulates regeneration, while Dandelion enhances bile flow and promotes detoxification, making these capsules effective for supporting liver function and overall digestive health.

582. Psyllium Husk and Oat Bran Daily Fiber Drink

Ingredients: 1 tablespoon Psyllium Husk, 1 tablespoon Oat Bran, 1 cup warm water.
Preparation: Mix Psyllium Husk and Oat Bran into the warm water, stirring until

fully dissolved.

Suggested Usage: Drink once daily, followed by an additional glass of water to support bowel regularity.

Benefits: Psyllium Husk and Oat Bran provide a balanced mix of soluble and insoluble fiber, which absorbs water and forms bulk in the stool, promoting smooth, regular bowel movements and supporting overall digestive health.

583. Marshmallow Root and Licorice Soothing Gut Gel

Ingredients: 1 tablespoon Marshmallow Root powder, 1 tablespoon Licorice Root powder, 1 cup water.

Preparation: Mix Marshmallow Root and Licorice powders into water, stirring until a gel-like consistency forms. Store in a glass jar.

Suggested Usage: Take 1 tablespoon up to twice daily to coat the gut lining and reduce inflammation.

Benefits: Marshmallow Root and Licorice Root are rich in mucilage, which coats and protects the mucous membranes of the digestive tract, making this gel highly effective for managing conditions like gastritis, acid reflux, and colitis.

584. Ginger and Peppermint Bloating Relief Capsules

Ingredients: 1 tablespoon Ginger powder, 1 tablespoon Peppermint powder, empty gel capsules.

Preparation: Mix Ginger and Peppermint powders thoroughly. Fill empty gel capsules with the mixture and seal.

Suggested Usage: Take 1 capsule up to twice daily to relieve bloating and promote digestion.

Benefits: Ginger and Peppermint are carminative herbs that relax the digestive tract, reduce gas, and stimulate digestion, making these capsules effective for alleviating bloating and post-meal discomfort.

585. Agrimony and Yarrow Intestinal Health Tea

Ingredients: 1 tablespoon dried Agrimony, 1 tablespoon dried Yarrow, 2 cups hot water.

Preparation: Steep Agrimony and Yarrow in hot water for 15 minutes. Strain and serve warm.

Suggested Usage: Drink 1 cup up to twice daily to support intestinal health and relieve diarrhea.

Benefits: Agrimony and Yarrow are astringent herbs that tone the digestive tract, reduce inflammation, and firm up stools, making this tea highly effective for managing diarrhea and promoting overall gut health.

586. Chamomile and Fennel Gas-Reducing Tea

Ingredients: 1 tablespoon dried Chamomile flowers, 1 tablespoon Fennel seeds, 2 cups hot water.

Preparation: Steep Chamomile and Fennel in hot water for 15 minutes. Strain and serve warm.

Suggested Usage: Drink 1 cup after meals to reduce gas and bloating.

Benefits: Chamomile and Fennel are gentle carminative herbs that promote the expulsion of gas, relax the digestive tract, and reduce bloating, making this tea ideal for post-meal discomfort and digestive support.

587. Holy Basil and Lemon Balm Adaptogen Tea

Ingredients: 1 tablespoon dried Holy Basil leaves, 1 tablespoon dried Lemon Balm leaves, 2 cups hot water.
Preparation: Steep Holy Basil and Lemon Balm in hot water for 15 minutes. Strain and serve warm.
Suggested Usage: Drink 1-2 cups daily to reduce stress and support adrenal health.
Benefits: Holy Basil and Lemon Balm are adaptogenic herbs that help the body cope with stress, balance cortisol levels, and reduce the impact of stress on the digestive system, making this tea effective for stress-induced digestive issues.

588. Milk Thistle and Yellow Dock Detox Capsules

Ingredients: 1 tablespoon Milk Thistle seed powder, 1 tablespoon Yellow Dock Root powder, empty gel capsules.
Preparation: Mix Milk Thistle and Yellow Dock powders thoroughly. Fill empty gel capsules with the mixture and seal.
Suggested Usage: Take 1 capsule daily to support liver function and promote detoxification.
Benefits: Milk Thistle protects and regenerates liver cells, while Yellow Dock enhances bile flow and supports digestion, making these capsules effective for promoting liver health and supporting the body's natural detoxification processes.

589. Turmeric and Black Pepper Anti-Inflammatory Capsules

Ingredients: 1 tablespoon Turmeric powder, 1 teaspoon Black Pepper powder, empty gel capsules.
Preparation: Mix Turmeric and Black Pepper powders thoroughly. Fill empty gel capsules with the mixture and seal.
Suggested Usage: Take 1 capsule up to twice daily to reduce inflammation and support overall health.
Benefits: Turmeric's active compound, curcumin, has potent anti-inflammatory properties, while Black Pepper enhances its bioavailability, making these capsules effective for managing inflammation and supporting overall health.

590. Ginger, Cardamom, and Cinnamon Digestion-Stimulating Tea

Ingredients: 1 tablespoon grated fresh Ginger, 1 teaspoon crushed Cardamom pods, 1 cinnamon stick, 2 cups hot water.
Preparation: Steep Ginger, Cardamom, and Cinnamon in hot water for 15 minutes. Strain and serve warm.
Suggested Usage: Drink 1 cup before meals to stimulate digestion and reduce bloating.
Benefits: Ginger, Cardamom, and Cinnamon are warming spices that stimulate the production of digestive enzymes and enhance digestive fire, making this tea effective for improving digestion and relieving symptoms of indigestion and gas.

Book 26: Natural Remedies for Acid Reflux

Acid reflux, often referred to as heartburn, is a common condition characterized by the backflow of stomach acid into the esophagus, resulting in a burning sensation in the chest or throat. If left unmanaged, it can lead to more serious conditions such as gastroesophageal reflux disease (GERD) and damage to the esophageal lining. Fortunately, a variety of natural remedies and lifestyle adjustments can help manage and prevent acid reflux without relying on conventional medications, which may have undesirable side effects when used long-term.

Herbs to Alleviate Heartburn

Several herbs have been traditionally used to address the symptoms of acid reflux by reducing stomach acidity, soothing the esophagus, and promoting healthy digestion. Understanding which herbs to use and how to incorporate them can provide substantial relief for those suffering from occasional or chronic heartburn.

One of the most effective herbs for reducing acid reflux is Licorice Root. Deglycyrrhizinated Licorice (DGL), a form of Licorice Root with the compound glycyrrhizin removed, is particularly effective for promoting the healing of the esophagus and reducing inflammation without the risk of raising blood pressure. Licorice helps increase the mucous coating in the esophagus, protecting it from the harsh effects of stomach acid.

Marshmallow Root is another powerful herb that forms a mucilaginous coating over the esophageal lining. Its high mucilage content provides a protective barrier, which helps reduce irritation and promote healing. This makes Marshmallow Root an excellent choice for those dealing with frequent reflux episodes that lead to esophageal discomfort.

Slippery Elm is a classic remedy for acid reflux. Like Marshmallow Root, Slippery Elm is rich in mucilage, a gel-like substance that coats and soothes the esophagus. It helps neutralize excess stomach acid and creates a protective layer that prevents further irritation, making it effective for both immediate relief and long-term healing of the digestive tract.

Another useful herb for managing acid reflux is Chamomile. This gentle herb has anti-inflammatory and calming properties, making it ideal for reducing stress-related reflux. Chamomile not only helps soothe the digestive tract but also supports relaxation, which can be particularly beneficial for individuals whose acid reflux is triggered by stress or anxiety.

Ginger, while traditionally used as a digestive aid, is also beneficial for managing acid reflux. Its anti-inflammatory properties help reduce the irritation and inflammation in the

225

esophagus, while its ability to stimulate digestion ensures that food moves through the stomach more efficiently, reducing the chances of acid buildup and backflow.

For those seeking to balance stomach acid levels naturally, Meadowsweet can be helpful. Unlike conventional antacids that neutralize stomach acid entirely, Meadowsweet works by buffering and balancing acidity in the stomach, preventing excessive acid production without disrupting digestion.

Recipes for Soothing Elixirs

Creating herbal elixirs tailored to the management of acid reflux can provide both immediate relief and long-term support. Elixirs combine the power of medicinal herbs with soothing bases like honey or Aloe Vera to offer comprehensive relief from symptoms while promoting healing.

Licorice and Marshmallow Soothing Syrup is a powerful remedy that combines two of the most effective herbs for managing acid reflux. The syrup's mucilage-rich nature forms a protective coating over the esophagus, while Licorice reduces inflammation and supports healing. To make this syrup, combine 1 tablespoon each of Licorice Root and Marshmallow Root with 2 cups of water. Simmer for 20 minutes, strain, and add 1 cup of raw honey. Take 1 tablespoon as needed, especially before meals.

For immediate relief, Aloe Vera and Ginger Acid-Soothing Elixir is highly effective. Aloe Vera juice is known for its cooling and anti-inflammatory properties, while Ginger enhances digestion and reduces the likelihood of acid backflow. Mix ½ cup of Aloe Vera juice with 1 tablespoon of freshly grated Ginger and 1 teaspoon of raw honey. Take 2-3 tablespoons before meals or whenever heartburn occurs.

Another potent recipe is the Slippery Elm and Chamomile Digestive Drink. Combine 1 tablespoon of Slippery Elm powder, 1 tablespoon of dried Chamomile flowers, and 2 cups of hot water. Steep for 15 minutes, then strain and add 1 teaspoon of raw honey. Drink 1 cup before meals to coat the esophagus and prevent irritation from stomach acid.

For a versatile and tasty remedy, try the Ginger and Licorice Digestive Tonic. This tonic combines the anti-inflammatory effects of Ginger with the esophagus-soothing properties of Licorice. To prepare, simmer 1 tablespoon of Licorice Root and 1 tablespoon of sliced fresh Ginger in 3 cups of water for 15 minutes. Strain, let cool slightly, and add 1 teaspoon of raw honey. Take ½ cup up to twice daily for ongoing support.

Lifestyle Changes to Prevent Reflux

In addition to herbal remedies, lifestyle changes are essential for managing and preventing acid reflux. Implementing strategies such as modifying eating habits, avoiding certain foods, and managing stress can help reduce the frequency and severity of reflux episodes.

Eating smaller, more frequent meals is crucial. Large meals can overload the stomach and increase the chances of acid reflux. Opting for smaller, more frequent meals helps reduce pressure on the stomach and minimizes acid production, thereby preventing the backflow of acid into the esophagus.

Identifying and avoiding trigger foods is another key strategy. Common culprits like spicy foods, citrus fruits, chocolate, caffeine, and fatty or fried foods can exacerbate reflux. Eliminating these foods from your diet, or consuming them in moderation, can significantly reduce symptoms.

For those who experience reflux at night, elevating the head of the bed by 6-8 inches can prevent stomach acid from flowing back into the esophagus while sleeping. Gravity plays a crucial role in keeping stomach contents in place, so this simple adjustment can greatly improve nighttime symptoms.

Maintaining a healthy weight is also essential, as excess weight, especially around the abdomen, can increase pressure on the stomach and lead to acid reflux. Achieving and maintaining a healthy weight can significantly reduce the risk of reflux and its associated complications.

In addition, it's advisable to avoid lying down immediately after eating. Gravity helps keep food and stomach acid in place, so waiting at least 2-3 hours after eating before lying down allows for complete digestion and reduces the likelihood of reflux.

Lastly, incorporating stress management practices into daily life is crucial. Stress is a common trigger for acid reflux and can exacerbate symptoms. Engaging in activities such as yoga, meditation, deep breathing exercises, or simply spending time in nature can help reduce stress levels. Integrating herbal relaxation aids such as Chamomile tea, Lavender essential oil, or Holy Basil supplements can further support relaxation and reduce the frequency of stress-related reflux episodes.

Book 27: Herbal Support for Liver Health

The liver is one of the body's most vital organs, responsible for filtering toxins, metabolizing nutrients, and maintaining overall metabolic health. As the main detoxification organ, the liver plays a key role in breaking down and eliminating harmful substances that enter the body through food, air, and water. Maintaining optimal liver function is essential for overall wellness, as a healthy liver is crucial for efficient digestion, balanced hormones, and robust immune function. Supporting liver health naturally through herbs is a safe and effective way to promote detoxification, enhance energy levels, and protect the liver from damage caused by environmental toxins and dietary excesses.

Detoxifying Herbs for Liver Function

Certain herbs have a long-standing reputation for their ability to promote liver detoxification, enhance bile production, and support the regeneration of liver cells. Incorporating these herbs into a regular wellness routine can help maintain a healthy liver, protect it from damage, and support its detoxification capacity.

Milk Thistle is one of the most well-known and researched liver-supportive herbs. Its active compound, silymarin, is a powerful antioxidant that helps protect liver cells from toxins and promotes the regeneration of damaged cells. Silymarin stabilizes cell membranes and supports the liver's ability to produce glutathione, a vital compound for detoxification. Milk Thistle is particularly effective for those with compromised liver function or those exposed to high levels of environmental toxins.

Dandelion Root is another potent herb for liver health. It stimulates bile production, which is necessary for digesting fats and removing waste products from the liver. Dandelion Root acts as a gentle diuretic, helping to flush toxins through the kidneys while also enhancing liver function. Its rich content of vitamins and minerals makes it a nourishing addition to any liver support regimen.

Burdock Root is traditionally used to cleanse the blood and support liver function. It contains inulin, a prebiotic fiber that helps nourish beneficial gut bacteria, and antioxidants that neutralize free radicals. Burdock Root is often combined with other liver-supportive herbs in detox blends because of its ability to promote healthy digestion, support liver detoxification, and clear skin conditions linked to liver health.

Artichoke Leaf, like Dandelion, is a powerful liver tonic that promotes bile flow, supporting the liver's role in breaking down fats and removing toxins. Its high antioxidant content helps protect liver cells from damage, making it a valuable herb for maintaining liver health and preventing oxidative stress.

Turmeric, with its active compound curcumin, is renowned for its potent anti-inflammatory and antioxidant properties. Curcumin has been shown to protect the liver from damage, reduce inflammation, and support the regeneration of liver cells. Turmeric's ability to enhance bile production and flow also makes it an excellent herb for improving digestion and supporting the liver's detoxification processes.

Schisandra Berry is an adaptogenic herb that has been used for centuries in Traditional Chinese Medicine to support liver health. Schisandra enhances liver detoxification pathways, improves the body's stress response, and promotes the regeneration of liver cells. Its high content of lignans and antioxidants makes Schisandra particularly effective for protecting the liver from toxins and enhancing overall resilience.

Other beneficial herbs for liver health include Yellow Dock Root, which stimulates bile production and promotes digestion, and Licorice Root, which has anti-inflammatory and hepatoprotective properties, making it useful for supporting the liver in times of stress or exposure to harmful substances.

Recipes for Liver-Boosting Tonics

Creating herbal liver tonics is a wonderful way to incorporate these powerful herbs into daily routines. Tonics can be enjoyed as part of a morning ritual or taken throughout the day to support ongoing detoxification and liver function.

One of the simplest and most effective tonics is the **Dandelion and Milk Thistle Liver Detox Tea**. To prepare, combine 1 tablespoon each of dried Dandelion Root and Milk Thistle seeds with 3 cups of water. Simmer gently for 20 minutes, then strain. This tea can be enjoyed up to twice daily to promote liver function and enhance detoxification. The combination of Dandelion and Milk Thistle helps stimulate bile production, supports liver cell regeneration, and promotes the elimination of toxins.

For those looking for a more comprehensive liver-supporting blend, the **Burdock and Artichoke Liver Tonic** is ideal. To prepare, combine 1 tablespoon each of dried Burdock Root and Artichoke Leaf with 2 cups of water. Simmer gently for 15 minutes, then strain. This tonic can be taken ½ cup at a time, up to twice daily, to support digestion, promote healthy liver function, and clear toxins. Burdock and Artichoke work synergistically to stimulate bile flow, cleanse the blood, and protect the liver from oxidative stress.

A powerful anti-inflammatory liver tonic is the **Turmeric and Ginger Golden Milk**. Combine 1 cup of unsweetened almond milk, 1 teaspoon of Turmeric powder, ½ teaspoon of Ginger powder, and a pinch of black pepper. Heat gently on the stove until warm, then add 1 teaspoon of raw honey if desired. Drink this golden milk in the evening to reduce liver inflammation, enhance detoxification, and support restful sleep. The addition of black pepper enhances the bioavailability of curcumin in Turmeric, making it a more potent liver-protective remedy.

For those who prefer a refreshing cold tonic, the **Schisandra and Lemon Detox Elixir** is an excellent choice. Steep 1 tablespoon of dried Schisandra Berries in 2 cups of hot water for 20 minutes. Strain and let cool, then add the juice of one lemon and a teaspoon of raw honey. This tonic can be consumed over ice throughout the day to promote liver health, reduce oxidative stress, and support energy levels.

Another easy-to-make remedy is the **Liver Cleanse Smoothie**. Blend 1 cup of chopped dandelion greens, 1 small beet, ½ cup of frozen berries, 1 tablespoon of freshly grated ginger, and 1 cup of coconut water. This vibrant smoothie can be consumed in the morning to kickstart liver detoxification and promote healthy bile flow. Beets are particularly beneficial for liver health due to their high content of betaine, which supports the detoxification of harmful substances and promotes healthy liver function.

Finally, consider the **Yellow Dock and Licorice Liver Support Elixir**. Combine 1 tablespoon each of Yellow Dock Root and Licorice Root with 3 cups of water. Simmer for 15 minutes, strain, and add 1 teaspoon of raw honey. This tonic can be taken 1-2 times daily to reduce inflammation, support bile production, and protect the liver from damage.

By integrating these herbal remedies and tonics into daily routines, individuals can support liver health naturally, enhance detoxification, and maintain optimal wellness. Regular use of liver-supportive herbs can protect the liver from the damaging effects of environmental toxins, promote the regeneration of healthy cells, and ensure the efficient elimination of waste products, making them an essential component of a holistic health regimen.

Remedies for Liver Health

591. Milk Thistle and Dandelion Liver Detox Tea

Ingredients: 1 tablespoon Milk Thistle seeds, 1 tablespoon dried Dandelion Root, 3 cups water.
Preparation: Simmer Milk Thistle seeds and Dandelion Root in water for 20 minutes. Strain and serve warm.
Suggested Usage: Drink 1 cup daily to support liver detoxification and promote overall liver health.

Benefits: Milk Thistle protects liver cells and supports their regeneration, while Dandelion stimulates bile production and aids in flushing toxins, making this tea ideal for liver detoxification.

592. Burdock Root and Yellow Dock Liver Cleanse Capsules

Ingredients: 1 tablespoon Burdock Root powder, 1 tablespoon Yellow Dock Root powder, empty gel capsules.

Preparation: Mix Burdock Root and Yellow Dock powders thoroughly. Fill empty capsules with the mixture and seal.

Suggested Usage: Take 1 capsule up to twice daily to support liver health and promote detoxification.

Benefits: Burdock Root and Yellow Dock stimulate bile production and support the elimination of waste products, making these capsules effective for enhancing liver function and maintaining healthy digestion.

593. Schisandra and Lemon Detox Elixir

Ingredients: 1 tablespoon dried Schisandra Berries, 2 cups hot water, juice of 1 lemon, 1 teaspoon raw honey.

Preparation: Steep Schisandra Berries in hot water for 20 minutes. Strain and add lemon juice and honey. Serve warm or over ice.

Suggested Usage: Drink 1 cup up to twice daily to support liver health and enhance detoxification.

Benefits: Schisandra Berries protect liver cells, enhance liver detoxification pathways, and improve energy levels, while lemon provides vitamin C and additional antioxidant support.

594. Turmeric and Ginger Golden Milk

Ingredients: 1 cup unsweetened almond milk, 1 teaspoon Turmeric powder, ½ teaspoon grated fresh Ginger, a pinch of black pepper, 1 teaspoon raw honey (optional).

Preparation: Warm the almond milk on the stove, then add Turmeric, Ginger, and black pepper. Stir until fully dissolved and remove from heat. Add honey if desired.

Suggested Usage: Drink 1 cup in the evening to reduce liver inflammation and promote detoxification.

Benefits: Turmeric's curcumin and Ginger's gingerol have powerful anti-inflammatory properties, making this drink effective for reducing liver inflammation and promoting overall liver health.

595. Dandelion Root and Artichoke Liver Tonic

Ingredients: 1 tablespoon dried Dandelion Root, 1 tablespoon dried Artichoke Leaf, 2 cups water.

Preparation: Simmer Dandelion Root and Artichoke Leaf in water for 20 minutes. Strain and serve warm.

Suggested Usage: Drink 1 cup daily to promote liver function and support digestion.

Benefits: Dandelion Root enhances bile production and supports detoxification, while Artichoke Leaf protects liver cells and stimulates digestion, making this tonic effective for maintaining a healthy liver.

596. Licorice Root and Ginger Liver Support Capsules

Ingredients: 1 tablespoon Licorice Root powder, 1 tablespoon Ginger powder, empty gel capsules.

Preparation: Mix Licorice Root and Ginger powders thoroughly. Fill empty gel capsules with the mixture and seal.

Suggested Usage: Take 1 capsule up to twice daily to reduce liver inflammation and support liver health.

Benefits: Licorice Root has anti-inflammatory properties and helps protect the liver from toxins, while Ginger stimulates digestion and enhances the absorption of nutrients.

597. Reishi and Schisandra Liver Protective Tincture

Ingredients: 1 tablespoon dried Reishi Mushroom, 1 tablespoon dried Schisandra Berries, 1 cup vodka or brandy (for tincture base).
Preparation: Combine Reishi and Schisandra with alcohol in a glass jar. Seal tightly and let steep for 4-6 weeks, shaking occasionally. Strain and store in a dark glass bottle.
Suggested Usage: Take ½ teaspoon up to twice daily to protect the liver and enhance resilience.
Benefits: Reishi and Schisandra are adaptogenic herbs that support liver function, enhance detoxification, and protect the liver from damage caused by environmental toxins.

598. Holy Basil and Milk Thistle Stress-Reducing Liver Capsules

Ingredients: 1 tablespoon Holy Basil powder, 1 tablespoon Milk Thistle seed powder, empty gel capsules.
Preparation: Mix Holy Basil and Milk Thistle powders thoroughly. Fill empty gel capsules with the mixture and seal.
Suggested Usage: Take 1 capsule daily to reduce stress and support liver health.
Benefits: Holy Basil helps balance cortisol levels and reduce the impact of stress on the liver, while Milk Thistle

supports liver regeneration and protects against toxins.

599. Beetroot and Ginger Liver Cleansing Smoothie

Ingredients: 1 small beet, 1 tablespoon grated fresh Ginger, 1 cup chopped dandelion greens, ½ cup frozen berries, 1 cup coconut water.
Preparation: Blend all ingredients until smooth. Serve immediately.
Suggested Usage: Drink in the morning to support liver detoxification and enhance bile flow.
Benefits: Beets are rich in betaine, which supports liver detoxification, while Ginger stimulates digestion, making this smoothie effective for promoting a healthy liver and digestive system.

600. Chicory Root and Peppermint Liver Support Tea

Ingredients: 1 tablespoon dried Chicory Root, 1 tablespoon dried Peppermint leaves, 2 cups hot water.
Preparation: Steep Chicory Root and Peppermint in hot water for 15 minutes. Strain and serve warm.
Suggested Usage: Drink 1 cup daily to support liver function and promote digestion.
Benefits: Chicory Root stimulates bile production and supports liver detoxification, while Peppermint soothes the digestive tract, making this tea ideal for maintaining liver and gut health.

601. Yellow Dock and Burdock Root Liver Health Tonic

Ingredients: 1 tablespoon dried Yellow Dock Root, 1 tablespoon dried Burdock Root, 4 cups water.

Preparation: Simmer Yellow Dock and Burdock Root in water for 30 minutes. Strain and serve warm.

Suggested Usage: Drink 1 cup daily to support liver detoxification and improve overall liver health.

Benefits: Yellow Dock and Burdock are powerful blood-purifying herbs that enhance liver function and support the elimination of toxins, making this tonic ideal for promoting liver health.

602. Artichoke Leaf and Rosemary Digestive Liver Tea

Ingredients: 1 tablespoon dried Artichoke Leaf, 1 tablespoon dried Rosemary, 2 cups hot water.

Preparation: Steep Artichoke Leaf and Rosemary in hot water for 15 minutes. Strain and serve warm.

Suggested Usage: Drink 1 cup before meals to stimulate digestion and support liver function.

Benefits: Artichoke Leaf promotes bile production and protects liver cells, while Rosemary enhances circulation and digestion, making this tea effective for improving both liver and digestive health.

603. Fennel and Dandelion Gut and Liver Support Tea

Ingredients: 1 tablespoon dried Fennel seeds, 1 tablespoon dried Dandelion Root, 2 cups hot water.

Preparation: Steep Fennel and Dandelion in hot water for 15 minutes. Strain and serve warm.

Suggested Usage: Drink 1 cup up to twice daily to support digestion and liver health.

Benefits: Fennel reduces gas and bloating, while Dandelion supports liver detoxification, making this tea ideal for promoting healthy digestion and a strong liver.

604. Turmeric and Black Pepper Anti-Inflammatory Capsules

Ingredients: 1 tablespoon Turmeric powder, 1 teaspoon Black Pepper powder, empty gel capsules.

Preparation: Mix Turmeric and Black Pepper powders thoroughly. Fill empty gel capsules with the mixture and seal.

Suggested Usage: Take 1 capsule up to twice daily to reduce inflammation and support liver health.

Benefits: Turmeric's curcumin has powerful anti-inflammatory properties, while Black Pepper enhances its bioavailability, making these capsules effective for managing liver inflammation and supporting overall liver health.

605. Triphala Liver Tonic Capsules

Ingredients: 1 tablespoon Triphala powder, empty gel capsules.

Preparation: Fill empty gel capsules with Triphala powder and seal.

Suggested Usage: Take 1 capsule up to twice daily to support liver detoxification and promote healthy digestion.

Benefits: Triphala is a traditional Ayurvedic blend that supports liver function, promotes regular bowel movements, and aids in detoxification, making it a valuable addition to any liver health regimen.

606. Nettle and Dandelion Mineral-Rich Liver Tonic

Ingredients: 1 tablespoon dried Nettle leaves, 1 tablespoon dried Dandelion Root, 2 cups hot water.
Preparation: Steep Nettle and Dandelion Root in hot water for 15 minutes. Strain and serve warm.
Suggested Usage: Drink 1 cup up to twice daily to nourish the liver and support detoxification.
Benefits: Nettle and Dandelion are rich in vitamins and minerals, promoting healthy liver function and supporting the body's detoxification pathways.

607. Reishi and Licorice Adaptogenic Liver Support Capsules

Ingredients: 1 tablespoon Reishi Mushroom powder, 1 tablespoon Licorice Root powder, empty gel capsules.
Preparation: Mix Reishi and Licorice powders thoroughly. Fill empty gel capsules with the mixture and seal.
Suggested Usage: Take 1 capsule up to twice daily to reduce liver stress and enhance resilience.
Benefits: Reishi and Licorice are adaptogens that support liver health, reduce stress, and promote liver cell regeneration, making these capsules ideal for comprehensive liver support.

608. Calendula and Dandelion Gut and Liver Tonic

Ingredients: 1 tablespoon dried Calendula flowers, 1 tablespoon dried Dandelion Root, 2 cups hot water.
Preparation: Steep Calendula and Dandelion Root in hot water for 15 minutes. Strain and serve warm.
Suggested Usage: Drink 1 cup daily to support liver detoxification and promote gut health.
Benefits: Calendula is a gentle anti-inflammatory herb that promotes gut and liver health, while Dandelion supports detoxification and bile flow, making this tonic effective for comprehensive digestive and liver support.

609. Ashwagandha and Schisandra Stress-Relief Liver Tincture

Ingredients: 1 tablespoon Ashwagandha Root, 1 tablespoon Schisandra Berries, 1 cup vodka or brandy.
Preparation: Combine Ashwagandha and Schisandra with alcohol in a glass jar. Seal tightly and let steep for 4-6 weeks, shaking occasionally. Strain and store in a dark glass bottle.
Suggested Usage: Take ½ teaspoon daily to reduce liver stress and support overall resilience.
Benefits: Ashwagandha and Schisandra are adaptogenic herbs that enhance the body's resistance to stress and support healthy liver function, making this tincture ideal for managing stress-related liver conditions.

610. Turmeric and Dandelion Detoxification Tea

Ingredients: 1 tablespoon grated fresh Turmeric, 1 tablespoon dried Dandelion

Root, 2 cups hot water.

Preparation: Steep Turmeric and Dandelion in hot water for 15 minutes. Strain and serve warm.

Suggested Usage: Drink 1 cup up to twice daily to reduce inflammation and support liver detoxification.

Benefits: Turmeric's curcumin reduces inflammation, while Dandelion stimulates bile production and enhances detoxification, making this tea highly effective for maintaining liver health.

611. Milk Thistle and Burdock Root Detox Capsules

Ingredients: 1 tablespoon Milk Thistle seed powder, 1 tablespoon Burdock Root powder, empty gel capsules.

Preparation: Mix Milk Thistle and Burdock powders thoroughly. Fill empty gel capsules with the mixture and seal.

Suggested Usage: Take 1 capsule up to twice daily to promote liver detoxification.

Benefits: Milk Thistle protects liver cells and supports regeneration, while Burdock Root cleanses the blood and enhances liver function, making these capsules ideal for supporting liver health.

612. Schisandra and Lemon Peel Liver Vitality Tea

Ingredients: 1 tablespoon dried Schisandra Berries, 1 teaspoon dried Lemon Peel, 2 cups hot water.

Preparation: Steep Schisandra Berries and Lemon Peel in hot water for 20 minutes. Strain and serve warm.

Suggested Usage: Drink 1 cup daily to enhance liver vitality and support detoxification.

Benefits: Schisandra is a potent liver tonic that enhances liver detoxification, while Lemon Peel adds a boost of vitamin C and antioxidants, making this tea ideal for promoting overall liver health.

613. Yellow Dock and Artichoke Leaf Liver Bitter Capsules

Ingredients: 1 tablespoon Yellow Dock Root powder, 1 tablespoon Artichoke Leaf powder, empty gel capsules.

Preparation: Mix Yellow Dock and Artichoke Leaf powders thoroughly. Fill empty gel capsules with the mixture and seal.

Suggested Usage: Take 1 capsule before meals to stimulate digestion and support liver function.

Benefits: Yellow Dock and Artichoke Leaf are powerful bitter herbs that stimulate bile production, enhance digestion, and support detoxification, making these capsules effective for maintaining healthy liver and digestive function.

614. Rosemary and Lemon Liver Cleansing Tea

Ingredients: 1 tablespoon dried Rosemary, zest of 1 lemon, 2 cups hot water.

Preparation: Steep Rosemary and Lemon zest in hot water for 15 minutes. Strain and serve warm.

Suggested Usage: Drink 1 cup daily to support liver health and improve circulation.

Benefits: Rosemary enhances circulation and stimulates digestion, while Lemon provides antioxidants that protect liver cells, making this tea ideal for cleansing the liver and promoting overall vitality.

615. Nettle and Calendula Liver Support Infusion

Ingredients: 1 tablespoon dried Nettle leaves, 1 tablespoon dried Calendula flowers, 2 cups hot water.
Preparation: Steep Nettle and Calendula in hot water for 15 minutes. Strain and serve warm.
Suggested Usage: Drink 1 cup daily to nourish the liver and support detoxification.
Benefits: Nettle is rich in minerals that support liver health, while Calendula reduces inflammation and promotes healing, making this infusion effective for supporting both the liver and overall well-being.

616. Holy Basil and Gotu Kola Liver Adaptogen Capsules

Ingredients: 1 tablespoon Holy Basil powder, 1 tablespoon Gotu Kola powder, empty gel capsules.
Preparation: Mix Holy Basil and Gotu Kola powders thoroughly. Fill empty gel capsules with the mixture and seal.
Suggested Usage: Take 1 capsule daily to reduce liver stress and enhance resilience.
Benefits: Holy Basil and Gotu Kola are adaptogens that help the liver cope with stress, reduce inflammation, and support liver cell regeneration, making these capsules effective for comprehensive liver health.

617. Dandelion and Ginger Liver Stimulating Tonic

Ingredients: 1 tablespoon dried Dandelion Root, 1 tablespoon grated fresh Ginger, 2 cups water.
Preparation: Simmer Dandelion and Ginger in water for 15 minutes. Strain and serve warm.
Suggested Usage: Drink 1 cup before meals to stimulate digestion and promote liver function.
Benefits: Dandelion enhances bile production and detoxification, while Ginger stimulates digestion and reduces inflammation, making this tonic effective for enhancing liver function and promoting overall health.

618. Lemon Balm and Peppermint Liver Soothing Tea

Ingredients: 1 tablespoon dried Lemon Balm leaves, 1 tablespoon dried Peppermint leaves, 2 cups hot water.
Preparation: Steep Lemon Balm and Peppermint in hot water for 15 minutes. Strain and serve warm.
Suggested Usage: Drink 1 cup up to twice daily to soothe the liver and promote digestion.
Benefits: Lemon Balm and Peppermint are gentle herbs that calm the digestive tract, reduce stress, and support liver health, making this tea ideal for managing digestive discomfort and promoting relaxation.

619. Licorice Root and Turmeric Anti-Inflammatory Liver Capsules

Ingredients: 1 tablespoon Licorice Root powder, 1 tablespoon Turmeric powder, empty gel capsules.
Preparation: Mix Licorice Root and Turmeric powders thoroughly. Fill empty gel capsules with the mixture and seal.
Suggested Usage: Take 1 capsule up to twice daily to reduce liver inflammation and support detoxification.
Benefits: Licorice Root and Turmeric are anti-inflammatory herbs that protect liver cells from damage and promote healing, making these capsules effective for reducing inflammation and enhancing liver health.

620. Burdock Root and Artichoke Liver Cleanse Elixir

Ingredients: 1 tablespoon dried Burdock Root, 1 tablespoon dried Artichoke Leaf, 3 cups water.
Preparation: Simmer Burdock Root and Artichoke Leaf in water for 30 minutes. Strain and let cool.
Suggested Usage: Drink ½ cup up to twice daily to support liver detoxification and enhance digestion.
Benefits: Burdock and Artichoke support bile production, cleanse the blood, and promote detoxification, making this elixir ideal for comprehensive liver health support.

621. Turmeric and Reishi Mushroom Liver Support Tincture

Ingredients: 1 tablespoon dried Reishi Mushroom, 1 tablespoon Turmeric Root, 1 cup vodka or brandy (for tincture base).
Preparation: Combine Reishi and Turmeric with alcohol in a glass jar. Seal tightly and let steep for 4-6 weeks, shaking occasionally. Strain and store in a dark glass bottle.
Suggested Usage: Take ½ teaspoon up to twice daily to support liver health and promote resilience.
Benefits: Reishi and Turmeric have strong anti-inflammatory and hepatoprotective properties, making this tincture highly effective for supporting liver function and protecting the liver from damage.

622. Ashwagandha and Holy Basil Liver Detox Capsules

Ingredients: 1 tablespoon Ashwagandha Root powder, 1 tablespoon Holy Basil powder, empty gel capsules.
Preparation: Mix Ashwagandha and Holy Basil powders thoroughly. Fill empty gel capsules with the mixture and seal.
Suggested Usage: Take 1 capsule daily to support liver detoxification and reduce stress.
Benefits: Ashwagandha and Holy Basil are adaptogenic herbs that reduce the impact of stress on the liver, enhance liver detoxification, and promote overall health and well-being.

623. Dandelion and Schisandra Immune-Supporting Liver Tea

Ingredients: 1 tablespoon dried Dandelion Root, 1 tablespoon dried Schisandra Berries, 2 cups hot water.
Preparation: Steep Dandelion and Schisandra in hot water for 20 minutes. Strain and serve warm.
Suggested Usage: Drink 1 cup daily to support liver health and boost the immune

system.

Benefits: Dandelion supports liver detoxification, while Schisandra enhances liver function and provides immune support, making this tea ideal for promoting overall health and vitality.

624. Turmeric and Yellow Dock Blood Cleanse Capsules

Ingredients: 1 tablespoon Turmeric powder, 1 tablespoon Yellow Dock Root powder, empty gel capsules.
Preparation: Mix Turmeric and Yellow Dock powders thoroughly. Fill empty gel capsules with the mixture and seal.
Suggested Usage: Take 1 capsule up to twice daily to promote liver function and support blood detoxification.
Benefits: Turmeric and Yellow Dock cleanse the blood, reduce inflammation, and support liver detoxification, making these capsules effective for enhancing liver health and promoting overall detoxification.

625. Ginger, Lemon, and Beetroot Liver Cleansing Juice

Ingredients: 1 small beet, 1 tablespoon grated fresh Ginger, juice of 1 lemon, 1 cup water.
Preparation: Blend all ingredients until smooth. Serve immediately.
Suggested Usage: Drink in the morning to support liver detoxification and promote bile flow.
Benefits: Beets are rich in betaine, which supports liver detoxification, while Ginger and Lemon enhance digestion and reduce inflammation, making this juice effective for maintaining liver health.

626. Reishi Mushroom and Licorice Liver Protective Elixir

Ingredients: 1 tablespoon dried Reishi Mushroom, 1 tablespoon Licorice Root, 3 cups water.
Preparation: Simmer Reishi and Licorice Root in water for 30 minutes. Strain and serve warm.
Suggested Usage: Drink 1 cup daily to reduce liver inflammation and support overall health.
Benefits: Reishi and Licorice are adaptogens that protect the liver, reduce inflammation, and promote healing, making this elixir ideal for protecting the liver from stress and environmental toxins.

627. Schisandra and Ashwagandha Adaptogen Liver Tonic

Ingredients: 1 tablespoon Schisandra Berries, 1 tablespoon Ashwagandha Root, 2 cups hot water.
Preparation: Steep Schisandra and Ashwagandha in hot water for 20 minutes. Strain and serve warm.
Suggested Usage: Drink 1 cup daily to reduce liver stress and enhance detoxification.
Benefits: Schisandra and Ashwagandha support the liver's ability to cope with stress, enhance detoxification, and promote overall health, making this tonic ideal for maintaining a healthy liver.

628. Burdock Root and Licorice Immune-Supporting Liver Tea

Ingredients: 1 tablespoon dried Burdock Root, 1 tablespoon Licorice Root, 2 cups hot water.
Preparation: Simmer Burdock and Licorice in water for 20 minutes. Strain and serve warm.
Suggested Usage: Drink 1 cup daily to support liver function and boost immunity.
Benefits: Burdock and Licorice cleanse the blood, enhance liver function, and support the immune system, making this tea ideal for promoting both liver health and overall immunity.

629. Triphala and Schisandra Liver Health Capsules

Ingredients: 1 tablespoon Triphala powder, 1 tablespoon Schisandra Berry powder, empty gel capsules.
Preparation: Mix Triphala and Schisandra powders thoroughly. Fill empty gel capsules with the mixture and seal.
Suggested Usage: Take 1 capsule up to twice daily to support liver detoxification and promote liver health.
Benefits: Triphala and Schisandra support the liver's detoxification pathways, promote the regeneration of liver cells, and protect the liver from damage, making these capsules ideal for comprehensive liver health.

630. Milk Thistle and Schisandra Berry Liver Support Tincture

Ingredients: 1 tablespoon Milk Thistle seeds, 1 tablespoon Schisandra Berries, 1 cup vodka or brandy.
Preparation: Combine Milk Thistle and

Schisandra with alcohol in a glass jar. Seal tightly and let steep for 4-6 weeks, shaking occasionally. Strain and store in a dark glass bottle.
Suggested Usage: Take ½ teaspoon up to twice daily to protect liver cells and enhance detoxification.
Benefits: Milk Thistle and Schisandra are potent hepatoprotective herbs that support liver regeneration and detoxification, making this tincture highly effective for promoting liver health.

631. Turmeric and Holy Basil Liver-Protecting Tea

Ingredients: 1 tablespoon grated fresh Turmeric, 1 tablespoon dried Holy Basil, 2 cups hot water.
Preparation: Steep Turmeric and Holy Basil in hot water for 15 minutes. Strain and serve warm.
Suggested Usage: Drink 1 cup daily to reduce liver inflammation and support detoxification.
Benefits: Turmeric and Holy Basil are powerful anti-inflammatory herbs that protect the liver from oxidative stress and promote liver regeneration, making this tea effective for maintaining liver health and resilience.

632. Dandelion and Fennel Digestive Liver Tea

Ingredients: 1 tablespoon dried Dandelion Root, 1 tablespoon Fennel seeds, 2 cups hot water.
Preparation: Steep Dandelion Root and Fennel in hot water for 15 minutes. Strain and serve warm.
Suggested Usage: Drink 1 cup up to twice

daily to support liver health and improve digestion.

Benefits: Dandelion enhances bile production, which promotes liver detoxification and healthy digestion, while Fennel reduces gas and bloating, making this tea ideal for supporting overall liver and digestive function.

633. Calendula and Nettle Liver Restorative Infusion

Ingredients: 1 tablespoon dried Calendula flowers, 1 tablespoon dried Nettle leaves, 3 cups hot water.
Preparation: Steep Calendula and Nettle in hot water for 20 minutes. Strain and serve warm.
Suggested Usage: Drink 1 cup daily to nourish the liver and promote healing.
Benefits: Calendula has gentle anti-inflammatory properties that promote healing and reduce irritation, while Nettle is rich in minerals that support liver function and overall wellness, making this infusion effective for comprehensive liver support.

634. Lemon Balm and Licorice Root Liver Balancing Tea

Ingredients: 1 tablespoon dried Lemon Balm leaves, 1 tablespoon dried Licorice Root, 2 cups hot water.
Preparation: Steep Lemon Balm and Licorice Root in hot water for 15 minutes. Strain and serve warm.
Suggested Usage: Drink 1 cup up to twice daily to reduce liver inflammation and promote balance.
Benefits: Lemon Balm helps calm the nervous system and reduce stress, while

Licorice Root supports liver health and protects against inflammation, making this tea ideal for managing stress-related liver issues.

635. Schisandra Berry and Milk Thistle Liver Antioxidant Capsules

Ingredients: 1 tablespoon Schisandra Berry powder, 1 tablespoon Milk Thistle seed powder, empty gel capsules.
Preparation: Mix Schisandra and Milk Thistle powders thoroughly. Fill empty gel capsules with the mixture and seal.
Suggested Usage: Take 1 capsule daily to protect liver cells and enhance detoxification.
Benefits: Schisandra and Milk Thistle are powerful antioxidants that support liver cell regeneration and promote detoxification, making these capsules ideal for long-term liver support.

636. Gotu Kola and Reishi Mushroom Liver Tonic Tea

Ingredients: 1 tablespoon dried Gotu Kola leaves, 1 tablespoon dried Reishi Mushroom, 2 cups hot water.
Preparation: Steep Gotu Kola and Reishi in hot water for 15 minutes. Strain and serve warm.
Suggested Usage: Drink 1 cup daily to reduce liver stress and promote healing.
Benefits: Gotu Kola and Reishi are adaptogenic herbs that support liver health, promote the regeneration of liver cells, and enhance resilience, making this tea ideal for maintaining liver health and vitality.

637. Dandelion and Ashwagandha Hormone-Balancing Liver Capsules

Ingredients: 1 tablespoon Dandelion Root powder, 1 tablespoon Ashwagandha Root powder, empty gel capsules.
Preparation: Mix Dandelion and Ashwagandha powders thoroughly. Fill empty gel capsules with the mixture and seal.
Suggested Usage: Take 1 capsule daily to support liver detoxification and balance hormones.
Benefits: Dandelion supports liver function and hormone metabolism, while Ashwagandha helps balance cortisol levels, making these capsules effective for maintaining a healthy liver and balanced hormones.

638. Burdock and Calendula Liver Regeneration Tea

Ingredients: 1 tablespoon dried Burdock Root, 1 tablespoon dried Calendula flowers, 2 cups hot water.
Preparation: Steep Burdock Root and Calendula in hot water for 15 minutes. Strain and serve warm.
Suggested Usage: Drink 1 cup daily to promote liver regeneration and support overall liver health.
Benefits: Burdock Root is a blood purifier that supports liver detoxification, while Calendula reduces inflammation and promotes healing, making this tea ideal for supporting liver regeneration and overall health.

639. Yellow Dock and Holy Basil Liver Detox Capsules

Ingredients: 1 tablespoon Yellow Dock Root powder, 1 tablespoon Holy Basil powder, empty gel capsules.
Preparation: Mix Yellow Dock and Holy Basil powders thoroughly. Fill empty gel capsules with the mixture and seal.
Suggested Usage: Take 1 capsule up to twice daily to enhance liver detoxification and reduce stress.
Benefits: Yellow Dock supports bile production and promotes detoxification, while Holy Basil helps the liver cope with stress, making these capsules effective for comprehensive liver support.

640. Reishi Mushroom and Nettle Liver Health Tea

Ingredients: 1 tablespoon dried Reishi Mushroom, 1 tablespoon dried Nettle leaves, 3 cups hot water.
Preparation: Steep Reishi and Nettle in hot water for 20 minutes. Strain and serve warm.
Suggested Usage: Drink 1 cup daily to reduce liver inflammation and support detoxification.
Benefits: Reishi reduces liver inflammation and supports resilience, while Nettle provides essential minerals that promote liver function, making this tea ideal for maintaining a healthy liver and promoting overall well-being.

Book 28: Probiotics and Fermented Foods

Probiotics, often referred to as "good bacteria," are essential microorganisms that play a critical role in maintaining a balanced and healthy digestive system. These beneficial bacteria reside primarily in the gut and are responsible for supporting digestion, enhancing nutrient absorption, strengthening the immune system, and protecting against harmful pathogens. Understanding the role of probiotics and incorporating them into daily health routines can be transformative for digestive wellness and overall health. In recent years, the incorporation of herbal medicine into probiotic and fermented food practices has gained popularity, as the combination of herbs and probiotics can amplify the health benefits of both. This chapter explores the relationship between probiotics and herbal medicine, provides recipes for herbal-infused fermented foods, and explains how fermentation can enhance digestive health.

Understanding Probiotics in Herbal Medicine

Probiotics are live microorganisms that, when taken in adequate amounts, confer a health benefit on the host. The most common probiotic strains belong to the Lactobacillus and Bifidobacterium families, both of which are found naturally in the human digestive tract and play an essential role in maintaining the delicate balance of the gut microbiome. When this balance is disrupted by factors such as poor diet, stress, or antibiotics, it can lead to digestive disorders, weakened immunity, and increased susceptibility to infections. This is where probiotics step in, helping to restore the balance of the gut microbiota and promote overall digestive health.

Herbs play a complementary role in supporting probiotic health and ensuring that these beneficial microorganisms thrive in the digestive tract. Prebiotics, a type of fiber found in certain herbs, serve as food for probiotics and are necessary for their growth and activity. Chicory Root, Dandelion Root, and Burdock Root are excellent sources of prebiotic fibers such as inulin, which nourish and sustain healthy gut bacteria. Consuming these herbs alongside probiotics enhances the survival and colonization of beneficial bacteria in the gut.

Additionally, certain herbs like Chamomile, Fennel, and Licorice Root have been shown to support a healthy digestive environment by reducing inflammation, protecting the mucosal lining of the gut, and preventing the overgrowth of harmful bacteria. The combination of herbs and probiotics offers a synergistic effect, where the herbs create a favorable environment for probiotics, and the probiotics enhance the herbs' ability to support digestion and immunity.

One of the most powerful ways to incorporate both herbs and probiotics into a diet is through fermentation. Fermentation is a natural process in which bacteria, yeast, or other microorganisms break down sugars and starches in food, producing beneficial compounds such as lactic acid, enzymes, and vitamins. This process not only preserves food but also increases its nutritional value and makes it easier to digest. When herbs are included in fermented foods, they infuse these probiotic-rich foods with their own unique health benefits, creating potent functional foods that nourish the body on multiple levels.

Recipes for Fermented Herbal Foods

Creating fermented herbal foods at home is a wonderful way to support digestive health while enjoying delicious, nutrient-dense dishes. Many traditional fermented foods like sauerkraut, kimchi, and yogurt can be elevated with the addition of medicinal herbs, enhancing their flavor and therapeutic properties. Herbal-infused ferments can provide targeted support for digestive disorders, boost immunity, and promote a healthy gut microbiome.

One simple recipe is **Herbal Sauerkraut with Dill and Garlic**. To make this, shred one medium head of cabbage and mix it with 2 tablespoons of sea salt. Add 1 tablespoon of dried Dill, 3 cloves of minced garlic, and 1 tablespoon of dried Chamomile flowers. Pack the mixture tightly into a jar, ensuring that the cabbage is submerged in its own brine. Cover with a lid and let ferment at room temperature for 1-2 weeks, then store in the refrigerator. Dill and Chamomile have calming properties that support digestion and reduce bloating, while garlic offers antimicrobial benefits that prevent the growth of harmful bacteria.

Another probiotic-rich recipe is **Fermented Carrots with Ginger and Turmeric**. Slice 4 large carrots into sticks and place them in a jar. Add 1 tablespoon of grated fresh Ginger, 1 teaspoon of grated fresh Turmeric, and 1 teaspoon of sea salt. Fill the jar with filtered water, ensuring that the carrots are completely submerged. Cover with a lid and let ferment for 5-7 days. Turmeric and Ginger support liver function, reduce inflammation, and enhance the body's natural detoxification pathways, making this a delicious and therapeutic addition to meals.

For those looking to make a probiotic beverage, **Herbal Kvass with Beetroot and Dandelion Root** is an excellent choice. Combine 2 medium beets (diced), 1 tablespoon of dried Dandelion Root, 1 tablespoon of grated fresh Ginger, and 1 teaspoon of sea salt in a large jar. Fill the jar with filtered water, cover, and let ferment for 3-5 days. This earthy, slightly tangy beverage supports liver detoxification, improves bile flow, and promotes a healthy gut microbiome.

Yogurt can also be infused with herbs to create a gut-soothing and anti-inflammatory treat. To make **Chamomile and Lemon Balm Infused Yogurt**, prepare plain yogurt as usual and, before the final cooling stage, add 1 tablespoon each of dried Chamomile flowers and Lemon Balm leaves. Allow the herbs to infuse for 30 minutes, then strain them out before refrigerating the yogurt. Chamomile and Lemon Balm soothe the digestive tract, reduce stress, and promote relaxation, making this yogurt ideal for calming an irritated gut.

For a more adventurous recipe, try **Spiced Herbal Kimchi with Holy Basil and Ginger**. Chop 1 medium head of Napa cabbage and mix with 1 tablespoon of sea salt. Add 1 tablespoon of grated Ginger, 1 teaspoon of dried Holy Basil leaves, and 1 tablespoon of gochugaru (Korean red chili flakes). Pack the mixture tightly into a jar, ensuring that the cabbage is submerged in its own brine. Ferment at room temperature for 1-2 weeks, then store in the refrigerator. Holy Basil supports stress reduction and balances cortisol levels, while Ginger and chili flakes enhance circulation and digestion.

Enhancing Digestive Health with Fermentation

Fermented foods are beneficial for digestive health because the fermentation process enhances the bioavailability of nutrients, increases the production of vitamins (such as vitamin K and B vitamins), and generates enzymes that aid in the breakdown of food. Regular consumption of fermented foods can improve nutrient absorption, support immune function, and prevent the overgrowth of pathogenic bacteria. Including herbs in fermented foods adds another layer of therapeutic benefit, as the herbs provide targeted support for digestive health and create a synergistic effect that enhances the overall efficacy of the probiotic food.

Herbs like Dill, Fennel, and Caraway are excellent choices for digestive health and can be added to any vegetable ferment. These carminative herbs help reduce gas, bloating, and digestive discomfort, making ferments more tolerable for those with sensitive digestive systems. Antimicrobial herbs such as Garlic, Thyme, and Oregano can also be added to ferments to support immune health and prevent spoilage.

Combining probiotics, herbs, and fermented foods is a powerful strategy for optimizing digestive health. The probiotics help restore and maintain a healthy gut microbiome, the herbs provide targeted support and healing for the digestive tract, and the fermentation process makes all of these nutrients more bioavailable and easier for the body to utilize. With regular use, fermented herbal foods can transform digestive health, boost immunity, and promote overall wellness.

Book 29: Herbal Aids for Appetite Control

Maintaining a healthy appetite balance is essential for effective weight management and overall wellness. Many individuals struggle with controlling their appetite and managing cravings, which can lead to overeating and weight gain. Herbal remedies offer a natural approach to regulating appetite, curbing cravings, and promoting a sense of fullness, making them valuable tools for those seeking to achieve or maintain a healthy weight. The key to using herbs for appetite control lies in understanding their ability to influence hunger and satiety signals, support healthy digestion, and balance blood sugar levels.

Natural Appetite Suppressants

Several herbs have been traditionally used as appetite suppressants due to their ability to reduce the desire to eat, control cravings, and promote a sense of satiety. Unlike synthetic appetite suppressants, which may come with undesirable side effects, herbal remedies tend to work gently and holistically, making them safer for long-term use.

One of the most effective appetite-suppressing herbs is **Hoodia Gordonii**, a succulent plant traditionally used by the indigenous people of the Kalahari Desert to suppress hunger during long hunting trips. Hoodia contains a compound called P57, which is believed to affect the hypothalamus, the part of the brain that regulates hunger, thereby reducing appetite and promoting a feeling of fullness.

Another well-known appetite suppressant is **Garcinia Cambogia**, a tropical fruit whose rind contains hydroxycitric acid (HCA), a compound that is thought to increase serotonin levels and reduce the desire to eat. HCA also inhibits the enzyme citrate lyase, which the body uses to make fat, making Garcinia Cambogia popular for weight management.

Fennel Seed is another herb that can help reduce appetite. Fennel is rich in dietary fiber and has a mild diuretic effect, which can help reduce bloating and promote a feeling of fullness. Consuming Fennel tea before meals can help curb appetite and reduce the likelihood of overeating.

Gymnema Sylvestre, an herb commonly used in Ayurvedic medicine, has the unique ability to block the receptors on the tongue that are responsible for tasting sweetness. This reduces the appeal of sugary foods, making it easier to control sugar cravings and reduce caloric intake.

Yerba Mate, a traditional South American tea, is also known for its appetite-suppressing properties. Yerba Mate contains compounds such as theobromine and caffeine, which promote energy and enhance metabolism, while also reducing hunger and promoting a sense of satiety.

Green Tea Extract is another popular appetite suppressant. It contains catechins and caffeine, which work together to increase thermogenesis and fat oxidation, making it effective for both appetite control and weight loss. Consuming Green Tea before meals can reduce appetite and increase metabolism, promoting healthy weight management.

Herbs to Balance Hunger and Satiety

In addition to appetite suppressants, certain herbs can help regulate hunger signals and promote a sense of fullness, making them useful for those who struggle with frequent hunger or food cravings. These herbs work by influencing the hormones and neurotransmitters that regulate hunger and satiety, such as leptin, ghrelin, and serotonin.

Fenugreek, a spice commonly used in Indian cuisine, is rich in soluble fiber, which swells in the stomach and promotes a feeling of fullness. Consuming Fenugreek before meals can help reduce hunger and prevent overeating.

Psyllium Husk is another herb that supports satiety. Psyllium is a form of soluble fiber that absorbs water in the stomach, forming a gel-like substance that slows digestion and promotes a prolonged feeling of fullness. This makes Psyllium particularly effective for managing appetite and reducing overall caloric intake.

Caralluma Fimbriata is a succulent herb traditionally used in India to suppress appetite and increase endurance. It works by influencing hunger-regulating hormones, including ghrelin, which is known as the "hunger hormone." By reducing ghrelin levels, Caralluma Fimbriata helps reduce appetite and promote a sense of fullness.

Slippery Elm and **Marshmallow Root** are both mucilaginous herbs that create a soothing, gelatinous texture when combined with water. This mucilage can coat the stomach and promote a feeling of satiety, making these herbs useful for reducing hunger and managing appetite.

Bitter Melon, an herb commonly used in Asian cuisine, helps regulate blood sugar levels, reducing hunger spikes and preventing cravings for sugary foods. By balancing blood sugar levels, Bitter Melon can support a steady appetite and promote healthy eating habits.

Remedies for Appetite Control

Creating herbal remedies that support appetite control involves combining herbs that suppress appetite, promote satiety, and enhance digestion. These remedies can be used as teas, tinctures, capsules, or smoothies to provide effective, natural support for healthy weight management.

For those looking for a pre-meal tonic to reduce hunger, **Gymnema and Green Tea Appetite Control Tea** is ideal. To prepare, combine 1 tablespoon of dried Gymnema leaves and 1 teaspoon of Green Tea in 2 cups of hot water. Steep for 10 minutes, strain, and drink 30 minutes before meals. This tea reduces sugar cravings, promotes fullness, and boosts metabolism, making it effective for reducing overall caloric intake.

Another option is **Fennel and Psyllium Pre-Meal Satiety Drink**. Mix 1 teaspoon of Fennel Seed powder and 1 teaspoon of Psyllium Husk in 1 cup of water. Stir well and drink immediately, followed by an additional glass of water. This drink expands in the stomach, promoting a feeling of fullness and reducing the likelihood of overeating.

For those struggling with sugar cravings, **Gymnema and Holy Basil Sweet Craving Tincture** is a powerful remedy. Combine 1 tablespoon each of Gymnema and Holy Basil with 1 cup of vodka or brandy in a glass jar. Let steep for 4-6 weeks, shaking occasionally. Strain and store in a dark glass bottle. Take ½ teaspoon when sugar cravings strike to reduce the desire for sweets and balance blood sugar levels.

Yerba Mate and Garcinia Cambogia Appetite Suppressant Tea is another effective remedy. To prepare, combine 1 tablespoon of Yerba Mate leaves and 1 teaspoon of Garcinia Cambogia powder in 2 cups of hot water. Steep for 10 minutes, strain, and drink mid-morning to reduce appetite and enhance metabolism.

For a more comprehensive remedy, try **Hoodia and Fenugreek Appetite Balancing Capsules**. Mix 1 tablespoon of Hoodia powder and 1 tablespoon of Fenugreek powder, then fill empty gel capsules with the mixture. Take 1 capsule up to twice daily before meals to reduce hunger and promote fullness.

Incorporating these herbal remedies into a daily routine can provide effective, natural support for appetite control, making it easier to maintain a healthy weight and reduce the likelihood of overeating.

Book 30: Natural Remedies for Food Allergies

Food allergies are becoming increasingly common and can significantly impact the quality of life for those affected. When an individual with a food allergy consumes a triggering substance, the immune system overreacts, releasing chemicals such as histamine that cause inflammation and symptoms ranging from mild hives and itching to more severe reactions like difficulty breathing or anaphylaxis. Managing food allergies typically involves strict avoidance of the allergen, but certain herbs can provide additional support by alleviating symptoms, reducing inflammation, and supporting the immune system. This chapter explores how herbal remedies can complement traditional management strategies for food allergies and presents options for creating allergy-friendly meals.

Herbs to Manage Allergic Reactions to Food

Certain herbs have natural antihistamine, anti-inflammatory, and immune-modulating properties that can help mitigate the symptoms of food allergies. By reducing the body's allergic response and supporting the health of the digestive and immune systems, these herbs can provide relief from symptoms such as itching, swelling, and gastrointestinal discomfort.

One of the most effective herbs for managing allergic reactions is **Stinging Nettle**. Nettle is a natural antihistamine that blocks histamine receptors, thereby reducing the severity of allergic reactions. It can be taken as a tea, tincture, or capsule to alleviate symptoms such as itching, hives, and nasal congestion. Nettle's high mineral content also supports the overall health of the immune system.

Quercetin, a flavonoid found in many herbs such as **Chamomile** and **Elderberry**, is another powerful natural antihistamine that stabilizes mast cells and prevents the release of histamine. Quercetin's anti-inflammatory properties make it useful for reducing swelling and alleviating symptoms of food allergies. It can be taken as a supplement or consumed through quercetin-rich foods and herbs.

Butterbur is another herb known for its ability to reduce histamine and support respiratory health. It is particularly effective for managing allergy-related asthma and respiratory symptoms. However, it's important to use only certified "PA-free" Butterbur products, as the raw plant contains pyrrolizidine alkaloids (PAs) that can be toxic to the liver.

For digestive support, **Chamomile** is an excellent choice. Chamomile has antispasmodic and anti-inflammatory properties that can soothe gastrointestinal symptoms associated with food allergies, such as cramping, bloating, and diarrhea. Drinking Chamomile tea before or after a meal can help calm the digestive tract and prevent discomfort.

Licorice Root is another herb that supports the health of the digestive and immune systems. Its anti-inflammatory properties help reduce gut inflammation, which is often present in individuals with food sensitivities. Licorice also promotes the healing of the mucous membranes in the digestive tract, making it beneficial for managing symptoms like acid reflux and stomach pain.

For those dealing with skin-related allergy symptoms, **Calendula** is highly effective. Calendula has natural anti-inflammatory and wound-healing properties that soothe irritated skin, reduce itching, and promote the healing of rashes and hives. It can be used topically as a cream or salve or taken internally as a tea to support overall skin health.

Turmeric is another versatile herb that supports allergy management through its potent anti-inflammatory effects. Curcumin, the active compound in Turmeric, inhibits the release of inflammatory compounds and supports the health of the immune system. Taking Turmeric with black pepper enhances the absorption of curcumin, making it more effective for reducing inflammation and managing allergy symptoms.

Recipes for Allergy-Friendly Meals

Creating allergy-friendly meals that are free of common allergens such as dairy, gluten, nuts, and soy can be challenging. However, incorporating herbs into these meals not only enhances their flavor but also provides therapeutic benefits that support the immune and digestive systems. The following recipes are designed to be both delicious and safe for those with food allergies, making them suitable for a wide range of dietary needs.

Chamomile and Ginger Infused Quinoa Salad is a light, refreshing dish that is free of common allergens and packed with anti-inflammatory herbs. To prepare, rinse 1 cup of quinoa thoroughly and cook it in 2 cups of water along with 1 tablespoon of dried Chamomile flowers and 1 tablespoon of freshly grated Ginger. Once the quinoa is cooked, remove the Chamomile flowers and fluff the quinoa with a fork. Add chopped cucumbers, shredded carrots, and a handful of fresh mint leaves. Dress with lemon juice and olive oil, and serve chilled. Chamomile and Ginger calm the digestive tract, while mint adds a cooling, anti-inflammatory touch.

For a nourishing breakfast option, try **Turmeric and Nettle Porridge**. Combine ½ cup of gluten-free oats, 1 cup of unsweetened almond milk, 1 teaspoon of Turmeric powder, and 1 tablespoon of dried Nettle leaves in a small saucepan. Bring to a simmer, stirring frequently until the oats are tender and creamy. Remove from heat, strain out the Nettle leaves, and top with fresh berries and a drizzle of honey. This warming porridge supports immune health, reduces inflammation, and provides a gentle energy boost.

Another excellent recipe is **Licorice and Marshmallow Root Gut-Healing Soup**. This soothing soup is ideal for those with digestive discomfort or food sensitivities. To prepare, simmer 1 tablespoon each of Licorice Root and Marshmallow Root in 4 cups of vegetable broth for 20 minutes. Strain out the herbs, then add 1 cup of chopped sweet potatoes, 1 cup of chopped carrots, and 1 cup of shredded cabbage. Simmer until the vegetables are tender. Season with salt, pepper, and fresh thyme, and enjoy warm. Licorice and Marshmallow Root soothe the gut lining and reduce inflammation, making this soup ideal for supporting digestive health.

For a sweet treat, consider **Calendula and Chamomile Anti-Allergy Gummies**. To prepare, steep 1 tablespoon each of dried Calendula and Chamomile flowers in 1 cup of hot water for 15 minutes. Strain and mix with 2 tablespoons of gelatin and 1 tablespoon of raw honey. Pour the mixture into a silicone mold and refrigerate until set. These gummies can be enjoyed as a soothing, anti-inflammatory snack that helps reduce allergy symptoms.

For a refreshing beverage, **Nettle and Peppermint Iced Tea** is a perfect choice. Steep 1 tablespoon of dried Nettle leaves and 1 tablespoon of dried Peppermint in 4 cups of hot water for 20 minutes. Strain and pour over ice. Add a splash of lemon juice and a teaspoon of honey if desired. This mineral-rich tea supports immune health and reduces inflammation, making it a great addition to an allergy-friendly diet.

Enhancing Digestive Health and Immunity through Herbal Remedies

While managing food allergies often involves strict avoidance of allergens, incorporating herbs that support the health of the immune and digestive systems can significantly improve outcomes. Many food allergies are linked to gut health, as a compromised digestive system can increase the likelihood of developing food sensitivities. By using herbs that heal the gut, reduce inflammation, and support immune balance, it is possible to reduce the severity of allergic reactions and enhance overall health.

Herbs such as **Slippery Elm**, **Marshmallow Root**, and **Licorice Root** coat and protect the mucous membranes in the gut, preventing allergens from crossing the gut barrier and triggering an immune response. **Turmeric**, **Ginger**, and **Nettle** reduce systemic inflammation, support detoxification, and enhance resilience, making them invaluable for managing food allergies. By combining these herbs with an allergy-friendly diet and appropriate lifestyle changes, individuals can create a holistic approach to managing food allergies naturally.

Remedies for Food Allergies

541. Stinging Nettle Anti-Allergy Capsules

Ingredients: 1 tablespoon dried Nettle leaf powder, empty gel capsules.
Preparation: Fill empty capsules with

Nettle leaf powder and seal.

Suggested Usage: Take 1 capsule up to twice daily to reduce allergy symptoms.

Benefits: Nettle is a natural antihistamine that helps block histamine receptors, reducing allergic reactions such as itching, sneezing, and hives.

542. Chamomile and Ginger Anti-Inflammatory Tea

Ingredients: 1 tablespoon dried Chamomile flowers, 1 teaspoon grated fresh Ginger, 2 cups hot water.

Preparation: Steep Chamomile and Ginger in hot water for 15 minutes. Strain and serve warm.

Suggested Usage: Drink 1 cup up to twice daily to reduce inflammation and soothe the digestive tract.

Benefits: Chamomile and Ginger are anti-inflammatory herbs that calm the digestive system, reduce inflammation, and alleviate allergy-related discomfort.

543. Quercetin and Nettle Histamine-Blocking Capsules

Ingredients: 1 tablespoon Quercetin powder, 1 tablespoon dried Nettle leaf powder, empty gel capsules.

Preparation: Mix Quercetin and Nettle powders thoroughly. Fill empty capsules and seal.

Suggested Usage: Take 1 capsule up to twice daily to prevent allergic reactions.

Benefits: Quercetin stabilizes mast cells, preventing histamine release, while Nettle provides additional antihistamine support, making these capsules effective for managing seasonal allergies.

544. Butterbur and Elderflower Allergy Relief Tea

Ingredients: 1 tablespoon dried Butterbur, 1 tablespoon dried Elderflower, 2 cups hot water.

Preparation: Steep Butterbur and Elderflower in hot water for 15 minutes. Strain and serve warm.

Suggested Usage: Drink 1 cup daily to relieve allergy symptoms, particularly respiratory issues.

Benefits: Butterbur reduces histamine production and supports respiratory health, while Elderflower alleviates congestion and soothes the sinuses, making this tea effective for allergy relief.

545. Turmeric and Ginger Anti-Inflammatory Tonic

Ingredients: 1 teaspoon Turmeric powder, ½ teaspoon grated fresh Ginger, a pinch of black pepper, 1 cup hot water.

Preparation: Combine all ingredients in hot water and stir until fully dissolved. Serve warm.

Suggested Usage: Drink 1 cup daily to reduce inflammation and support immune health.

Benefits: Turmeric and Ginger are powerful anti-inflammatory herbs that reduce inflammation throughout the body, while black pepper enhances the absorption of curcumin, making this tonic ideal for managing allergy-related inflammation.

546. Licorice Root and Marshmallow Gut-Healing Powder

Ingredients: 1 tablespoon Licorice Root powder, 1 tablespoon Marshmallow Root powder.

Preparation: Mix Licorice Root and Marshmallow powders thoroughly. Store in an airtight container.

Suggested Usage: Mix ½ teaspoon of the powder in warm water and drink up to twice daily to soothe the digestive tract.

Benefits: Licorice Root and Marshmallow soothe the mucous membranes of the digestive tract, reduce inflammation, and promote healing, making this powder ideal for managing gastrointestinal symptoms associated with food allergies.

547. Reishi and Schisandra Immune-Modulating Capsules

Ingredients: 1 tablespoon Reishi Mushroom powder, 1 tablespoon Schisandra Berry powder, empty gel capsules.

Preparation: Mix Reishi and Schisandra powders thoroughly. Fill empty capsules and seal.

Suggested Usage: Take 1 capsule up to twice daily to enhance immune function and reduce allergy sensitivity.

Benefits: Reishi and Schisandra are adaptogens that balance the immune response, making these capsules effective for supporting overall immune health and reducing the severity of allergic reactions.

548. Calendula and Chamomile Anti-Inflammatory Salve

Ingredients: 1 tablespoon dried Calendula flowers, 1 tablespoon dried Chamomile flowers, ½ cup coconut oil, 1 tablespoon beeswax.

Preparation: Infuse Calendula and Chamomile in melted coconut oil for 30 minutes on low heat. Strain and add beeswax. Stir until melted, then pour into a glass jar and let cool.

Suggested Usage: Apply to irritated skin as needed to reduce itching and promote healing.

Benefits: Calendula and Chamomile soothe inflamed skin, reduce itching, and promote healing, making this salve ideal for treating hives, rashes, and other allergy-related skin irritations.

549. Peppermint and Lemon Balm Anti-Spasm Tea

Ingredients: 1 tablespoon dried Peppermint leaves, 1 tablespoon dried Lemon Balm leaves, 2 cups hot water.

Preparation: Steep Peppermint and Lemon Balm in hot water for 15 minutes. Strain and serve warm.

Suggested Usage: Drink 1 cup daily to soothe digestive discomfort and reduce bloating.

Benefits: Peppermint and Lemon Balm have antispasmodic properties that relax the digestive tract, making this tea ideal for alleviating symptoms such as cramping and bloating associated with food allergies.

550. Holy Basil and Nettle Adaptogen Capsules

Ingredients: 1 tablespoon Holy Basil powder, 1 tablespoon Nettle leaf powder, empty gel capsules.

Preparation: Mix Holy Basil and Nettle powders thoroughly. Fill empty capsules and seal.

Suggested Usage: Take 1 capsule up to twice daily to reduce stress and enhance immune function.

Benefits: Holy Basil and Nettle are adaptogenic herbs that support the body's stress response and modulate the immune system, making these capsules effective for managing stress-related allergy symptoms.

551. Fennel and Ginger Anti-Bloat Capsules

Ingredients: 1 tablespoon Fennel seed powder, 1 tablespoon Ginger powder, empty gel capsules.

Preparation: Mix Fennel and Ginger powders thoroughly. Fill empty capsules and seal.

Suggested Usage: Take 1 capsule up to twice daily to reduce bloating and promote digestion.

Benefits: Fennel and Ginger relieve gas and bloating, reduce inflammation, and promote healthy digestion, making these capsules effective for managing digestive discomfort associated with food allergies.

552. Quercetin and Bromelain Anti-Allergy Tincture

Ingredients: 1 tablespoon Quercetin powder, 1 tablespoon Bromelain powder, 1 cup vodka or brandy.

Preparation: Combine Quercetin and Bromelain with alcohol in a glass jar. Seal tightly and let steep for 4-6 weeks, shaking occasionally. Strain and store in a dark glass bottle.

Suggested Usage: Take ½ teaspoon daily to reduce allergy symptoms.

Benefits: Quercetin stabilizes mast cells and prevents histamine release, while Bromelain reduces inflammation, making this tincture highly effective for managing seasonal and food-related allergies.

553. Lemon Balm and Skullcap Anti-Anxiety Tea

Ingredients: 1 tablespoon dried Lemon Balm leaves, 1 tablespoon dried Skullcap, 2 cups hot water.

Preparation: Steep Lemon Balm and Skullcap in hot water for 15 minutes. Strain and serve warm.

Suggested Usage: Drink 1 cup daily to reduce anxiety and promote relaxation.

Benefits: Lemon Balm and Skullcap calm the nervous system and reduce stress, making this tea ideal for managing anxiety-related allergy flare-ups.

554. Licorice Root and Calendula Skin-Soothing Lotion

Ingredients: 1 tablespoon Licorice Root powder, 1 tablespoon Calendula flowers, ½ cup shea butter, 2 tablespoons olive oil.

Preparation: Infuse Licorice and Calendula in olive oil over low heat for 30 minutes. Strain and mix with melted shea butter. Pour into a jar and let cool.

Suggested Usage: Apply to irritated skin as needed to reduce redness and promote healing.

Benefits: Licorice and Calendula reduce inflammation, calm irritated skin, and promote healing, making this lotion ideal for soothing allergy-related skin conditions.

555. Butterbur and Nettle Sinus-Clearing Capsules

Ingredients: 1 tablespoon Butterbur powder, 1 tablespoon dried Nettle leaf powder, empty gel capsules.
Preparation: Mix Butterbur and Nettle powders thoroughly. Fill empty capsules with the mixture and seal.
Suggested Usage: Take 1 capsule up to twice daily to reduce sinus congestion and manage seasonal allergies.
Benefits: Butterbur and Nettle are natural antihistamines that reduce inflammation and clear sinus congestion, making these capsules effective for managing allergy-related respiratory symptoms.

556. Reishi and Holy Basil Stress-Relieving Tea

Ingredients: 1 tablespoon dried Reishi Mushroom, 1 tablespoon dried Holy Basil leaves, 2 cups hot water.
Preparation: Steep Reishi and Holy Basil in hot water for 15 minutes. Strain and serve warm.
Suggested Usage: Drink 1 cup up to twice daily to reduce stress and enhance resilience.
Benefits: Reishi and Holy Basil are adaptogenic herbs that balance the body's stress response, reduce inflammation, and support immune health, making this tea ideal for managing stress-induced allergy symptoms.

557. Turmeric and Licorice Anti-Inflammatory Capsules

Ingredients: 1 tablespoon Turmeric powder, 1 tablespoon Licorice Root powder, empty gel capsules.
Preparation: Mix Turmeric and Licorice powders thoroughly. Fill empty capsules with the mixture and seal.
Suggested Usage: Take 1 capsule up to twice daily to reduce inflammation and support immune function.
Benefits: Turmeric and Licorice have potent anti-inflammatory properties that reduce systemic inflammation, support liver health, and promote immune balance, making these capsules ideal for managing allergy-related inflammation.

558. Dandelion and Burdock Liver-Support Capsules

Ingredients: 1 tablespoon Dandelion Root powder, 1 tablespoon Burdock Root powder, empty gel capsules.
Preparation: Mix Dandelion and Burdock powders thoroughly. Fill empty capsules with the mixture and seal.
Suggested Usage: Take 1 capsule daily to promote liver detoxification and support overall health.
Benefits: Dandelion and Burdock cleanse the liver, support bile production, and promote detoxification, making these capsules ideal for enhancing liver health and overall wellness.

559. Chamomile and Ginger Digestive Comfort Tea

Ingredients: 1 tablespoon dried Chamomile flowers, 1 teaspoon grated fresh Ginger, 2 cups hot water.
Preparation: Steep Chamomile and Ginger in hot water for 15 minutes. Strain

and serve warm.

Suggested Usage: Drink 1 cup up to twice daily to soothe the digestive tract and reduce discomfort.

Benefits: Chamomile and Ginger are calming and anti-inflammatory herbs that reduce gas, bloating, and nausea, making this tea ideal for managing digestive discomfort associated with food sensitivities.

560. Skullcap and Valerian Nerve-Soothing Capsules

Ingredients: 1 tablespoon Skullcap powder, 1 tablespoon Valerian Root powder, empty gel capsules.

Preparation: Mix Skullcap and Valerian powders thoroughly. Fill empty capsules with the mixture and seal.

Suggested Usage: Take 1 capsule daily to reduce anxiety and support restful sleep.

Benefits: Skullcap and Valerian calm the nervous system, reduce stress, and promote relaxation, making these capsules ideal for managing anxiety and stress-related allergies.

561. Calendula and Plantain Anti-Itch Lotion

Ingredients: 1 tablespoon dried Calendula flowers, 1 tablespoon dried Plantain leaves, ½ cup shea butter, 2 tablespoons olive oil.

Preparation: Infuse Calendula and Plantain in olive oil over low heat for 30 minutes. Strain and mix with melted shea butter. Pour into a jar and let cool.

Suggested Usage: Apply to irritated skin as needed to reduce itching and promote healing.

Benefits: Calendula and Plantain have anti-inflammatory and soothing properties that reduce itching and promote skin healing, making this lotion ideal for treating hives and rashes.

562. Milk Thistle and Nettle Liver Detox Tea

Ingredients: 1 tablespoon Milk Thistle seeds, 1 tablespoon dried Nettle leaves, 2 cups hot water.

Preparation: Steep Milk Thistle and Nettle in hot water for 15 minutes. Strain and serve warm.

Suggested Usage: Drink 1 cup daily to support liver detoxification and promote overall health.

Benefits: Milk Thistle protects liver cells and promotes detoxification, while Nettle provides minerals and supports liver function, making this tea ideal for enhancing liver health.

563. Slippery Elm and Marshmallow Root Gut-Coating Syrup

Ingredients: 1 tablespoon Slippery Elm powder, 1 tablespoon Marshmallow Root powder, 1 cup warm water.

Preparation: Mix Slippery Elm and Marshmallow Root powders in warm water until a thick syrup forms.

Suggested Usage: Take 1 teaspoon up to twice daily to soothe the digestive tract.

Benefits: Slippery Elm and Marshmallow Root coat and protect the mucous membranes of the digestive tract, reduce inflammation, and promote healing, making this syrup effective for managing gastrointestinal symptoms associated with food allergies.

564. Astragalus and Schisandra Immune-Boosting Tea

Ingredients: 1 tablespoon dried Astragalus Root, 1 tablespoon dried Schisandra Berries, 2 cups hot water.
Preparation: Steep Astragalus and Schisandra in hot water for 20 minutes. Strain and serve warm.
Suggested Usage: Drink 1 cup daily to support immune function and enhance resilience.
Benefits: Astragalus and Schisandra are adaptogenic herbs that support immune health, balance the body's stress response, and enhance energy levels, making this tea ideal for reducing allergy sensitivity and boosting overall health.

565. Licorice and Turmeric Anti-Inflammatory Tea

Ingredients: 1 tablespoon dried Licorice Root, 1 teaspoon Turmeric powder, 2 cups hot water.
Preparation: Steep Licorice and Turmeric in hot water for 15 minutes. Strain and serve warm.
Suggested Usage: Drink 1 cup up to twice daily to reduce inflammation and support digestive health.
Benefits: Licorice and Turmeric reduce systemic inflammation, promote gut health, and protect against allergy-related inflammation, making this tea effective for managing symptoms of food allergies.

566. Nettle and Elderflower Antihistamine Tea

Ingredients: 1 tablespoon dried Nettle leaves, 1 tablespoon dried Elderflower, 2 cups hot water.
Preparation: Steep Nettle and Elderflower in hot water for 15 minutes. Strain and serve warm.
Suggested Usage: Drink 1 cup daily to reduce allergy symptoms and promote respiratory health.
Benefits: Nettle and Elderflower are natural antihistamines that reduce histamine levels and alleviate respiratory symptoms, making this tea ideal for managing seasonal and food-related allergies.

567. Ginger and Fennel Digestive Soothing Tonic

Ingredients: 1 tablespoon grated fresh Ginger, 1 teaspoon Fennel seeds, 2 cups water.
Preparation: Simmer Ginger and Fennel seeds in water for 10 minutes. Strain and serve warm.
Suggested Usage: Drink 1 cup up to twice daily to relieve gas and bloating.
Benefits: Ginger and Fennel are digestive herbs that soothe the gastrointestinal tract, reduce gas, and alleviate cramping, making this tonic ideal for managing digestive symptoms associated with food allergies.

568. Chamomile and Lemon Balm Calming Elixir

Ingredients: 1 tablespoon dried Chamomile flowers, 1 tablespoon dried Lemon Balm leaves, 1 cup hot water.
Preparation: Steep Chamomile and Lemon Balm in hot water for 15 minutes. Strain and serve warm.
Suggested Usage: Drink 1 cup daily to reduce anxiety and promote relaxation.
Benefits: Chamomile and Lemon Balm calm the nervous system, reduce stress, and promote emotional balance, making this elixir ideal for managing anxiety-related allergy flare-ups.

569. Ashwagandha and Holy Basil Stress-Reducing Capsules

Ingredients: 1 tablespoon Ashwagandha Root powder, 1 tablespoon Holy Basil powder, empty gel capsules.
Preparation: Mix Ashwagandha and Holy Basil powders thoroughly. Fill empty capsules with the mixture and seal.
Suggested Usage: Take 1 capsule up to twice daily to support stress management and enhance resilience.
Benefits: Ashwagandha and Holy Basil are adaptogenic herbs that reduce the impact of stress on the immune system, making these capsules effective for managing stress-induced allergy symptoms.

570. Burdock Root and Yellow Dock Blood-Cleansing Tea

Ingredients: 1 tablespoon dried Burdock Root, 1 tablespoon dried Yellow Dock Root, 2 cups hot water.
Preparation: Simmer Burdock Root and Yellow Dock Root in hot water for 15 minutes. Strain and serve warm.

Suggested Usage: Drink 1 cup daily to promote blood purification and liver detoxification.
Benefits: Burdock and Yellow Dock cleanse the blood, support liver function, and enhance detoxification, making this tea ideal for reducing the toxic load that can trigger allergic reactions.

571. Schisandra and Reishi Mushroom Immune Tonic

Ingredients: 1 tablespoon dried Schisandra Berries, 1 tablespoon dried Reishi Mushroom, 2 cups hot water.
Preparation: Simmer Schisandra and Reishi in water for 20 minutes. Strain and serve warm.
Suggested Usage: Drink 1 cup daily to support immune health and reduce allergy sensitivity.
Benefits: Schisandra and Reishi are adaptogenic herbs that balance the immune response, reduce inflammation, and enhance resilience, making this tonic ideal for reducing the severity of allergic reactions.

572. Calendula and Oatmeal Anti-Itch Skin Bath Soak

Ingredients: 1 tablespoon dried Calendula flowers, ½ cup colloidal oatmeal, 4 cups hot water.
Preparation: Steep Calendula and oatmeal in hot water for 15 minutes. Strain and add the liquid to a warm bath.
Suggested Usage: Soak in the bath for 20 minutes to reduce skin irritation and itching.
Benefits: Calendula and oatmeal soothe irritated skin, reduce inflammation, and

promote healing, making this bath soak ideal for managing hives, rashes, and other allergy-related skin conditions.

573. Milk Thistle and Dandelion Liver Cleanse Capsules

Ingredients: 1 tablespoon Milk Thistle seed powder, 1 tablespoon Dandelion Root powder, empty gel capsules.
Preparation: Mix Milk Thistle and Dandelion powders thoroughly. Fill empty capsules and seal.
Suggested Usage: Take 1 capsule up to twice daily to promote liver detoxification and support liver health.
Benefits: Milk Thistle and Dandelion enhance liver function, support bile production, and promote detoxification, making these capsules effective for reducing the toxic burden that can exacerbate allergies.

574. Marshmallow Root and Aloe Vera Gut-Healing Gel

Ingredients: 1 tablespoon Marshmallow Root powder, 2 tablespoons Aloe Vera gel.
Preparation: Mix Marshmallow Root powder and Aloe Vera gel thoroughly until a smooth consistency is achieved.
Suggested Usage: Take 1 teaspoon up to twice daily to coat and soothe the digestive tract.
Benefits: Marshmallow Root and Aloe Vera reduce inflammation, coat the mucous membranes, and promote healing, making this gel ideal for managing gastrointestinal symptoms associated with food allergies.

575. Holy Basil and Nettle Adrenal Support Capsules

Ingredients: 1 tablespoon Holy Basil powder, 1 tablespoon Nettle leaf powder, empty gel capsules.
Preparation: Mix Holy Basil and Nettle powders thoroughly. Fill empty capsules and seal.
Suggested Usage: Take 1 capsule up to twice daily to reduce stress and support adrenal health.
Benefits: Holy Basil and Nettle are adaptogens that reduce stress and support adrenal function, making these capsules ideal for managing stress-related immune imbalances and allergy symptoms.

576. Peppermint and Chamomile Anti-Spasm Tea

Ingredients: 1 tablespoon dried Peppermint leaves, 1 tablespoon dried Chamomile flowers, 2 cups hot water.
Preparation: Steep Peppermint and Chamomile in hot water for 15 minutes. Strain and serve warm.
Suggested Usage: Drink 1 cup up to twice daily to relieve digestive spasms and reduce gas.
Benefits: Peppermint and Chamomile relax the muscles of the digestive tract, reduce spasms, and alleviate cramping, making this tea ideal for managing digestive symptoms associated with food sensitivities.

577. Slippery Elm and Licorice Throat-Coating Lozenges

Ingredients: 1 tablespoon Slippery Elm powder, 1 tablespoon Licorice Root powder, 1 tablespoon honey, enough water to form a dough.
Preparation: Mix all ingredients together until a thick dough forms. Roll into small balls and flatten. Allow to dry for 24 hours before use.
Suggested Usage: Dissolve 1 lozenge in the mouth as needed to soothe the throat.
Benefits: Slippery Elm and Licorice coat the throat, reduce inflammation, and promote healing, making these lozenges effective for soothing allergy-related throat irritation and discomfort.

578. Nettle and Lemon Peel Vitamin C Tea

Ingredients: 1 tablespoon dried Nettle leaves, 1 teaspoon dried Lemon Peel, 2 cups hot water.
Preparation: Steep Nettle and Lemon Peel in hot water for 15 minutes. Strain and serve warm.
Suggested Usage: Drink 1 cup daily to boost immune health and reduce allergy symptoms.
Benefits: Nettle and Lemon Peel are rich in vitamins and antioxidants that support immune health, reduce histamine levels, and alleviate allergy-related symptoms, making this tea ideal for comprehensive allergy support.

579. Ginger and Turmeric Inflammation Relief Capsules

Ingredients: 1 tablespoon Ginger powder, 1 tablespoon Turmeric powder, empty gel capsules.
Preparation: Mix Ginger and Turmeric

powders thoroughly. Fill empty capsules and seal.
Suggested Usage: Take 1 capsule up to twice daily to reduce inflammation and support immune health.
Benefits: Ginger and Turmeric are potent anti-inflammatory herbs that reduce systemic inflammation, promote healthy digestion, and support immune function, making these capsules ideal for managing allergy-related inflammation and discomfort.

580. Valerian and Skullcap Sleep Support Tea

Ingredients: 1 tablespoon dried Valerian Root, 1 tablespoon dried Skullcap, 2 cups hot water.
Preparation: Steep Valerian and Skullcap in hot water for 15 minutes. Strain and serve warm.
Suggested Usage: Drink 1 cup before bedtime to promote relaxation and restful sleep.
Benefits: Valerian and Skullcap are calming nervines that reduce anxiety and promote relaxation, making this tea ideal for managing sleep disturbances associated with allergies and stress.

581. Lemon Balm and Fennel Nerve-Calming Capsules

Ingredients: 1 tablespoon Lemon Balm powder, 1 tablespoon Fennel seed powder, empty gel capsules.
Preparation: Mix Lemon Balm and Fennel powders thoroughly. Fill empty capsules and seal.
Suggested Usage: Take 1 capsule up to twice daily to reduce anxiety and calm

digestive discomfort.

Benefits: Lemon Balm and Fennel reduce nervous tension, calm the digestive system, and promote relaxation, making these capsules ideal for managing stress-related digestive symptoms.

582. Calendula and Plantain Skin-Healing Cream

Ingredients: 1 tablespoon dried Calendula flowers, 1 tablespoon dried Plantain leaves, ½ cup shea butter, 2 tablespoons coconut oil.

Preparation: Infuse Calendula and Plantain in melted coconut oil over low heat for 30 minutes. Strain and mix with melted shea butter. Pour into a jar and let cool.

Suggested Usage: Apply to irritated skin as needed to reduce itching and promote healing.

Benefits: Calendula and Plantain soothe inflamed skin, reduce itching, and support healing, making this cream ideal for treating allergy-related rashes and dermatitis.

583. Reishi and Schisandra Adaptogen Capsules

Ingredients: 1 tablespoon Reishi Mushroom powder, 1 tablespoon Schisandra Berry powder, empty gel capsules.

Preparation: Mix Reishi and Schisandra powders thoroughly. Fill empty capsules and seal.

Suggested Usage: Take 1 capsule daily to support immune function and enhance resilience.

Benefits: Reishi and Schisandra are adaptogens that balance the body's stress response and support immune health, making these capsules ideal for reducing allergy sensitivity and enhancing overall health.

584. Chamomile and Lavender Anti-Allergy Sleep Tea

Ingredients: 1 tablespoon dried Chamomile flowers, 1 teaspoon dried Lavender flowers, 2 cups hot water.

Preparation: Steep Chamomile and Lavender in hot water for 15 minutes. Strain and serve warm.

Suggested Usage: Drink 1 cup before bedtime to promote relaxation and support allergy relief.

Benefits: Chamomile and Lavender calm the nervous system, reduce histamine release, and promote restful sleep, making this tea ideal for managing nighttime allergy symptoms and improving sleep quality.

585. Butterbur and Quercetin Respiratory Support Capsules

Ingredients: 1 tablespoon Butterbur powder, 1 tablespoon Quercetin powder, empty gel capsules.

Preparation: Mix Butterbur and Quercetin powders thoroughly. Fill empty capsules and seal.

Suggested Usage: Take 1 capsule up to twice daily to reduce respiratory allergy symptoms.

Benefits: Butterbur reduces inflammation and prevents the release of histamine, while Quercetin stabilizes mast cells, making these capsules effective for managing respiratory allergies such as asthma and hay fever.

586. Holy Basil and Schisandra Adrenal Support Tonic

Ingredients: 1 tablespoon dried Holy Basil leaves, 1 tablespoon dried Schisandra Berries, 2 cups hot water.
Preparation: Steep Holy Basil and Schisandra in hot water for 15 minutes. Strain and serve warm.
Suggested Usage: Drink 1 cup daily to reduce stress and support adrenal health.
Benefits: Holy Basil and Schisandra are adaptogens that balance the body's stress response, reduce inflammation, and support adrenal function, making this tonic ideal for managing stress-related immune imbalances and reducing allergy sensitivity.

587. Peppermint and Ginger Digestive Soothing Tea

Ingredients: 1 tablespoon dried Peppermint leaves, 1 teaspoon grated fresh Ginger, 2 cups hot water.
Preparation: Steep Peppermint and Ginger in hot water for 15 minutes. Strain and serve warm.
Suggested Usage: Drink 1 cup up to twice daily to relieve digestive discomfort and promote healthy digestion.
Benefits: Peppermint and Ginger soothe the digestive tract, reduce gas, and promote healthy digestion, making this tea effective for managing digestive symptoms associated with food allergies.

588. Ashwagandha and Licorice Root Stress-Reducing Capsules

Ingredients: 1 tablespoon Ashwagandha Root powder, 1 tablespoon Licorice Root powder, empty gel capsules.
Preparation: Mix Ashwagandha and Licorice powders thoroughly. Fill empty capsules and seal.
Suggested Usage: Take 1 capsule daily to reduce stress and support immune health.
Benefits: Ashwagandha and Licorice are adaptogenic herbs that reduce stress, support adrenal health, and enhance immune resilience, making these capsules ideal for reducing allergy sensitivity and managing stress-related allergy symptoms.

589. Nettle and Elderflower Sinus-Clearing Tea

Ingredients: 1 tablespoon dried Nettle leaves, 1 tablespoon dried Elderflower, 2 cups hot water.
Preparation: Steep Nettle and Elderflower in hot water for 15 minutes. Strain and serve warm.
Suggested Usage: Drink 1 cup up to twice daily to reduce sinus congestion and alleviate respiratory symptoms.
Benefits: Nettle and Elderflower are natural antihistamines that reduce sinus congestion and soothe the respiratory system, making this tea ideal for managing allergy-related sinus issues.

590. Milk Thistle and Turmeric Liver Support Elixir

Ingredients: 1 tablespoon Milk Thistle seeds, 1 teaspoon Turmeric powder, 2 cups hot water.

Preparation: Steep Milk Thistle and Turmeric in hot water for 15 minutes. Strain and serve warm.

Suggested Usage: Drink 1 cup daily to support liver detoxification and promote overall health.

Benefits: Milk Thistle and Turmeric protect liver cells, promote detoxification, and reduce inflammation, making this elixir ideal for enhancing liver health and supporting overall wellness.

591. Calendula and Marshmallow Root Soothing Skin Spray

Ingredients: 1 tablespoon dried Calendula flowers, 1 tablespoon dried Marshmallow Root, 2 cups water.

Preparation: Simmer Calendula and Marshmallow Root in water for 20 minutes. Strain and pour into a spray bottle.

Suggested Usage: Spray onto irritated skin as needed to reduce itching and promote healing.

Benefits: Calendula and Marshmallow Root have anti-inflammatory and soothing properties that reduce irritation and promote skin healing, making this spray effective for managing hives, rashes, and other allergy-related skin conditions.

Book 31: Natural Stress Relief

In today's fast-paced world, managing stress and anxiety is crucial for maintaining overall health and well-being. Chronic stress can negatively impact mental, emotional, and physical health, leading to issues such as insomnia, fatigue, weakened immunity, and even cardiovascular problems. Herbal remedies have long been used to support the body in times of stress, offering a natural way to calm the nervous system, enhance resilience, and promote emotional balance. This chapter delves into various herbs that combat stress and anxiety, along with complementary relaxation techniques to create a comprehensive approach to stress relief and mental wellness.

Herbs to Combat Stress and Anxiety

Many herbs, often referred to as "adaptogens" and "nervines," have been used traditionally to support the body's response to stress and alleviate symptoms of anxiety. Adaptogens are herbs that enhance the body's ability to adapt to physical, mental, and environmental stressors by regulating the stress hormones cortisol and adrenaline. They build resilience and promote a sense of balance in the body and mind. Nervines, on the other hand, are herbs that specifically target the nervous system, promoting relaxation, reducing anxiety, and alleviating tension.

One of the most widely known adaptogenic herbs is **Ashwagandha**. This powerful herb, used in Ayurvedic medicine, is known for its ability to lower cortisol levels and enhance the body's resistance to stress. Studies have shown that Ashwagandha can reduce symptoms of anxiety and improve sleep quality, making it an excellent choice for managing chronic stress and supporting overall well-being. Ashwagandha can be taken in capsule form or as a tea or tincture to promote a calm and balanced state of mind.

Another effective adaptogen is **Rhodiola Rosea**. Rhodiola is particularly beneficial for combating mental fatigue, improving focus, and reducing stress-induced burnout. It works by balancing neurotransmitters in the brain, such as serotonin and dopamine, which play a key role in regulating mood and emotional stability. Rhodiola is best taken as a standardized extract to ensure consistent results.

For a more calming adaptogen, **Holy Basil (Tulsi)** is highly recommended. Known as the "Queen of Herbs" in Ayurveda, Holy Basil supports the body's stress response, balances cortisol levels, and promotes mental clarity and relaxation. Holy Basil can be taken as a tea throughout the day to alleviate anxiety and promote a state of calm alertness.

For those who need help with acute anxiety and nervous tension, **Passionflower** is an effective nervine that gently relaxes the nervous system and reduces anxiety. Passionflower contains compounds that increase the levels of gamma-aminobutyric acid (GABA) in the brain, a neurotransmitter that inhibits overactivity and promotes relaxation. It is particularly useful for those who experience anxiety-related insomnia or agitation. Passionflower can be taken as a tea or tincture, especially before bedtime, to promote restful sleep.

Another popular nervine is **Chamomile**. Chamomile has mild sedative properties that soothe the nervous system, alleviate anxiety, and promote relaxation without causing drowsiness. It is ideal for managing daily stress and anxiety and can be consumed as a calming tea or applied topically in the form of essential oil for aromatherapy.

Lemon Balm is another excellent nervine herb that calms the mind, reduces nervousness, and alleviates symptoms of mild to moderate anxiety. It is often combined with other calming herbs like Chamomile and Lavender to create a powerful, relaxing blend. Lemon Balm tea can be enjoyed throughout the day to maintain emotional balance and reduce stress.

For those dealing with adrenal fatigue and stress-related exhaustion, **Licorice Root** can provide support. Licorice Root is an adaptogen that helps maintain healthy cortisol levels and supports adrenal gland function, making it ideal for those who experience burnout and chronic stress. However, Licorice Root should be used with caution, as it can raise blood pressure in some individuals.

Finally, **Skullcap** is a nervine that helps to calm frazzled nerves, reduce tension, and alleviate stress-induced headaches. Skullcap is particularly beneficial for those who experience anxiety-related muscle tension and spasms. It can be taken as a tea or tincture to promote relaxation and reduce physical tension.

Relaxation Techniques with Herbal Support

Incorporating relaxation techniques into a daily routine is essential for managing stress and promoting mental and emotional well-being. When paired with herbal remedies, these practices can be even more effective at reducing anxiety, calming the mind, and enhancing overall resilience to stress.

One of the most accessible and effective relaxation techniques is **deep breathing**. Deep breathing activates the parasympathetic nervous system, which counteracts the "fight or flight" response triggered by stress. To enhance this practice, use **Lavender Essential Oil**. Lavender has calming and anxiolytic properties that reduce anxiety and promote relaxation. Add a few drops of Lavender essential oil to a diffuser or inhale directly before beginning a deep breathing session. This combination can quickly calm the mind and promote a sense of peace.

Meditation is another powerful tool for reducing stress and anxiety. Pairing meditation with adaptogenic herbs such as **Holy Basil Tea** can deepen the practice by calming the mind and reducing mental chatter. To create a meditative atmosphere, prepare a cup of Holy Basil tea, find a quiet space, and focus on your breathing. Allow the calming effects of the tea to permeate your body, helping you enter a state of calm focus.

For those who prefer physical activity to release stress, **yoga** is an excellent choice. Yoga combines physical postures, breathwork, and meditation to promote relaxation and reduce anxiety. Drinking a cup of **Ashwagandha and Lemon Balm Tea** before or after a yoga session can enhance the relaxing effects of the practice, reduce muscle tension, and support overall mental balance.

For individuals who experience difficulty sleeping due to stress, creating a bedtime ritual with calming herbs can promote restful sleep and alleviate anxiety. Start by preparing a **Chamomile and Passionflower Sleep Tea** to relax the mind and body. Then, take a warm bath infused with **Lavender and Epsom Salt**. The Epsom salts relax tense muscles, while Lavender reduces stress and promotes sleep. After the bath, engage in a brief meditation or journaling session to release any lingering thoughts before bed. This combination of herbal support and calming practices can greatly improve sleep quality and reduce nighttime anxiety.

Another effective relaxation technique is **aromatherapy**. Essential oils like **Lavender, Chamomile, and Bergamot** can be used in a diffuser or applied topically (diluted in a carrier oil) to calm the mind, reduce anxiety, and create a peaceful atmosphere. For added benefit, pair aromatherapy with an herbal tea blend like **Chamomile, Lemon Balm, and Skullcap** to create a multi-sensory relaxation experience that soothes both the body and mind.

For those looking for a creative outlet, **journaling** is an excellent way to process emotions, release mental tension, and gain clarity. Before beginning a journaling session, drink a cup of **Lemon Balm and Skullcap Tea** to reduce anxiety and promote focus. This herbal blend calms the nervous system, allowing for deeper introspection and emotional release during the journaling process.

By combining these herbal remedies and relaxation techniques, individuals can create a personalized stress management plan that addresses their unique needs and enhances overall mental and emotional well-being. This holistic approach not only alleviates symptoms of stress and anxiety but also builds resilience, promotes a sense of balance, and supports long-term health and vitality.

Remedies for Stress Relief

592. Ashwagandha Stress-Reducing Capsules

Ingredients: 1 tablespoon Ashwagandha Root powder, empty gel capsules.
Preparation: Fill empty capsules with Ashwagandha powder and seal.

The Complete Collection of Barbara O'Neill   Jacqueline Bridge

Suggested Usage: Take 1 capsule up to twice daily to reduce stress and enhance resilience.

Benefits: Ashwagandha is an adaptogen that helps lower cortisol levels, reducing stress and anxiety while promoting overall emotional balance.

593. Holy Basil and Lemon Balm Calming Tea

Ingredients: 1 tablespoon dried Holy Basil leaves, 1 tablespoon dried Lemon Balm leaves, 2 cups hot water.

Preparation: Steep Holy Basil and Lemon Balm in hot water for 15 minutes. Strain and serve warm.

Suggested Usage: Drink 1 cup up to twice daily to promote relaxation and reduce anxiety.

Benefits: Holy Basil and Lemon Balm calm the nervous system, reduce anxiety, and balance the stress response, making this tea ideal for reducing tension and promoting a sense of calm.

594. Chamomile and Lavender Sleep Support Elixir

Ingredients: 1 tablespoon dried Chamomile flowers, 1 teaspoon dried Lavender flowers, 2 cups hot water.

Preparation: Steep Chamomile and Lavender in hot water for 15 minutes. Strain and serve warm.

Suggested Usage: Drink 1 cup before bedtime to promote restful sleep and reduce nighttime anxiety.

Benefits: Chamomile and Lavender have mild sedative properties that calm the nervous system, reduce anxiety, and promote restful sleep, making this elixir ideal for managing insomnia and anxiety.

595. Passionflower and Skullcap Anxiety-Relief Tincture

Ingredients: 1 tablespoon dried Passionflower, 1 tablespoon dried Skullcap, 1 cup vodka or brandy.

Preparation: Combine herbs and alcohol in a glass jar. Seal tightly and let steep for 4-6 weeks, shaking occasionally. Strain and store in a dark glass bottle.

Suggested Usage: Take ½ teaspoon up to twice daily to reduce anxiety and promote relaxation.

Benefits: Passionflower and Skullcap calm the nervous system, reduce anxiety, and promote emotional balance, making this tincture ideal for managing stress-induced anxiety.

596. Reishi and Schisandra Adaptogenic Tonic

Ingredients: 1 tablespoon dried Reishi Mushroom, 1 tablespoon dried Schisandra Berries, 2 cups hot water.

Preparation: Simmer Reishi and Schisandra in hot water for 20 minutes. Strain and serve warm.

Suggested Usage: Drink 1 cup daily to enhance resilience and support immune health.

Benefits: Reishi and Schisandra are adaptogens that balance the body's stress response, support adrenal health, and promote overall emotional stability, making this tonic ideal for enhancing resilience to stress.

266

597. Lemon Balm and Valerian Anti-Anxiety Tea

Ingredients: 1 tablespoon dried Lemon Balm leaves, 1 teaspoon dried Valerian Root, 2 cups hot water.
Preparation: Steep Lemon Balm and Valerian in hot water for 15 minutes. Strain and serve warm.
Suggested Usage: Drink 1 cup up to twice daily to reduce anxiety and promote relaxation.
Benefits: Lemon Balm and Valerian calm the nervous system, reduce nervous tension, and alleviate symptoms of mild to moderate anxiety, making this tea effective for managing daily stress.

598. Tulsi and Rhodiola Adrenal Support Capsules

Ingredients: 1 tablespoon Tulsi (Holy Basil) powder, 1 tablespoon Rhodiola Root powder, empty gel capsules.
Preparation: Mix Tulsi and Rhodiola powders thoroughly. Fill empty capsules with the mixture and seal.
Suggested Usage: Take 1 capsule up to twice daily to support adrenal health and reduce stress.
Benefits: Tulsi and Rhodiola enhance the body's stress response, reduce fatigue, and support adrenal health, making these capsules ideal for reducing stress-induced exhaustion.

599. Ginger and Chamomile Digestive Calming Tea

Ingredients: 1 tablespoon dried Chamomile flowers, 1 teaspoon grated fresh Ginger, 2 cups hot water.
Preparation: Steep Chamomile and Ginger in hot water for 15 minutes. Strain and serve warm.
Suggested Usage: Drink 1 cup up to twice daily to reduce digestive discomfort and promote relaxation.
Benefits: Chamomile and Ginger soothe the digestive tract, reduce nausea, and alleviate stress-related digestive symptoms, making this tea ideal for promoting digestive and emotional balance.

600. Skullcap and Lemon Balm Nervine Capsules

Ingredients: 1 tablespoon Skullcap powder, 1 tablespoon Lemon Balm powder, empty gel capsules.
Preparation: Mix Skullcap and Lemon Balm powders thoroughly. Fill empty capsules with the mixture and seal.
Suggested Usage: Take 1 capsule daily to reduce nervous tension and promote relaxation.
Benefits: Skullcap and Lemon Balm are nervines that calm the nervous system, reduce anxiety, and promote emotional stability, making these capsules ideal for managing stress and anxiety.

601. Holy Basil and Ashwagandha Stress-Balancing Capsules

Ingredients: 1 tablespoon Holy Basil powder, 1 tablespoon Ashwagandha powder, empty gel capsules.
Preparation: Mix Holy Basil and Ashwagandha powders thoroughly. Fill empty capsules and seal.
Suggested Usage: Take 1 capsule up to

twice daily to reduce stress and enhance resilience.

Benefits: Holy Basil and Ashwagandha are adaptogens that support adrenal health, balance the stress response, and promote overall well-being, making these capsules ideal for reducing stress and enhancing emotional stability.

602. Lavender and Lemon Balm Relaxation Tea

Ingredients: 1 tablespoon dried Lavender flowers, 1 tablespoon dried Lemon Balm leaves, 2 cups hot water.
Preparation: Steep Lavender and Lemon Balm in hot water for 15 minutes. Strain and serve warm.
Suggested Usage: Drink 1 cup up to twice daily to promote relaxation and reduce anxiety.
Benefits: Lavender and Lemon Balm calm the nervous system, reduce anxiety, and promote relaxation, making this tea ideal for managing stress and enhancing mental clarity.

603. Passionflower and Valerian Bedtime Tea

Ingredients: 1 tablespoon dried Passionflower, 1 teaspoon dried Valerian Root, 2 cups hot water.
Preparation: Steep Passionflower and Valerian in hot water for 15 minutes. Strain and serve warm.
Suggested Usage: Drink 1 cup before bedtime to promote restful sleep and reduce nighttime anxiety.
Benefits: Passionflower and Valerian reduce anxiety, calm the nervous system, and promote restful sleep, making this tea

ideal for managing insomnia and anxiety-induced sleep disturbances.

604. Skullcap and Oatstraw Nerve Tonic

Ingredients: 1 tablespoon dried Skullcap, 1 tablespoon dried Oatstraw, 2 cups hot water.
Preparation: Steep Skullcap and Oatstraw in hot water for 15 minutes. Strain and serve warm.
Suggested Usage: Drink 1 cup daily to calm the nervous system and reduce tension.
Benefits: Skullcap and Oatstraw are nervines that promote emotional balance, reduce anxiety, and nourish the nervous system, making this tonic ideal for managing stress and promoting a sense of calm.

605. Chamomile, Lavender, and Skullcap Bedtime Elixir

Ingredients: 1 tablespoon dried Chamomile flowers, 1 teaspoon dried Lavender flowers, 1 teaspoon dried Skullcap, 2 cups hot water.
Preparation: Steep Chamomile, Lavender, and Skullcap in hot water for 15 minutes. Strain and serve warm.
Suggested Usage: Drink 1 cup before bedtime to promote restful sleep and reduce nighttime anxiety.
Benefits: Chamomile, Lavender, and Skullcap are calming herbs that promote relaxation and reduce anxiety, making this elixir ideal for managing insomnia and nighttime restlessness.

606. Lemon Balm and Ginger Digestive Ease Tea

Ingredients: 1 tablespoon dried Lemon Balm leaves, 1 teaspoon grated fresh Ginger, 2 cups hot water.
Preparation: Steep Lemon Balm and Ginger in hot water for 15 minutes. Strain and serve warm.
Suggested Usage: Drink 1 cup up to twice daily to alleviate digestive discomfort and reduce bloating.
Benefits: Lemon Balm and Ginger soothe the digestive tract, reduce gas, and promote healthy digestion, making this tea effective for managing stress-related digestive issues.

607. Reishi and Rhodiola Immune-Enhancing Capsules

Ingredients: 1 tablespoon Reishi Mushroom powder, 1 tablespoon Rhodiola Root powder, empty gel capsules.
Preparation: Mix Reishi and Rhodiola powders thoroughly. Fill empty capsules and seal.
Suggested Usage: Take 1 capsule daily to support immune function and enhance resilience.
Benefits: Reishi and Rhodiola are adaptogens that support immune health, balance the body's stress response, and promote overall vitality, making these capsules ideal for reducing stress and enhancing immune resilience.

608. Lavender and Holy Basil Stress Relief Capsules

Ingredients: 1 tablespoon dried Lavender powder, 1 tablespoon Holy Basil powder, empty gel capsules.
Preparation: Mix Lavender and Holy Basil powders thoroughly. Fill empty capsules and seal.
Suggested Usage: Take 1 capsule daily to reduce anxiety and promote relaxation.
Benefits: Lavender and Holy Basil calm the nervous system, balance the stress response, and promote emotional stability, making these capsules ideal for managing daily stress.

609. Lemon Balm and Peppermint Nervous Tension Tea

Ingredients: 1 tablespoon dried Lemon Balm leaves, 1 tablespoon dried Peppermint leaves, 2 cups hot water.
Preparation: Steep Lemon Balm and Peppermint in hot water for 15 minutes. Strain and serve warm.
Suggested Usage: Drink 1 cup up to twice daily to reduce nervous tension and promote relaxation.
Benefits: Lemon Balm and Peppermint calm the nervous system, reduce anxiety, and alleviate digestive tension, making this tea ideal for managing stress and promoting mental clarity.

610. Valerian and Skullcap Nerve-Calming Capsules

Ingredients: 1 tablespoon Valerian Root powder, 1 tablespoon Skullcap powder, empty gel capsules.
Preparation: Mix Valerian and Skullcap powders thoroughly. Fill empty capsules and seal.
Suggested Usage: Take 1 capsule daily to

reduce anxiety and promote relaxation.

Benefits: Valerian and Skullcap are nervines that calm the nervous system, reduce stress, and promote restful sleep, making these capsules ideal for managing anxiety and tension.

611. Oatstraw and Chamomile Relaxation Tea

Ingredients: 1 tablespoon dried Oatstraw, 1 tablespoon dried Chamomile flowers, 2 cups hot water.

Preparation: Steep Oatstraw and Chamomile in hot water for 15 minutes. Strain and serve warm.

Suggested Usage: Drink 1 cup up to twice daily to promote relaxation and reduce stress.

Benefits: Oatstraw and Chamomile nourish the nervous system, reduce anxiety, and promote relaxation, making this tea ideal for managing stress and enhancing emotional stability.

612. Rhodiola and Ginseng Energy Support Capsules

Ingredients: 1 tablespoon Rhodiola Root powder, 1 tablespoon Ginseng Root powder, empty gel capsules.

Preparation: Mix Rhodiola and Ginseng powders thoroughly. Fill empty capsules and seal.

Suggested Usage: Take 1 capsule daily to support energy levels and reduce fatigue.

Benefits: Rhodiola and Ginseng are adaptogens that enhance physical and mental energy, reduce stress-induced fatigue, and promote resilience, making these capsules ideal for managing energy levels during stressful periods.

613. Chamomile and Ginger Calming Tonic

Ingredients: 1 tablespoon dried Chamomile flowers, 1 teaspoon grated fresh Ginger, 2 cups hot water.

Preparation: Steep Chamomile and Ginger in hot water for 15 minutes. Strain and serve warm.

Suggested Usage: Drink 1 cup up to twice daily to reduce anxiety and promote relaxation.

Benefits: Chamomile and Ginger calm the nervous system, reduce anxiety, and promote healthy digestion, making this tonic ideal for managing stress-related digestive issues.

614. Passionflower and Lemon Balm Sleep Capsules

Ingredients: 1 tablespoon Passionflower powder, 1 tablespoon Lemon Balm powder, empty gel capsules.

Preparation: Mix Passionflower and Lemon Balm powders thoroughly. Fill empty capsules and seal.

Suggested Usage: Take 1 capsule before bedtime to promote restful sleep and reduce nighttime anxiety.

Benefits: Passionflower and Lemon Balm promote relaxation, reduce anxiety, and support restful sleep, making these capsules ideal for managing insomnia and nighttime anxiety.

615. Schisandra and Ashwagandha Adrenal Support Tonic

Ingredients: 1 tablespoon dried Schisandra Berries, 1 tablespoon dried

Ashwagandha Root, 2 cups hot water.
Preparation: Simmer Schisandra and Ashwagandha in water for 20 minutes. Strain and serve warm.
Suggested Usage: Drink 1 cup daily to support adrenal health and enhance resilience.
Benefits: Schisandra and Ashwagandha are adaptogens that balance the body's stress response, support adrenal function, and promote overall vitality, making this tonic ideal for managing chronic stress.

616. Skullcap and Peppermint Headache Relief Tea

Ingredients: 1 tablespoon dried Skullcap, 1 tablespoon dried Peppermint leaves, 2 cups hot water.
Preparation: Steep Skullcap and Peppermint in hot water for 15 minutes. Strain and serve warm.
Suggested Usage: Drink 1 cup at the onset of a headache or as needed to reduce tension and relieve headaches.
Benefits: Skullcap and Peppermint have antispasmodic and relaxing properties that reduce muscle tension, alleviate headaches, and promote relaxation, making this tea effective for stress-induced headaches.

617. Holy Basil and Reishi Adaptogen Tea

Ingredients: 1 tablespoon dried Holy Basil leaves, 1 tablespoon dried Reishi Mushroom, 2 cups hot water.
Preparation: Steep Holy Basil and Reishi in hot water for 20 minutes. Strain and serve warm.
Suggested Usage: Drink 1 cup up to twice daily to reduce stress and support immune function.
Benefits: Holy Basil and Reishi balance the body's stress response, reduce anxiety, and support adrenal health, making this tea ideal for managing chronic stress and enhancing resilience.

618. Lemon Balm, Chamomile, and Lavender Calm Elixir

Ingredients: 1 tablespoon dried Lemon Balm leaves, 1 tablespoon dried Chamomile flowers, 1 teaspoon dried Lavender flowers, 2 cups hot water.
Preparation: Steep Lemon Balm, Chamomile, and Lavender in hot water for 15 minutes. Strain and serve warm.
Suggested Usage: Drink 1 cup up to twice daily to reduce anxiety and promote relaxation.
Benefits: Lemon Balm, Chamomile, and Lavender calm the nervous system, promote emotional stability, and reduce anxiety, making this elixir ideal for managing stress and enhancing emotional balance.

619. Ashwagandha and Valerian Root Nerve-Soothing Tea

Ingredients: 1 tablespoon dried Ashwagandha Root, 1 teaspoon dried Valerian Root, 2 cups hot water.
Preparation: Simmer Ashwagandha and Valerian in hot water for 15 minutes. Strain and serve warm.
Suggested Usage: Drink 1 cup before bedtime to reduce anxiety and promote restful sleep.
Benefits: Ashwagandha and Valerian reduce anxiety, calm the nervous system,

and promote restful sleep, making this tea ideal for managing stress and anxiety-induced sleep disturbances.

620. Licorice and Holy Basil Adrenal Support Capsules

Ingredients: 1 tablespoon Licorice Root powder, 1 tablespoon Holy Basil powder, empty gel capsules.
Preparation: Mix Licorice and Holy Basil powders thoroughly. Fill empty capsules and seal.
Suggested Usage: Take 1 capsule daily to support adrenal health and reduce stress.
Benefits: Licorice and Holy Basil balance the body's stress response, support adrenal health, and promote emotional stability, making these capsules ideal for managing adrenal fatigue and chronic stress.

621. Schisandra and Rhodiola Adaptogenic Tea

Ingredients: 1 tablespoon dried Schisandra Berries, 1 tablespoon Rhodiola Root, 2 cups hot water.
Preparation: Simmer Schisandra and Rhodiola in water for 15 minutes. Strain and serve warm.
Suggested Usage: Drink 1 cup daily to enhance resilience and reduce stress-induced fatigue.
Benefits: Schisandra and Rhodiola are adaptogens that support energy levels, reduce mental and physical fatigue, and promote emotional balance, making this tea ideal for managing stress and enhancing vitality.

622. Skullcap and Lemon Balm Anti-Anxiety Capsules

Ingredients: 1 tablespoon Skullcap powder, 1 tablespoon Lemon Balm powder, empty gel capsules.
Preparation: Mix Skullcap and Lemon Balm powders thoroughly. Fill empty capsules and seal.
Suggested Usage: Take 1 capsule up to twice daily to reduce anxiety and promote relaxation.
Benefits: Skullcap and Lemon Balm are nervines that calm the nervous system, reduce anxiety, and promote emotional stability, making these capsules ideal for managing stress and anxiety.

623. Chamomile and Lavender Nighttime Tea

Ingredients: 1 tablespoon dried Chamomile flowers, 1 teaspoon dried Lavender flowers, 2 cups hot water.
Preparation: Steep Chamomile and Lavender in hot water for 15 minutes. Strain and serve warm.
Suggested Usage: Drink 1 cup before bedtime to promote restful sleep and reduce nighttime anxiety.
Benefits: Chamomile and Lavender calm the nervous system, reduce anxiety, and promote restful sleep, making this tea ideal for managing nighttime anxiety and promoting a good night's sleep.

624. Ashwagandha and Rhodiola Anti-Stress Capsules

Ingredients: 1 tablespoon Ashwagandha Root powder, 1 tablespoon Rhodiola Root

powder, empty gel capsules.

Preparation: Mix Ashwagandha and Rhodiola powders thoroughly. Fill empty capsules and seal.

Suggested Usage: Take 1 capsule daily to reduce stress and enhance resilience.

Benefits: Ashwagandha and Rhodiola balance the body's stress response, reduce anxiety, and enhance energy levels, making these capsules ideal for managing chronic stress and fatigue.

625. Chamomile and Lemon Balm Emotional Balance Tea

Ingredients: 1 tablespoon dried Chamomile flowers, 1 tablespoon dried Lemon Balm leaves, 2 cups hot water.

Preparation: Steep Chamomile and Lemon Balm in hot water for 15 minutes. Strain and serve warm.

Suggested Usage: Drink 1 cup up to twice daily to promote emotional balance and reduce anxiety.

Benefits: Chamomile and Lemon Balm calm the nervous system, reduce anxiety, and promote emotional stability, making this tea ideal for managing stress and supporting mental wellness.

626. Skullcap and Passionflower Nervous System Tonic

Ingredients: 1 tablespoon dried Skullcap, 1 tablespoon dried Passionflower, 2 cups hot water.

Preparation: Steep Skullcap and Passionflower in hot water for 15 minutes. Strain and serve warm.

Suggested Usage: Drink 1 cup daily to calm the nervous system and reduce anxiety.

Benefits: Skullcap and Passionflower reduce anxiety, promote relaxation, and support the nervous system, making this tonic ideal for managing stress and anxiety-induced nervous tension.

627. Holy Basil and Ashwagandha Adaptogen Tonic

Ingredients: 1 tablespoon dried Holy Basil leaves, 1 tablespoon Ashwagandha Root, 2 cups hot water.

Preparation: Simmer Holy Basil and Ashwagandha in hot water for 15 minutes. Strain and serve warm.

Suggested Usage: Drink 1 cup up to twice daily to enhance resilience and reduce stress.

Benefits: Holy Basil and Ashwagandha are adaptogens that balance the body's stress response, reduce anxiety, and promote overall vitality, making this tonic ideal for managing chronic stress.

628. Passionflower and Hops Relaxation Elixir

Ingredients: 1 tablespoon dried Passionflower, 1 tablespoon dried Hops, 2 cups hot water.

Preparation: Steep Passionflower and Hops in hot water for 15 minutes. Strain and serve warm.

Suggested Usage: Drink 1 cup before bedtime to reduce anxiety and promote restful sleep.

Benefits: Passionflower and Hops are calming herbs that promote relaxation and support restful sleep, making this elixir ideal for managing insomnia and nighttime anxiety.

629. Chamomile and Lemon Balm Soothing Tea

Ingredients: 1 tablespoon dried Chamomile flowers, 1 tablespoon dried Lemon Balm leaves, 2 cups hot water.
Preparation: Steep Chamomile and Lemon Balm in hot water for 15 minutes. Strain and serve warm.
Suggested Usage: Drink 1 cup up to twice daily to promote relaxation and reduce anxiety.
Benefits: Chamomile and Lemon Balm are calming herbs that soothe the nervous system, reduce stress, and promote emotional balance, making this tea ideal for managing daily anxiety and stress.

630. Oatstraw and Holy Basil Stress Relief Tea

Ingredients: 1 tablespoon dried Oatstraw, 1 tablespoon dried Holy Basil leaves, 2 cups hot water.
Preparation: Steep Oatstraw and Holy Basil in hot water for 15 minutes. Strain and serve warm.
Suggested Usage: Drink 1 cup up to twice daily to reduce stress and support adrenal health.
Benefits: Oatstraw and Holy Basil nourish the nervous system, balance the body's stress response, and reduce anxiety, making this tea ideal for managing chronic stress and enhancing mental well-being.

631. Lavender and Passionflower Calm-Enhancing Capsules

Ingredients: 1 tablespoon Lavender powder, 1 tablespoon Passionflower powder, empty gel capsules.
Preparation: Mix Lavender and Passionflower powders thoroughly. Fill empty capsules and seal.
Suggested Usage: Take 1 capsule up to twice daily to reduce anxiety and promote relaxation.
Benefits: Lavender and Passionflower calm the nervous system, reduce anxiety, and promote emotional stability, making these capsules ideal for managing stress and supporting mental calmness.

632. Ashwagandha and Reishi Stress-Balancing Capsules

Ingredients: 1 tablespoon Ashwagandha powder, 1 tablespoon Reishi Mushroom powder, empty gel capsules.
Preparation: Mix Ashwagandha and Reishi powders thoroughly. Fill empty capsules and seal.
Suggested Usage: Take 1 capsule daily to reduce stress and support immune health.
Benefits: Ashwagandha and Reishi are adaptogens that enhance the body's ability to cope with stress, support adrenal function, and boost immune resilience, making these capsules ideal for managing stress and fatigue.

633. Lemon Balm and Skullcap Nerve Support Capsules

Ingredients: 1 tablespoon Lemon Balm powder, 1 tablespoon Skullcap powder, empty gel capsules.
Preparation: Mix Lemon Balm and Skullcap powders thoroughly. Fill empty capsules and seal.
Suggested Usage: Take 1 capsule up to twice daily to reduce anxiety and support

the nervous system.

Benefits: Lemon Balm and Skullcap calm the nervous system, reduce nervous tension, and promote emotional balance, making these capsules ideal for managing stress and anxiety-related symptoms.

634. Passionflower, Skullcap, and Valerian Sleep Tea

Ingredients: 1 tablespoon dried Passionflower, 1 tablespoon dried Skullcap, 1 teaspoon dried Valerian Root, 2 cups hot water.

Preparation: Steep Passionflower, Skullcap, and Valerian in hot water for 15 minutes. Strain and serve warm.

Suggested Usage: Drink 1 cup before bedtime to promote restful sleep and reduce anxiety.

Benefits: Passionflower, Skullcap, and Valerian calm the nervous system, reduce anxiety, and promote restful sleep, making this tea ideal for managing insomnia and nighttime anxiety.

635. Reishi and Schisandra Adaptogenic Tea

Ingredients: 1 tablespoon dried Reishi Mushroom, 1 tablespoon dried Schisandra Berries, 2 cups hot water.

Preparation: Simmer Reishi and Schisandra in water for 20 minutes. Strain and serve warm.

Suggested Usage: Drink 1 cup daily to reduce stress and enhance resilience.

Benefits: Reishi and Schisandra are adaptogenic herbs that balance the body's stress response, support adrenal health, and promote overall vitality, making this tea ideal for managing chronic stress and enhancing mental well-being.

636. Lemon Balm and Valerian Nerve-Soothing Capsules

Ingredients: 1 tablespoon Lemon Balm powder, 1 tablespoon Valerian Root powder, empty gel capsules.

Preparation: Mix Lemon Balm and Valerian powders thoroughly. Fill empty capsules and seal.

Suggested Usage: Take 1 capsule up to twice daily to reduce anxiety and promote relaxation.

Benefits: Lemon Balm and Valerian calm the nervous system, reduce nervous tension, and promote restful sleep, making these capsules ideal for managing anxiety and insomnia.

637. Lavender and Holy Basil Relaxation Capsules

Ingredients: 1 tablespoon Lavender powder, 1 tablespoon Holy Basil powder, empty gel capsules.

Preparation: Mix Lavender and Holy Basil powders thoroughly. Fill empty capsules and seal.

Suggested Usage: Take 1 capsule up to twice daily to reduce stress and promote relaxation.

Benefits: Lavender and Holy Basil calm the nervous system, reduce stress, and promote emotional stability, making these capsules ideal for managing daily anxiety and enhancing mental clarity.

638. Skullcap and Chamomile Emotional Balance Tea

Ingredients: 1 tablespoon dried Skullcap, 1 tablespoon dried Chamomile flowers, 2 cups hot water.

Preparation: Steep Skullcap and Chamomile in hot water for 15 minutes. Strain and serve warm.

Suggested Usage: Drink 1 cup up to twice daily to promote emotional balance and reduce stress.

Benefits: Skullcap and Chamomile calm the nervous system, reduce anxiety, and promote emotional stability, making this tea ideal for managing stress and supporting mental clarity.

639. Rhodiola and Schisandra Adaptogen Elixir

Ingredients: 1 tablespoon dried Rhodiola Root, 1 tablespoon dried Schisandra Berries, 2 cups hot water.

Preparation: Simmer Rhodiola and Schisandra in water for 20 minutes. Strain and serve warm.

Suggested Usage: Drink 1 cup daily to enhance resilience and reduce fatigue.

Benefits: Rhodiola and Schisandra are adaptogens that enhance energy levels, reduce stress-induced fatigue, and support adrenal health, making this elixir ideal for managing chronic stress and fatigue.

640. Chamomile, Lemon Balm, and Holy Basil Tea

Ingredients: 1 tablespoon dried Chamomile flowers, 1 tablespoon dried Lemon Balm leaves, 1 tablespoon dried Holy Basil leaves, 2 cups hot water.

Preparation: Steep Chamomile, Lemon Balm, and Holy Basil in hot water for 15 minutes. Strain and serve warm.

Suggested Usage: Drink 1 cup up to twice daily to reduce stress and promote emotional balance.

Benefits: Chamomile, Lemon Balm, and Holy Basil calm the nervous system, reduce anxiety, and promote emotional stability, making this tea ideal for managing daily stress and enhancing mental clarity.

641. Lavender and Skullcap Anti-Anxiety Capsules

Ingredients: 1 tablespoon Lavender powder, 1 tablespoon Skullcap powder, empty gel capsules.

Preparation: Mix Lavender and Skullcap powders thoroughly. Fill empty capsules and seal.

Suggested Usage: Take 1 capsule up to twice daily to reduce anxiety and promote relaxation.

Benefits: Lavender and Skullcap are calming herbs that reduce anxiety, promote relaxation, and support emotional stability, making these capsules ideal for managing stress and promoting mental well-being.

Book 32: Herbs for Anxiety and Depression

Managing anxiety and depression can be challenging, and many people seek natural solutions that provide relief without the side effects associated with pharmaceuticals. Herbs have been used for centuries to support mental health, enhance mood, and promote emotional stability. These plant allies work through various mechanisms, such as modulating neurotransmitters, balancing hormones, and reducing inflammation. In this chapter, we explore some of the most effective herbs for managing anxiety and depression, along with specific herbal blends designed to support emotional balance and overall well-being.

Natural Treatments for Mood Disorders

Herbs that support mood balance can be divided into three main categories: adaptogens, nervines, and antidepressant herbs. **Adaptogens** help the body adapt to stress, regulate the hormonal response, and support adrenal function, which is crucial for maintaining mental and physical energy. **Nervines** specifically target the nervous system, promoting relaxation, reducing anxiety, and enhancing resilience to emotional stress. Finally, **antidepressant herbs** work by balancing neurotransmitters, such as serotonin and dopamine, which are essential for regulating mood and emotional health.

One of the most well-known herbs for managing anxiety and mild depression is **St. John's Wort**. This herb has been extensively studied for its antidepressant effects and is often used as a natural alternative to conventional antidepressants. St. John's Wort works by increasing serotonin, dopamine, and norepinephrine levels in the brain, which can elevate mood and improve emotional stability. However, it is essential to use St. John's Wort with caution, as it can interact with certain medications, such as SSRIs and oral contraceptives.

Another powerful herb for emotional balance is **Rhodiola Rosea**. Rhodiola is an adaptogen that enhances the body's resistance to stress, reduces mental fatigue, and promotes a balanced mood. It works by modulating the activity of neurotransmitters like serotonin and dopamine, making it particularly useful for individuals experiencing stress-induced anxiety and depression. Rhodiola is best used in the morning, as it can be stimulating for some people.

Ashwagandha is another adaptogen with profound effects on anxiety and depression. It lowers cortisol levels, reduces stress, and supports adrenal health, making it ideal for individuals with anxiety related to chronic stress or adrenal fatigue. Ashwagandha also has a mild mood-boosting effect and can enhance overall emotional resilience. It can be taken in the form of capsules, tinctures, or as a tea for long-term support.

For those dealing with anxiety, **Passionflower** is an excellent choice. Passionflower is a nervine that calms the nervous system, reduces anxiety, and promotes relaxation without causing drowsiness. It works by increasing the levels of gamma-aminobutyric acid (GABA) in the brain, a neurotransmitter that inhibits overactivity and promotes a sense of calm. Passionflower can be taken as a tea, tincture, or in capsule form, especially before bedtime to reduce nighttime anxiety.

Lavender is another powerful nervine herb known for its calming and anxiolytic properties. Studies have shown that Lavender essential oil is effective at reducing symptoms of anxiety and improving sleep quality. Lavender can be used in various forms, including aromatherapy, teas, and topical applications, making it a versatile option for managing anxiety and stress.

For individuals with mild to moderate depression, **Saffron** can be highly effective. Saffron has been shown to increase serotonin and dopamine levels, thereby elevating mood and reducing depressive symptoms. It is particularly beneficial for those experiencing seasonal affective disorder (SAD) or mood imbalances related to hormonal changes. Saffron can be taken as a supplement or added to culinary dishes for daily support.

Another herb that supports emotional balance is **Lemon Balm**. Lemon Balm is a gentle nervine that reduces anxiety, promotes relaxation, and enhances cognitive function. It can be used alone or combined with other calming herbs like Chamomile or Lavender to create soothing teas or tinctures that support emotional stability.

Holy Basil, or Tulsi, is an adaptogen and nervine that supports the nervous system, reduces anxiety, and enhances resilience to stress. Holy Basil is particularly useful for individuals who experience mood imbalances due to chronic stress or adrenal fatigue. It can be taken as a tea, tincture, or in capsule form to promote emotional balance and support mental clarity.

Herbal Blends for Emotional Balance

Creating herbal blends that target anxiety and depression can enhance the effectiveness of each herb by combining their unique properties. The following are some specific blends designed to promote emotional stability and support mental well-being:

Calm Mind Tea: This soothing blend combines Lemon Balm, Chamomile, and Skullcap to reduce anxiety and promote relaxation. Lemon Balm calms the nervous system, Chamomile reduces anxiety and promotes a gentle sense of peace, and Skullcap supports emotional stability by reducing nervous tension. This tea can be enjoyed throughout the day or before bedtime to enhance relaxation and reduce anxiety-related symptoms.

Mood-Lifting Elixir: Combining St. John's Wort, Rhodiola, and Saffron creates a powerful mood-enhancing blend that supports neurotransmitter balance and reduces symptoms of depression. St. John's Wort elevates serotonin and dopamine levels, Rhodiola reduces fatigue and stress, and Saffron enhances mood and promotes emotional well-being. This elixir can be taken daily to manage mild to moderate depression and support emotional balance.

Stress Relief Capsules: A combination of Ashwagandha, Holy Basil, and Reishi Mushroom works synergistically to balance the stress response, support adrenal health, and enhance resilience. Ashwagandha reduces cortisol levels and supports emotional balance, Holy Basil calms the nervous system and enhances mental clarity, and Reishi promotes immune health and overall vitality. This blend is ideal for those dealing with chronic stress and stress-induced anxiety.

Sleep Support Tea: Passionflower, Valerian Root, and Lavender combine to create a powerful sleep-promoting tea that reduces nighttime anxiety and enhances restful sleep. Passionflower increases GABA levels in the brain, Valerian reduces anxiety and promotes relaxation, and Lavender enhances sleep quality and reduces stress. This tea is best consumed 30-60 minutes before bedtime to promote restful and uninterrupted sleep.

Emotional Balance Tincture: This blend of Skullcap, Lemon Balm, and Holy Basil creates a soothing tincture that calms the mind, reduces anxiety, and enhances resilience. Skullcap and Lemon Balm reduce nervous tension, while Holy Basil balances the body's stress response, making this tincture ideal for managing emotional instability and enhancing mental clarity.

Nervine Elixir: Combine Chamomile, Passionflower, and Lavender to create a calming nervine elixir that promotes relaxation, reduces anxiety, and supports restful sleep. Chamomile and Lavender soothe the nervous system, while Passionflower promotes relaxation and reduces anxiety, making this elixir ideal for managing daily stress and supporting restful sleep.

Adaptogenic Tea for Resilience: A blend of Rhodiola, Holy Basil, and Schisandra enhances the body's ability to cope with stress, balances mood, and promotes emotional resilience. Rhodiola reduces stress and mental fatigue, Holy Basil supports adrenal health and mental clarity, and Schisandra enhances resilience to both physical and emotional stressors, making this tea an excellent choice for those looking to build overall mental and emotional strength.

Each of these herbal combinations offers a unique approach to managing anxiety and depression. By selecting herbs that complement each other, these blends not only address the symptoms but also target the underlying causes of mood imbalances. When combined with lifestyle modifications, such as regular exercise, adequate sleep, and mindfulness practices, these herbal solutions can play a significant role in supporting mental and emotional well-being.

Remedies for Anxiety and Depression

642. St. John's Wort Mood-Lifting Capsules

Ingredients: 1 tablespoon St. John's Wort powder, empty gel capsules.
Preparation: Fill empty capsules with St. John's Wort powder and seal.
Suggested Usage: Take 1 capsule up to twice daily to improve mood and reduce depressive symptoms.
Benefits: St. John's Wort increases serotonin and dopamine levels, promoting emotional stability and reducing symptoms of mild to moderate depression.

643. Lemon Balm and Lavender Calming Tea

Ingredients: 1 tablespoon dried Lemon Balm leaves, 1 teaspoon dried Lavender flowers, 2 cups hot water.
Preparation: Steep Lemon Balm and Lavender in hot water for 15 minutes. Strain and serve warm.
Suggested Usage: Drink 1 cup up to twice daily to reduce anxiety and promote relaxation.
Benefits: Lemon Balm and Lavender calm the nervous system, reduce anxiety, and promote a sense of peace, making this tea ideal for managing stress and enhancing emotional well-being.

644. Holy Basil and Rhodiola Adaptogenic Elixir

Ingredients: 1 tablespoon dried Holy Basil leaves, 1 tablespoon dried Rhodiola Root, 2 cups hot water.
Preparation: Simmer Holy Basil and Rhodiola in hot water for 15 minutes. Strain and serve warm.
Suggested Usage: Drink 1 cup up to twice daily to support stress management and improve resilience.
Benefits: Holy Basil and Rhodiola balance the body's stress response, reduce mental fatigue, and enhance emotional stability, making this elixir ideal for managing anxiety and stress.

645. Chamomile and Passionflower Sleep Support Tincture

Ingredients: 1 tablespoon dried Chamomile flowers, 1 tablespoon dried Passionflower, 1 cup vodka or brandy.
Preparation: Combine Chamomile and Passionflower in a glass jar. Add alcohol, seal, and let steep for 4-6 weeks, shaking occasionally. Strain and store in a dark bottle.
Suggested Usage: Take ½ teaspoon before bedtime to promote restful sleep and reduce nighttime anxiety.
Benefits: Chamomile and Passionflower calm the nervous system, reduce anxiety, and promote restful sleep, making this tincture effective for managing insomnia and stress-related sleep disturbances.

646. Skullcap and Valerian Nerve-Soothing Capsules

Ingredients: 1 tablespoon Skullcap powder, 1 tablespoon Valerian Root powder, empty gel capsules.
Preparation: Mix Skullcap and Valerian powders thoroughly. Fill empty capsules and seal.
Suggested Usage: Take 1 capsule daily to reduce anxiety and promote relaxation.
Benefits: Skullcap and Valerian calm the nervous system, reduce nervous tension, and promote restful sleep, making these capsules ideal for managing stress-induced anxiety.

647. Ashwagandha and Schisandra Stress Relief Capsules

Ingredients: 1 tablespoon Ashwagandha powder, 1 tablespoon Schisandra Berry powder, empty gel capsules.
Preparation: Mix Ashwagandha and Schisandra powders thoroughly. Fill empty capsules and seal.
Suggested Usage: Take 1 capsule up to twice daily to reduce stress and promote emotional resilience.
Benefits: Ashwagandha and Schisandra are adaptogens that support adrenal health, balance the body's stress response, and promote emotional stability, making these capsules effective for managing chronic stress.

648. Saffron and Lavender Antidepressant Tea

Ingredients: 1 pinch Saffron threads, 1 teaspoon dried Lavender flowers, 2 cups hot water.
Preparation: Steep Saffron and Lavender in hot water for 15 minutes. Strain and serve warm.
Suggested Usage: Drink 1 cup daily to elevate mood and reduce symptoms of mild depression.
Benefits: Saffron and Lavender balance neurotransmitters, reduce anxiety, and promote emotional stability, making this tea effective for managing mood disorders.

649. Reishi and Rhodiola Stress-Balancing Capsules

Ingredients: 1 tablespoon Reishi Mushroom powder, 1 tablespoon Rhodiola Root powder, empty gel capsules.
Preparation: Mix Reishi and Rhodiola powders thoroughly. Fill empty capsules and seal.
Suggested Usage: Take 1 capsule daily to enhance resilience and support emotional stability.
Benefits: Reishi and Rhodiola are adaptogens that reduce stress-induced fatigue, support adrenal health, and enhance overall mental well-being, making these capsules ideal for managing chronic stress.

650. Passionflower and Lemon Balm Anti-Anxiety Tea

Ingredients: 1 tablespoon dried Passionflower, 1 tablespoon dried Lemon Balm, 2 cups hot water.
Preparation: Steep Passionflower and Lemon Balm in hot water for 15 minutes. Strain and serve warm.
Suggested Usage: Drink 1 cup up to twice

daily to reduce anxiety and promote emotional stability.

Benefits: Passionflower and Lemon Balm calm the nervous system, reduce nervous tension, and promote emotional balance, making this tea effective for managing daily stress.

651. Holy Basil and Licorice Adrenal Support Capsules

Ingredients: 1 tablespoon Holy Basil powder, 1 tablespoon Licorice Root powder, empty gel capsules.
Preparation: Mix Holy Basil and Licorice powders thoroughly. Fill empty capsules and seal.
Suggested Usage: Take 1 capsule daily to support adrenal function and balance stress hormones.
Benefits: Holy Basil and Licorice enhance adrenal health, reduce fatigue, and promote emotional stability, making these capsules ideal for managing chronic stress and adrenal fatigue.

652. Skullcap and Hops Bedtime Tincture

Ingredients: 1 tablespoon dried Skullcap, 1 tablespoon dried Hops, 1 cup vodka or brandy.
Preparation: Combine Skullcap and Hops in a glass jar. Add alcohol, seal, and let steep for 4-6 weeks, shaking occasionally. Strain and store in a dark bottle.
Suggested Usage: Take ½ teaspoon before bedtime to promote restful sleep and reduce nighttime anxiety.
Benefits: Skullcap and Hops calm the nervous system, reduce anxiety, and promote deep, restful sleep, making this tincture effective for managing insomnia and nighttime anxiety.

653. Lemon Balm and Peppermint Digestive Ease Tea

Ingredients: 1 tablespoon dried Lemon Balm leaves, 1 tablespoon dried Peppermint leaves, 2 cups hot water.
Preparation: Steep Lemon Balm and Peppermint in hot water for 15 minutes. Strain and serve warm.
Suggested Usage: Drink 1 cup after meals to promote digestion and reduce anxiety-related digestive symptoms.
Benefits: Lemon Balm and Peppermint calm the digestive tract, reduce gas, and promote healthy digestion, making this tea effective for managing stress-related digestive issues.

654. St. John's Wort and Saffron Mood Stabilizing Capsules

Ingredients: 1 tablespoon St. John's Wort powder, 1 tablespoon Saffron powder, empty gel capsules.
Preparation: Mix St. John's Wort and Saffron powders thoroughly. Fill empty capsules and seal.
Suggested Usage: Take 1 capsule daily to enhance mood and reduce depressive symptoms.
Benefits: St. John's Wort and Saffron elevate mood, balance neurotransmitters, and reduce symptoms of mild to moderate depression, making these capsules effective for managing mood disorders naturally.

655. Lavender and Holy Basil Relaxation Capsules

Ingredients: 1 tablespoon dried Lavender powder, 1 tablespoon Holy Basil powder, empty gel capsules.
Preparation: Mix Lavender and Holy Basil powders thoroughly. Fill empty capsules and seal.
Suggested Usage: Take 1 capsule up to twice daily to reduce anxiety and promote relaxation.
Benefits: Lavender and Holy Basil calm the nervous system, reduce anxiety, and promote emotional stability, making these capsules ideal for managing stress and supporting mental calmness.

656. Chamomile and Valerian Sleep-Enhancing Elixir

Ingredients: 1 tablespoon dried Chamomile flowers, 1 teaspoon dried Valerian Root, 1 cup hot water.
Preparation: Steep Chamomile and Valerian in hot water for 15 minutes. Strain and serve warm.
Suggested Usage: Drink 1 cup before bedtime to promote restful sleep and reduce nighttime anxiety.
Benefits: Chamomile and Valerian have mild sedative properties that help calm the mind and promote deep, restful sleep, making this elixir effective for those with insomnia and sleep disturbances.

657. Rhodiola and Ginseng Energy-Boosting Capsules

Ingredients: 1 tablespoon Rhodiola Root powder, 1 tablespoon Ginseng Root powder, empty gel capsules.
Preparation: Mix Rhodiola and Ginseng powders thoroughly. Fill empty capsules and seal.
Suggested Usage: Take 1 capsule daily to enhance energy levels and reduce fatigue.
Benefits: Rhodiola and Ginseng are adaptogens that boost physical and mental energy, reduce stress-induced fatigue, and promote resilience, making these capsules ideal for enhancing vitality during periods of high stress.

658. Lemon Balm and Skullcap Nervine Tonic

Ingredients: 1 tablespoon dried Lemon Balm leaves, 1 tablespoon dried Skullcap, 2 cups hot water.
Preparation: Steep Lemon Balm and Skullcap in hot water for 15 minutes. Strain and serve warm.
Suggested Usage: Drink 1 cup up to twice daily to reduce anxiety and promote relaxation.
Benefits: Lemon Balm and Skullcap calm the nervous system, reduce nervous tension, and promote emotional stability, making this tonic ideal for managing daily anxiety and stress.

659. Holy Basil and Ashwagandha Calm Capsules

Ingredients: 1 tablespoon Holy Basil powder, 1 tablespoon Ashwagandha Root powder, empty gel capsules.
Preparation: Mix Holy Basil and Ashwagandha powders thoroughly. Fill empty capsules and seal.
Suggested Usage: Take 1 capsule daily to reduce stress and enhance resilience.

Benefits: Holy Basil and Ashwagandha are adaptogens that balance the body's stress response, reduce anxiety, and promote overall vitality, making these capsules ideal for managing chronic stress and enhancing mental well-being.

660. Chamomile, Lavender, and Skullcap Sleep Tea

Ingredients: 1 tablespoon dried Chamomile flowers, 1 teaspoon dried Lavender flowers, 1 teaspoon dried Skullcap, 2 cups hot water.
Preparation: Steep Chamomile, Lavender, and Skullcap in hot water for 15 minutes. Strain and serve warm.
Suggested Usage: Drink 1 cup before bedtime to promote restful sleep and reduce nighttime anxiety.
Benefits: Chamomile, Lavender, and Skullcap calm the nervous system, reduce anxiety, and promote restful sleep, making this tea ideal for managing insomnia and nighttime stress.

661. St. John's Wort and Rhodiola Depression Relief Elixir

Ingredients: 1 tablespoon dried St. John's Wort, 1 tablespoon dried Rhodiola Root, 1 cup vodka or brandy.
Preparation: Combine herbs and alcohol in a glass jar. Seal tightly and let steep for 4-6 weeks, shaking occasionally. Strain and store in a dark glass bottle.
Suggested Usage: Take ½ teaspoon up to twice daily to reduce depressive symptoms and enhance mood.
Benefits: St. John's Wort and Rhodiola balance neurotransmitters, reduce depressive symptoms, and promote emotional stability, making this elixir ideal for managing mild to moderate depression.

662. Reishi Mushroom and Holy Basil Mood Stabilizing Capsules

Ingredients: 1 tablespoon Reishi Mushroom powder, 1 tablespoon Holy Basil powder, empty gel capsules.
Preparation: Mix Reishi and Holy Basil powders thoroughly. Fill empty capsules and seal.
Suggested Usage: Take 1 capsule daily to enhance emotional balance and support mental resilience.
Benefits: Reishi and Holy Basil calm the nervous system, support adrenal health, and promote emotional stability, making these capsules ideal for managing mood disorders and stress-related anxiety.

663. Passionflower and Lemon Balm Nervine Capsules

Ingredients: 1 tablespoon Passionflower powder, 1 tablespoon Lemon Balm powder, empty gel capsules.
Preparation: Mix Passionflower and Lemon Balm powders thoroughly. Fill empty capsules and seal.
Suggested Usage: Take 1 capsule up to twice daily to reduce anxiety and promote emotional stability.
Benefits: Passionflower and Lemon Balm calm the nervous system, reduce anxiety, and promote a sense of peace, making these capsules ideal for managing stress and supporting emotional balance.

664. Saffron and Licorice Antidepressant Tea

Ingredients: 1 pinch Saffron threads, 1 teaspoon Licorice Root, 2 cups hot water.
Preparation: Steep Saffron and Licorice Root in hot water for 15 minutes. Strain and serve warm.
Suggested Usage: Drink 1 cup daily to elevate mood and reduce depressive symptoms.
Benefits: Saffron and Licorice balance neurotransmitters, reduce anxiety, and promote emotional stability, making this tea effective for managing mild to moderate depression.

665. Skullcap and Oatstraw Nerve Restoring Tincture

Ingredients: 1 tablespoon dried Skullcap, 1 tablespoon dried Oatstraw, 1 cup vodka or brandy.
Preparation: Combine herbs and alcohol in a glass jar. Seal tightly and let steep for 4-6 weeks, shaking occasionally. Strain and store in a dark glass bottle.
Suggested Usage: Take ½ teaspoon up to twice daily to reduce nervous tension and promote emotional stability.
Benefits: Skullcap and Oatstraw support the nervous system, reduce anxiety, and promote emotional stability, making this tincture ideal for managing chronic stress and anxiety.

666. Rhodiola and Holy Basil Stress-Balancing Capsules

Ingredients: 1 tablespoon Rhodiola Root powder, 1 tablespoon Holy Basil powder, empty gel capsules.
Preparation: Mix Rhodiola and Holy Basil powders thoroughly. Fill empty capsules and seal.
Suggested Usage: Take 1 capsule daily to enhance resilience and reduce stress-induced fatigue.
Benefits: Rhodiola and Holy Basil are adaptogens that enhance the body's stress response, reduce fatigue, and promote emotional balance, making these capsules ideal for managing chronic stress and anxiety-induced exhaustion.

667. Lemon Balm and Chamomile Emotional Balance Tea

Ingredients: 1 tablespoon dried Lemon Balm leaves, 1 tablespoon dried Chamomile flowers, 2 cups hot water.
Preparation: Steep Lemon Balm and Chamomile in hot water for 15 minutes. Strain and serve warm.
Suggested Usage: Drink 1 cup up to twice daily to promote emotional stability and reduce anxiety.
Benefits: Lemon Balm and Chamomile calm the nervous system, reduce anxiety, and promote emotional balance, making this tea ideal for managing stress and supporting mental wellness.

668. Valerian and Passionflower Anxiety-Relief Tea

Ingredients: 1 tablespoon dried Valerian Root, 1 tablespoon dried Passionflower, 2 cups hot water.
Preparation: Steep Valerian and Passionflower in hot water for 15 minutes. Strain and serve warm.
Suggested Usage: Drink 1 cup before

bedtime to reduce anxiety and promote restful sleep.

Benefits: Valerian and Passionflower promote relaxation, reduce anxiety, and support restful sleep, making this tea effective for managing anxiety-related sleep disturbances.

669. Chamomile and Skullcap Nervous System Calming Capsules

Ingredients: 1 tablespoon Chamomile powder, 1 tablespoon Skullcap powder, empty gel capsules.
Preparation: Mix Chamomile and Skullcap powders thoroughly. Fill empty capsules and seal.
Suggested Usage: Take 1 capsule daily to reduce nervous tension and promote relaxation.
Benefits: Chamomile and Skullcap calm the nervous system, reduce anxiety, and promote emotional stability, making these capsules ideal for managing stress-induced anxiety.

670. Saffron and St. John's Wort Mood-Enhancing Tea

Ingredients: 1 pinch Saffron threads, 1 tablespoon dried St. John's Wort, 2 cups hot water.
Preparation: Steep Saffron and St. John's Wort in hot water for 15 minutes. Strain and serve warm.
Suggested Usage: Drink 1 cup daily to improve mood and reduce symptoms of mild depression.
Benefits: Saffron and St. John's Wort elevate mood, balance neurotransmitters, and promote emotional stability, making

this tea effective for managing mild to moderate depression.

671. Holy Basil and Lavender Adaptogen Elixir

Ingredients: 1 tablespoon dried Holy Basil leaves, 1 teaspoon dried Lavender flowers, 2 cups hot water.
Preparation: Steep Holy Basil and Lavender in hot water for 15 minutes. Strain and serve warm.
Suggested Usage: Drink 1 cup up to twice daily to reduce stress and promote relaxation.
Benefits: Holy Basil and Lavender calm the nervous system, balance the body's stress response, and promote emotional stability, making this elixir ideal for managing stress and anxiety.

672. Lemon Balm, Lavender, and Chamomile Bedtime Tea

Ingredients: 1 tablespoon dried Lemon Balm leaves, 1 teaspoon dried Lavender flowers, 1 tablespoon dried Chamomile flowers, 2 cups hot water.
Preparation: Steep Lemon Balm, Lavender, and Chamomile in hot water for 15 minutes. Strain and serve warm.
Suggested Usage: Drink 1 cup before bedtime to promote restful sleep and reduce nighttime anxiety.
Benefits: Lemon Balm, Lavender, and Chamomile calm the nervous system, reduce anxiety, and promote restful sleep, making this tea ideal for managing insomnia and nighttime restlessness.

673. Rhodiola and Schisandra Anti-Stress Tonic

Ingredients: 1 tablespoon dried Rhodiola Root, 1 tablespoon dried Schisandra Berries, 2 cups hot water.
Preparation: Simmer Rhodiola and Schisandra in water for 15 minutes. Strain and serve warm.
Suggested Usage: Drink 1 cup daily to reduce stress and support mental resilience.
Benefits: Rhodiola and Schisandra balance the body's stress response, reduce mental fatigue, and promote emotional stability, making this tonic effective for managing stress and enhancing cognitive function.

674. Passionflower and Valerian Emotional Balance Tea

Ingredients: 1 tablespoon dried Passionflower, 1 teaspoon dried Valerian Root, 2 cups hot water.
Preparation: Steep Passionflower and Valerian in hot water for 15 minutes. Strain and serve warm.
Suggested Usage: Drink 1 cup before bedtime to promote relaxation and reduce anxiety.
Benefits: Passionflower and Valerian reduce anxiety, calm the nervous system, and promote restful sleep, making this tea ideal for managing anxiety-related mood imbalances.

675. Chamomile and Skullcap Anxiety-Soothing Capsules

Ingredients: 1 tablespoon Chamomile powder, 1 tablespoon Skullcap powder, empty gel capsules.
Preparation: Mix Chamomile and Skullcap powders thoroughly. Fill empty capsules and seal.
Suggested Usage: Take 1 capsule up to twice daily to reduce anxiety and promote emotional stability.
Benefits: Chamomile and Skullcap calm the nervous system, reduce anxiety, and promote emotional balance, making these capsules effective for managing daily stress.

676. Reishi and Holy Basil Immune-Enhancing Capsules

Ingredients: 1 tablespoon Reishi Mushroom powder, 1 tablespoon Holy Basil powder, empty gel capsules.
Preparation: Mix Reishi and Holy Basil powders thoroughly. Fill empty capsules and seal.
Suggested Usage: Take 1 capsule daily to support immune function and promote emotional stability.
Benefits: Reishi and Holy Basil calm the nervous system, support immune health, and enhance emotional balance, making these capsules ideal for managing stress-induced immune imbalances.

677. St. John's Wort and Skullcap Mood-Balancing Tea

Ingredients: 1 tablespoon dried St. John's Wort, 1 tablespoon dried Skullcap, 2 cups hot water.
Preparation: Steep St. John's Wort and Skullcap in hot water for 15 minutes. Strain and serve warm.

Suggested Usage: Drink 1 cup daily to reduce depressive symptoms and promote emotional balance.
Benefits: St. John's Wort and Skullcap elevate mood, calm the nervous system, and promote emotional stability, making this tea ideal for managing mild to moderate depression.

678. Lemon Balm and Lavender Relaxation Capsules

Ingredients: 1 tablespoon Lemon Balm powder, 1 tablespoon Lavender powder, empty gel capsules.
Preparation: Mix Lemon Balm and Lavender powders thoroughly. Fill empty capsules and seal.
Suggested Usage: Take 1 capsule up to twice daily to reduce anxiety and promote relaxation.
Benefits: Lemon Balm and Lavender calm the nervous system, reduce anxiety, and promote a sense of peace, making these capsules ideal for managing stress and enhancing mental clarity.

679. Saffron and Rhodiola Adaptogen Elixir

Ingredients: 1 pinch Saffron threads, 1 tablespoon dried Rhodiola Root, 1 cup hot water.
Preparation: Simmer Rhodiola Root in hot water for 15 minutes. Remove from heat, add Saffron, and steep for another 5 minutes. Strain and serve warm.
Suggested Usage: Drink 1 cup daily to enhance mood and reduce stress-induced fatigue.
Benefits: Saffron and Rhodiola support emotional balance, enhance mental clarity, and reduce symptoms of mild depression, making this elixir effective for managing chronic stress and low energy.

680. Chamomile and Skullcap Anti-Anxiety Tea

Ingredients: 1 tablespoon dried Chamomile flowers, 1 tablespoon dried Skullcap, 2 cups hot water.
Preparation: Steep Chamomile and Skullcap in hot water for 15 minutes. Strain and serve warm.
Suggested Usage: Drink 1 cup up to twice daily to reduce anxiety and promote relaxation.
Benefits: Chamomile and Skullcap calm the nervous system, reduce nervous tension, and promote emotional stability, making this tea ideal for managing daily anxiety and supporting mental clarity.

681. Holy Basil and Passionflower Emotional Balance Capsules

Ingredients: 1 tablespoon Holy Basil powder, 1 tablespoon Passionflower powder, empty gel capsules.
Preparation: Mix Holy Basil and Passionflower powders thoroughly. Fill empty capsules and seal.
Suggested Usage: Take 1 capsule daily to reduce anxiety and promote emotional stability.
Benefits: Holy Basil and Passionflower calm the nervous system, support emotional balance, and reduce symptoms of anxiety, making these capsules effective for managing stress-related mood imbalances.

682. Valerian and Hops Bedtime Tonic

Ingredients: 1 tablespoon dried Valerian Root, 1 tablespoon dried Hops, 2 cups hot water.
Preparation: Simmer Valerian and Hops in water for 15 minutes. Strain and serve warm.
Suggested Usage: Drink 1 cup before bedtime to promote restful sleep and reduce nighttime anxiety.
Benefits: Valerian and Hops promote deep relaxation, reduce anxiety, and enhance sleep quality, making this tonic effective for managing insomnia and nighttime restlessness.

683. Lemon Balm, Skullcap, and Valerian Sleep-Enhancing Tea

Ingredients: 1 tablespoon dried Lemon Balm leaves, 1 tablespoon dried Skullcap, 1 teaspoon dried Valerian Root, 2 cups hot water.
Preparation: Steep Lemon Balm, Skullcap, and Valerian in hot water for 15 minutes. Strain and serve warm.
Suggested Usage: Drink 1 cup before bedtime to promote restful sleep and reduce nighttime anxiety.
Benefits: Lemon Balm, Skullcap, and Valerian calm the nervous system, promote deep relaxation, and support restful sleep, making this tea ideal for managing anxiety-induced sleep disturbances.

684. Skullcap and Chamomile Anti-Stress Capsules

Ingredients: 1 tablespoon Skullcap powder, 1 tablespoon Chamomile powder, empty gel capsules.
Preparation: Mix Skullcap and Chamomile powders thoroughly. Fill empty capsules and seal.
Suggested Usage: Take 1 capsule up to twice daily to reduce anxiety and promote emotional stability.
Benefits: Skullcap and Chamomile calm the nervous system, reduce anxiety, and promote emotional balance, making these capsules ideal for managing daily stress.

685. Ashwagandha and Licorice Adrenal Support Capsules

Ingredients: 1 tablespoon Ashwagandha Root powder, 1 tablespoon Licorice Root powder, empty gel capsules.
Preparation: Mix Ashwagandha and Licorice powders thoroughly. Fill empty capsules and seal.
Suggested Usage: Take 1 capsule daily to reduce stress and support adrenal health.
Benefits: Ashwagandha and Licorice balance the body's stress response, support adrenal function, and enhance emotional resilience, making these capsules ideal for managing chronic stress and adrenal fatigue.

686. Holy Basil and Rhodiola Mood Stabilizing Tea

Ingredients: 1 tablespoon dried Holy Basil leaves, 1 tablespoon dried Rhodiola Root, 2 cups hot water.
Preparation: Steep Holy Basil and Rhodiola in hot water for 15 minutes. Strain and serve warm.
Suggested Usage: Drink 1 cup daily to

support emotional balance and reduce stress.

Benefits: Holy Basil and Rhodiola balance the body's stress response, promote emotional stability, and reduce symptoms of anxiety and depression, making this tea effective for managing chronic stress.

687. Lavender and Lemon Balm Nervous System Calming Capsules

Ingredients: 1 tablespoon Lavender powder, 1 tablespoon Lemon Balm powder, empty gel capsules.
Preparation: Mix Lavender and Lemon Balm powders thoroughly. Fill empty capsules and seal.
Suggested Usage: Take 1 capsule daily to reduce anxiety and promote relaxation.
Benefits: Lavender and Lemon Balm calm the nervous system, reduce anxiety, and promote a sense of peace, making these capsules ideal for managing daily stress and enhancing mental clarity.

688. St. John's Wort and Reishi Depression Relief Capsules

Ingredients: 1 tablespoon St. John's Wort powder, 1 tablespoon Reishi Mushroom powder, empty gel capsules.
Preparation: Mix St. John's Wort and Reishi powders thoroughly. Fill empty capsules and seal.
Suggested Usage: Take 1 capsule daily to reduce depressive symptoms and promote emotional stability.
Benefits: St. John's Wort and Reishi support emotional balance, reduce symptoms of mild depression, and

promote overall mental resilience, making these capsules ideal for managing mood disorders.

689. Skullcap and Holy Basil Emotional Balance Tea

Ingredients: 1 tablespoon dried Skullcap, 1 tablespoon dried Holy Basil leaves, 2 cups hot water.
Preparation: Steep Skullcap and Holy Basil in hot water for 15 minutes. Strain and serve warm.
Suggested Usage: Drink 1 cup up to twice daily to promote emotional stability and reduce anxiety.
Benefits: Skullcap and Holy Basil calm the nervous system, reduce anxiety, and promote emotional balance, making this tea ideal for managing stress and supporting mental wellness.

690. Chamomile and Hops Sleep Support Elixir

Ingredients: 1 tablespoon dried Chamomile flowers, 1 tablespoon dried Hops, 1 cup hot water.
Preparation: Steep Chamomile and Hops in hot water for 15 minutes. Strain and serve warm.
Suggested Usage: Drink 1 cup before bedtime to promote restful sleep and reduce nighttime anxiety.
Benefits: Chamomile and Hops promote relaxation, reduce anxiety, and enhance sleep quality, making this elixir effective for managing insomnia and nighttime anxiety.

691. Lemon Balm and Skullcap Anxiety-Reducing Capsules

Ingredients: 1 tablespoon Lemon Balm powder, 1 tablespoon Skullcap powder, empty gel capsules.

Preparation: Mix Lemon Balm and Skullcap powders thoroughly. Fill empty capsules and seal.

Suggested Usage: Take 1 capsule up to twice daily to reduce anxiety and promote relaxation.

Benefits: Lemon Balm and Skullcap calm the nervous system, reduce anxiety, and promote emotional stability, making these capsules ideal for managing stress and supporting mental clarity.

Book 33: Enhancing Mental Clarity Naturally

Optimal cognitive function is essential for maintaining productivity, learning, and overall mental well-being. A variety of herbs have been used for centuries to support memory, focus, and mental clarity. These botanicals offer natural ways to enhance brain function, reduce mental fatigue, and protect against cognitive decline. In this chapter, we delve into the most effective herbs for boosting cognitive performance, providing strategies to incorporate them into daily routines to support mental sharpness and concentration.

Herbs to Boost Cognitive Function

There are numerous herbs known for their ability to enhance mental clarity and cognitive health. Each of these herbs works through unique mechanisms, such as improving blood flow to the brain, modulating neurotransmitter activity, or providing antioxidant protection to brain cells.

One of the most extensively researched herbs for cognitive health is **Ginkgo Biloba**. Known for its ability to increase cerebral blood flow, Ginkgo Biloba improves oxygen and nutrient delivery to the brain, resulting in better memory recall, sharper focus, and enhanced overall mental function. Ginkgo is also a powerful antioxidant, protecting brain cells from oxidative stress, which is crucial for preventing age-related cognitive decline.

Another potent herb for mental clarity is **Gotu Kola**. Often called the "herb of longevity," Gotu Kola is used in both Ayurvedic and traditional Chinese medicine to promote memory, reduce anxiety, and enhance mental clarity. It works by improving circulation, strengthening blood vessels, and supporting the health of brain tissue. Gotu Kola is often recommended for students, professionals, or anyone looking to enhance cognitive stamina and focus.

For enhancing memory and concentration, **Bacopa Monnieri** is one of the best-known herbs. Bacopa, also known as Brahmi, is revered in Ayurvedic medicine as a brain tonic that improves learning and cognitive performance. It works by supporting neurotransmitter function and protecting the brain from oxidative damage. Bacopa is especially effective for individuals experiencing age-related cognitive decline or those dealing with high levels of mental stress.

Rosemary is another herb that supports cognitive function and is known as the "herb of remembrance." This aromatic herb has been used since ancient times to stimulate cognitive function and improve memory. Rosemary contains compounds that increase cerebral blood flow, enhancing both focus and concentration. Interestingly, research has shown that even the aroma of Rosemary can improve cognitive performance, making it a versatile tool for boosting brain function.

Lion's Mane Mushroom is a powerful herb for brain health that has gained attention for its neuroprotective properties. Rich in compounds called hericenones and erinacines, Lion's Mane stimulates the production of nerve growth factor (NGF), a protein essential for the growth, maintenance, and survival of brain cells. Regular use of Lion's Mane can help improve memory, enhance focus, and protect against neurodegenerative diseases, making it a valuable herb for long-term brain health.

For combating mental fatigue and supporting mental resilience, **Rhodiola Rosea** is an excellent choice. Rhodiola is an adaptogenic herb that sharpens focus, reduces mental fatigue, and enhances memory recall, making it particularly useful during periods of high stress. It works by balancing stress hormones and enhancing the brain's capacity to perform under pressure, making it a go-to herb for enhancing mental clarity in stressful situations.

Ginseng, both American and Asian varieties, are well-known for their cognitive-enhancing properties. Ginseng is considered a natural stimulant that enhances energy levels, sharpens focus, and improves mental clarity. Unlike caffeine, Ginseng provides a steady boost in mental performance without causing jitters. It is especially beneficial for individuals experiencing mental fatigue or those looking to enhance overall cognitive performance.

Sage is another herb celebrated for its memory-enhancing effects. Traditionally used to improve memory and concentration, Sage works by modulating neurotransmitter activity and protecting brain cells from oxidative stress. Regular use of Sage can enhance mental clarity and prevent cognitive decline, making it a valuable herb for both young and older adults looking to maintain cognitive health.

Ashwagandha, a well-known adaptogen, also supports cognitive function by balancing stress hormones and protecting the brain from stress-induced damage. Ashwagandha's ability to reduce cortisol levels and promote mental resilience makes it a valuable herb for long-term cognitive health, especially for individuals dealing with high levels of chronic stress.

Lemon Balm is a gentle yet effective herb for promoting calm focus. It has been traditionally used to reduce anxiety, enhance mood, and promote mental clarity. Lemon Balm is an excellent addition to blends for improving concentration, making it ideal for situations where calm, sustained focus is needed.

By incorporating these herbs into daily routines, you can support optimal cognitive health, enhance focus, and protect against mental fatigue. Regular use of these botanicals can help maintain sharp mental clarity, promote long-term brain health, and improve overall cognitive performance.

Strategies for Enhancing Cognitive Function

Incorporating these herbs into a daily wellness routine can be done in various ways. Herbal teas, tinctures, and tonics are popular options for those looking for convenience and efficacy. For example, a simple tea combining Gotu Kola and Ginkgo Biloba can promote memory retention and enhance focus, while a tincture of Lion's Mane Mushroom and Rhodiola can provide a quick, concentrated boost in mental clarity and cognitive stamina.

Combining herbs that have complementary effects can also increase their efficacy. For instance, blending adaptogenic herbs like Rhodiola and Ashwagandha with brain-boosting herbs like Bacopa and Ginkgo creates a synergistic effect, enhancing focus, improving memory, and reducing stress simultaneously.

Dietary changes can also support cognitive function. Consuming a diet rich in healthy fats, such as omega-3s from fish oil or flaxseed, along with antioxidant-rich fruits and vegetables, provides the brain with essential nutrients needed for optimal performance. Herbs like Turmeric, which has strong anti-inflammatory and antioxidant properties, can be added to meals to support cognitive health and protect brain cells from oxidative damage.

Incorporating mindfulness practices, such as meditation and yoga, alongside herbal remedies can further enhance mental clarity and reduce stress. These practices improve focus, increase mental resilience, and promote a calm, centered mind. Using herbs like Lemon Balm, Holy Basil, or Chamomile in teas or tinctures before meditation can deepen the practice and enhance the overall effects on mental clarity and well-being.

By adopting a holistic approach that integrates these herbal strategies with healthy lifestyle practices, you can achieve and maintain peak cognitive performance, supporting mental clarity, focus, and long-term brain health.

Remedies for Mental Clarity

692. Ginkgo Biloba Memory Support Tea

Ingredients: 1 tablespoon dried Ginkgo Biloba leaves, 2 cups hot water.
Preparation: Steep Ginkgo leaves in hot water for 15 minutes. Strain and serve warm.

Suggested Usage: Drink 1 cup up to twice daily to support memory and cognitive function.
Benefits: Ginkgo Biloba enhances blood circulation to the brain, improving memory, mental sharpness, and overall cognitive performance. It is particularly effective for preventing age-related cognitive decline.

294

693. Gotu Kola and Rosemary Cognitive Boost Tea

Ingredients: 1 tablespoon dried Gotu Kola leaves, 1 tablespoon dried Rosemary, 2 cups hot water.
Preparation: Steep Gotu Kola and Rosemary in hot water for 15 minutes. Strain and serve warm.
Suggested Usage: Drink 1 cup daily to enhance mental clarity and concentration.
Benefits: Gotu Kola supports cognitive health and reduces anxiety, while Rosemary improves memory and focus, making this tea ideal for boosting overall mental performance.

694. Bacopa and Holy Basil Mental Clarity Capsules

Ingredients: 1 tablespoon Bacopa powder, 1 tablespoon Holy Basil powder, empty gel capsules.
Preparation: Mix Bacopa and Holy Basil powders thoroughly. Fill empty capsules and seal.
Suggested Usage: Take 1 capsule daily to enhance memory and promote mental clarity.
Benefits: Bacopa enhances learning, memory retention, and reduces mental fatigue, while Holy Basil calms the mind and supports focus, making these capsules ideal for enhancing cognitive clarity.

695. Lion's Mane and Ashwagandha Brain-Boosting Latte

Ingredients: 1 teaspoon Lion's Mane powder, 1 teaspoon Ashwagandha powder, 1 cup warm milk or plant-based milk.
Preparation: Mix Lion's Mane and Ashwagandha powders into warm milk. Stir until well combined.
Suggested Usage: Drink 1 cup in the morning to support mental clarity and reduce stress.
Benefits: Lion's Mane stimulates nerve growth factor, enhancing brain function, while Ashwagandha reduces cortisol levels, promoting a calm, focused mind.

696. Ginseng and Rhodiola Energy-Enhancing Capsules

Ingredients: 1 tablespoon Ginseng Root powder, 1 tablespoon Rhodiola Root powder, empty gel capsules.
Preparation: Mix Ginseng and Rhodiola powders thoroughly. Fill empty capsules and seal.
Suggested Usage: Take 1 capsule daily to enhance energy and reduce mental fatigue.
Benefits: Ginseng provides a natural boost in energy and mental clarity, while Rhodiola sharpens focus and reduces stress, making these capsules ideal for improving cognitive stamina.

697. Sage and Lemon Balm Focus Tea

Ingredients: 1 tablespoon dried Sage, 1 tablespoon dried Lemon Balm, 2 cups hot water.
Preparation: Steep Sage and Lemon Balm in hot water for 15 minutes. Strain and serve warm.
Suggested Usage: Drink 1 cup daily to promote mental clarity and reduce anxiety.
Benefits: Sage and Lemon Balm enhance

memory, reduce mental fog, and promote calm focus, making this tea ideal for improving concentration and cognitive health.

698. Rosemary and Peppermint Mental Sharpness Inhalation

Ingredients: 2 drops Rosemary essential oil, 2 drops Peppermint essential oil, bowl of hot water.
Preparation: Add essential oils to hot water. Lean over the bowl, cover your head with a towel, and inhale deeply for 5-10 minutes.
Suggested Usage: Use once daily to clear mental fog and improve focus.
Benefits: Rosemary and Peppermint enhance mental clarity, increase alertness, and stimulate cognitive function, making this inhalation effective for combating mental fatigue.

699. Rhodiola and Ginseng Concentration Tincture

Ingredients: 1 tablespoon dried Rhodiola Root, 1 tablespoon dried Ginseng Root, 1 cup vodka or brandy.
Preparation: Combine herbs and alcohol in a glass jar. Seal tightly and let steep for 4-6 weeks, shaking occasionally. Strain and store in a dark glass bottle.
Suggested Usage: Take ½ teaspoon in the morning to enhance focus and concentration.
Benefits: Rhodiola and Ginseng improve cognitive performance, reduce mental fatigue, and support mental clarity, making this tincture ideal for sustaining concentration during periods of high stress.

700. Gotu Kola and Ginkgo Biloba Cognitive Health Capsules

Ingredients: 1 tablespoon Gotu Kola powder, 1 tablespoon Ginkgo Biloba powder, empty gel capsules.
Preparation: Mix Gotu Kola and Ginkgo powders thoroughly. Fill empty capsules and seal.
Suggested Usage: Take 1 capsule up to twice daily to support cognitive health and memory.
Benefits: Gotu Kola enhances brain health and circulation, while Ginkgo Biloba improves memory and mental sharpness, making these capsules ideal for long-term cognitive support.

701. Brahmi and Lemon Balm Calm Focus Elixir

Ingredients: 1 tablespoon dried Brahmi, 1 tablespoon dried Lemon Balm, 2 cups hot water.
Preparation: Steep Brahmi and Lemon Balm in hot water for 15 minutes. Strain and serve warm.
Suggested Usage: Drink 1 cup daily to promote calm focus and enhance cognitive function.
Benefits: Brahmi enhances learning and memory retention, while Lemon Balm calms the nervous system, making this elixir ideal for maintaining focus and mental clarity.

702. Bacopa and Gotu Kola Memory Capsules

Ingredients: 1 tablespoon Bacopa powder, 1 tablespoon Gotu Kola powder, empty gel capsules.
Preparation: Mix Bacopa and Gotu Kola powders thoroughly. Fill empty capsules and seal.
Suggested Usage: Take 1 capsule daily to enhance memory and support cognitive health.
Benefits: Bacopa and Gotu Kola improve memory, reduce mental fatigue, and support long-term brain health, making these capsules ideal for students and professionals alike.

703. Schisandra and Rhodiola Anti-Stress Tea

Ingredients: 1 tablespoon dried Schisandra Berries, 1 tablespoon dried Rhodiola Root, 2 cups hot water.
Preparation: Steep Schisandra and Rhodiola in hot water for 15 minutes. Strain and serve warm.
Suggested Usage: Drink 1 cup up to twice daily to reduce stress and support mental clarity.
Benefits: Schisandra and Rhodiola balance the body's stress response, enhance cognitive performance, and promote mental clarity, making this tea ideal for managing stress and supporting focus.

704. Reishi and Lion's Mane Brain Function Capsules

Ingredients: 1 tablespoon Reishi Mushroom powder, 1 tablespoon Lion's Mane Mushroom powder, empty gel capsules.
Preparation: Mix Reishi and Lion's Mane powders thoroughly. Fill empty capsules and seal.
Suggested Usage: Take 1 capsule daily to support brain health and cognitive performance.
Benefits: Reishi and Lion's Mane promote nerve growth, enhance cognitive function, and protect against neurodegenerative conditions, making these capsules ideal for supporting long-term brain health.

705. Sage and Peppermint Cognitive Clarity Tea

Ingredients: 1 tablespoon dried Sage, 1 tablespoon dried Peppermint, 2 cups hot water.
Preparation: Steep Sage and Peppermint in hot water for 15 minutes. Strain and serve warm.
Suggested Usage: Drink 1 cup up to twice daily to enhance mental clarity and sharpen focus.
Benefits: Sage and Peppermint stimulate cognitive function, improve concentration, and promote mental clarity, making this tea ideal for boosting focus and memory.

706. Holy Basil and Ashwagandha Adaptogen Capsules

Ingredients: 1 tablespoon Holy Basil powder, 1 tablespoon Ashwagandha powder, empty gel capsules.
Preparation: Mix Holy Basil and Ashwagandha powders thoroughly. Fill empty capsules and seal.
Suggested Usage: Take 1 capsule daily to support stress resilience and mental clarity.
Benefits: Holy Basil and Ashwagandha

reduce cortisol levels, balance the body's stress response, and promote mental clarity, making these capsules ideal for managing stress and enhancing focus.

707. Gotu Kola and Bacopa Brain Tonic

Ingredients: 1 tablespoon dried Gotu Kola, 1 tablespoon dried Bacopa, 2 cups hot water.
Preparation: Steep Gotu Kola and Bacopa in hot water for 15 minutes. Strain and serve warm.
Suggested Usage: Drink 1 cup daily to enhance memory and promote cognitive function.
Benefits: Gotu Kola and Bacopa support brain health, reduce mental fatigue, and enhance memory retention, making this tonic ideal for maintaining mental sharpness.

708. Lemon Balm and Lavender Relaxation Tea for Focus

Ingredients: 1 tablespoon dried Lemon Balm, 1 teaspoon dried Lavender flowers, 2 cups hot water.
Preparation: Steep Lemon Balm and Lavender in hot water for 15 minutes. Strain and serve warm.
Suggested Usage: Drink 1 cup daily to reduce anxiety and promote calm focus.
Benefits: Lemon Balm and Lavender reduce stress and promote a sense of calm, making this tea ideal for situations that require a relaxed yet focused state of mind.

709. Ginkgo and Rhodiola Energy-Boosting Capsules

Ingredients: 1 tablespoon Ginkgo Biloba powder, 1 tablespoon Rhodiola Root powder, empty gel capsules.
Preparation: Mix Ginkgo and Rhodiola powders thoroughly. Fill empty capsules and seal.
Suggested Usage: Take 1 capsule daily to reduce mental fatigue and promote energy.
Benefits: Ginkgo improves circulation and oxygenation to the brain, while Rhodiola reduces mental fatigue and sharpens focus, making these capsules effective for sustaining cognitive performance.

710. Lion's Mane and Reishi Mushroom Nerve Regeneration Tea

Ingredients: 1 tablespoon dried Lion's Mane Mushroom, 1 tablespoon dried Reishi Mushroom, 2 cups hot water.
Preparation: Simmer Lion's Mane and Reishi in hot water for 20 minutes. Strain and serve warm.
Suggested Usage: Drink 1 cup daily to support nerve regeneration and cognitive health.
Benefits: Lion's Mane stimulates nerve growth factor, while Reishi supports cognitive function and emotional balance, making this tea ideal for long-term brain health.

711. Bacopa, Gotu Kola, and Brahmi Memory Tea

Ingredients: 1 tablespoon dried Bacopa, 1 tablespoon dried Gotu Kola, 1 tablespoon dried Brahmi, 2 cups hot water.

Preparation: Steep Bacopa, Gotu Kola, and Brahmi in hot water for 15 minutes. Strain and serve warm.

Suggested Usage: Drink 1 cup daily to support memory and cognitive performance.

Benefits: Bacopa, Gotu Kola, and Brahmi enhance learning, memory retention, and reduce mental fatigue, making this tea ideal for students and professionals.

712. Sage and Lemon Essential Oil Mental Clarity Spray

Ingredients: 10 drops Sage essential oil, 5 drops Lemon essential oil, 1 cup distilled water.

Preparation: Combine essential oils and water in a spray bottle. Shake well before each use.

Suggested Usage: Spray in the air or on pulse points as needed to enhance mental clarity and focus.

Benefits: Sage and Lemon essential oils stimulate cognitive function, clear mental fog, and promote sharp focus, making this spray ideal for quick mental refreshment.

713. Peppermint and Rosemary Focus-Enhancing Capsules

Ingredients: 1 tablespoon Peppermint powder, 1 tablespoon Rosemary powder, empty gel capsules.

Preparation: Mix Peppermint and Rosemary powders thoroughly. Fill empty capsules and seal.

Suggested Usage: Take 1 capsule daily to promote focus and mental sharpness.

Benefits: Peppermint and Rosemary increase alertness, sharpen focus, and

enhance cognitive performance, making these capsules effective for maintaining mental clarity.

714. Lion's Mane and Ginkgo Biloba Concentration Capsules

Ingredients: 1 tablespoon Lion's Mane powder, 1 tablespoon Ginkgo Biloba powder, empty gel capsules.

Preparation: Mix Lion's Mane and Ginkgo powders thoroughly. Fill empty capsules and seal.

Suggested Usage: Take 1 capsule daily to support concentration and cognitive health.

Benefits: Lion's Mane promotes nerve growth, while Ginkgo improves blood flow to the brain, making these capsules ideal for enhancing concentration and protecting brain health.

715. Rhodiola and Ginseng Stress-Resilience Capsules

Ingredients: 1 tablespoon Rhodiola Root powder, 1 tablespoon Ginseng Root powder, empty gel capsules.

Preparation: Mix Rhodiola and Ginseng powders thoroughly. Fill empty capsules and seal.

Suggested Usage: Take 1 capsule daily to reduce stress and promote mental clarity.

Benefits: Rhodiola and Ginseng enhance stress resilience, support focus, and reduce mental fatigue, making these capsules effective for managing high-stress situations.

716. Rosemary and Sage Mental Focus Capsules

Ingredients: 1 tablespoon Rosemary powder, 1 tablespoon Sage powder, empty gel capsules.
Preparation: Mix Rosemary and Sage powders thoroughly. Fill empty capsules and seal.
Suggested Usage: Take 1 capsule daily to enhance memory and mental clarity.
Benefits: Rosemary and Sage stimulate cognitive function, improve memory, and protect against cognitive decline, making these capsules ideal for maintaining sharp mental performance.

717. Holy Basil and Lemon Balm Calm Clarity Tea

Ingredients: 1 tablespoon dried Holy Basil leaves, 1 tablespoon dried Lemon Balm, 2 cups hot water.
Preparation: Steep Holy Basil and Lemon Balm in hot water for 15 minutes. Strain and serve warm.
Suggested Usage: Drink 1 cup daily to promote calm focus and reduce anxiety.
Benefits: Holy Basil and Lemon Balm reduce stress, promote emotional stability, and enhance cognitive clarity, making this tea effective for maintaining a calm and focused mind.

718. Ashwagandha and Ginseng Stress-Reduction Capsules

Ingredients: 1 tablespoon Ashwagandha Root powder, 1 tablespoon Ginseng Root powder, empty gel capsules.
Preparation: Mix Ashwagandha and Ginseng powders thoroughly. Fill empty capsules and seal.
Suggested Usage: Take 1 capsule daily to reduce stress and support mental energy.

Benefits: Ashwagandha and Ginseng balance the body's stress response, reduce mental fatigue, and promote resilience, making these capsules ideal for managing chronic stress.

719. Bacopa and Ginkgo Memory Elixir

Ingredients: 1 tablespoon dried Bacopa, 1 tablespoon dried Ginkgo Biloba, 2 cups hot water.
Preparation: Steep Bacopa and Ginkgo in hot water for 15 minutes. Strain and serve warm.
Suggested Usage: Drink 1 cup daily to support memory and cognitive function.
Benefits: Bacopa and Ginkgo enhance learning, improve memory recall, and protect brain health, making this elixir ideal for maintaining cognitive sharpness.

720. Gotu Kola and Peppermint Concentration Capsules

Ingredients: 1 tablespoon Gotu Kola powder, 1 tablespoon Peppermint powder, empty gel capsules.
Preparation: Mix Gotu Kola and Peppermint powders thoroughly. Fill empty capsules and seal.
Suggested Usage: Take 1 capsule daily to enhance concentration and cognitive performance.
Benefits: Gotu Kola supports brain health, while Peppermint increases alertness and mental clarity, making these capsules effective for promoting sustained focus and mental sharpness.

721. Ginseng and Schisandra Vitality-Enhancing Tea

Ingredients: 1 tablespoon dried Ginseng Root, 1 tablespoon dried Schisandra Berries, 2 cups hot water.
Preparation: Simmer Ginseng and Schisandra in hot water for 15 minutes. Strain and serve warm.
Suggested Usage: Drink 1 cup daily to boost energy levels and enhance mental vitality.
Benefits: Ginseng and Schisandra improve mental stamina, reduce fatigue, and support cognitive performance, making this tea ideal for enhancing overall vitality and mental sharpness.

722. Lemon Balm and Chamomile Mental Calm Capsules

Ingredients: 1 tablespoon Lemon Balm powder, 1 tablespoon Chamomile powder, empty gel capsules.
Preparation: Mix Lemon Balm and Chamomile powders thoroughly. Fill empty capsules and seal.
Suggested Usage: Take 1 capsule daily to promote relaxation and mental calm.
Benefits: Lemon Balm and Chamomile calm the nervous system, reduce anxiety, and promote mental clarity, making these capsules ideal for managing stress and supporting emotional balance.

723. Rosemary, Sage, and Thyme Memory Support Tea

Ingredients: 1 tablespoon dried Rosemary, 1 tablespoon dried Sage, 1 tablespoon dried Thyme, 2 cups hot water.
Preparation: Steep Rosemary, Sage, and Thyme in hot water for 15 minutes. Strain and serve warm.
Suggested Usage: Drink 1 cup up to twice daily to support memory and cognitive health.
Benefits: Rosemary, Sage, and Thyme stimulate cognitive function, enhance memory, and protect against cognitive decline, making this tea effective for maintaining mental sharpness and clarity.

724. Lion's Mane and Holy Basil Stress-Relief Tincture

Ingredients: 1 tablespoon dried Lion's Mane Mushroom, 1 tablespoon dried Holy Basil, 1 cup vodka or brandy.
Preparation: Combine herbs and alcohol in a glass jar. Seal tightly and let steep for 4-6 weeks, shaking occasionally. Strain and store in a dark bottle.
Suggested Usage: Take ½ teaspoon daily to reduce stress and enhance mental clarity.
Benefits: Lion's Mane stimulates nerve growth, while Holy Basil reduces cortisol levels, making this tincture effective for supporting brain health and reducing stress.

725. Lavender and Rosemary Focus Support Capsules

Ingredients: 1 tablespoon Lavender powder, 1 tablespoon Rosemary powder, empty gel capsules.
Preparation: Mix Lavender and Rosemary powders thoroughly. Fill empty capsules and seal.
Suggested Usage: Take 1 capsule daily to enhance focus and reduce mental fatigue.

Benefits: Lavender and Rosemary calm the mind, increase alertness, and sharpen focus, making these capsules ideal for maintaining concentration and mental clarity.

726. Lemon Balm and Holy Basil Stress-Reducing Tea

Ingredients: 1 tablespoon dried Lemon Balm leaves, 1 tablespoon dried Holy Basil leaves, 2 cups hot water.
Preparation: Steep Lemon Balm and Holy Basil in hot water for 15 minutes. Strain and serve warm.
Suggested Usage: Drink 1 cup up to twice daily to promote emotional stability and reduce stress.
Benefits: Lemon Balm and Holy Basil calm the nervous system, balance cortisol levels, and promote emotional stability, making this tea ideal for managing anxiety and enhancing focus.

727. Ashwagandha and Rhodiola Nerve Calming Elixir

Ingredients: 1 tablespoon dried Ashwagandha Root, 1 tablespoon dried Rhodiola Root, 2 cups hot water.
Preparation: Simmer Ashwagandha and Rhodiola in hot water for 20 minutes. Strain and serve warm.
Suggested Usage: Drink 1 cup daily to reduce stress and enhance mental clarity.
Benefits: Ashwagandha and Rhodiola balance stress hormones, reduce mental fatigue, and support mental resilience, making this elixir ideal for managing stress and supporting nerve health.

728. Bacopa, Ginkgo, and Gotu Kola Memory Tea

Ingredients: 1 tablespoon dried Bacopa, 1 tablespoon dried Ginkgo Biloba, 1 tablespoon dried Gotu Kola, 2 cups hot water.
Preparation: Steep Bacopa, Ginkgo, and Gotu Kola in hot water for 15 minutes. Strain and serve warm.
Suggested Usage: Drink 1 cup daily to support memory and cognitive performance.
Benefits: Bacopa, Ginkgo, and Gotu Kola enhance memory, improve mental sharpness, and protect brain cells from oxidative stress, making this tea effective for maintaining cognitive health.

729. Sage and Lemon Balm Cognitive Enhancement Tea

Ingredients: 1 tablespoon dried Sage, 1 tablespoon dried Lemon Balm, 2 cups hot water.
Preparation: Steep Sage and Lemon Balm in hot water for 15 minutes. Strain and serve warm.
Suggested Usage: Drink 1 cup up to twice daily to enhance focus and mental clarity.
Benefits: Sage and Lemon Balm improve cognitive function, reduce mental fog, and promote focus, making this tea ideal for enhancing mental sharpness.

730. Rhodiola and Schisandra Concentration Capsules

Ingredients: 1 tablespoon Rhodiola Root powder, 1 tablespoon Schisandra Berry powder, empty gel capsules.

Preparation: Mix Rhodiola and Schisandra powders thoroughly. Fill empty capsules and seal.

Suggested Usage: Take 1 capsule daily to promote concentration and cognitive resilience.

Benefits: Rhodiola and Schisandra reduce mental fatigue, support mental clarity, and promote sustained focus, making these capsules effective for enhancing concentration during high-stress periods.

731. Lemon Balm and Holy Basil Anxiety-Reducing Capsules

Ingredients: 1 tablespoon Lemon Balm powder, 1 tablespoon Holy Basil powder, empty gel capsules.

Preparation: Mix Lemon Balm and Holy Basil powders thoroughly. Fill empty capsules and seal.

Suggested Usage: Take 1 capsule daily to reduce anxiety and promote emotional stability.

Benefits: Lemon Balm and Holy Basil calm the nervous system, balance stress hormones, and promote a sense of peace, making these capsules ideal for managing stress and anxiety.

732. Lion's Mane, Reishi, and Ashwagandha Mental Clarity Tincture

Ingredients: 1 tablespoon dried Lion's Mane Mushroom, 1 tablespoon dried Reishi Mushroom, 1 tablespoon dried Ashwagandha Root, 1 cup vodka or brandy.

Preparation: Combine the herbs and alcohol in a glass jar. Seal tightly and let steep for 4-6 weeks, shaking occasionally.

Strain and store in a dark bottle.

Suggested Usage: Take ½ teaspoon daily to support mental clarity and reduce stress.

Benefits: Lion's Mane stimulates nerve growth factor, Reishi enhances brain function, and Ashwagandha reduces cortisol levels, making this tincture ideal for supporting cognitive performance and managing stress.

733. Peppermint and Gotu Kola Brain-Boosting Tea

Ingredients: 1 tablespoon dried Peppermint, 1 tablespoon dried Gotu Kola, 2 cups hot water.

Preparation: Steep Peppermint and Gotu Kola in hot water for 15 minutes. Strain and serve warm.

Suggested Usage: Drink 1 cup daily to enhance focus and promote mental clarity.

Benefits: Peppermint increases alertness and reduces mental fatigue, while Gotu Kola supports cognitive health, making this tea ideal for maintaining sharp mental performance.

734. Bacopa and Ginseng Memory Support Capsules

Ingredients: 1 tablespoon Bacopa powder, 1 tablespoon Ginseng powder, empty gel capsules.

Preparation: Mix Bacopa and Ginseng powders thoroughly. Fill empty capsules and seal.

Suggested Usage: Take 1 capsule daily to support memory and reduce mental fatigue.

Benefits: Bacopa enhances learning and memory retention, while Ginseng boosts energy levels and mental stamina, making these capsules ideal for promoting cognitive health and resilience.

735. Sage and Rosemary Focus Capsules

Ingredients: 1 tablespoon Sage powder, 1 tablespoon Rosemary powder, empty gel capsules.

Preparation: Mix Sage and Rosemary powders thoroughly. Fill empty capsules and seal.

Suggested Usage: Take 1 capsule daily to enhance focus and mental sharpness.

Benefits: Sage and Rosemary stimulate cognitive function, improve memory, and protect against cognitive decline, making these capsules effective for maintaining mental sharpness.

736. Brahmi and Lemon Balm Memory Tea

Ingredients: 1 tablespoon dried Brahmi, 1 tablespoon dried Lemon Balm, 2 cups hot water.

Preparation: Steep Brahmi and Lemon Balm in hot water for 15 minutes. Strain and serve warm.

Suggested Usage: Drink 1 cup daily to promote memory and mental clarity.

Benefits: Brahmi enhances learning and memory retention, while Lemon Balm calms the mind, making this tea ideal for maintaining focus and mental sharpness.

737. Ginkgo and Rhodiola Anti-Fatigue Elixir

Ingredients: 1 tablespoon dried Ginkgo Biloba, 1 tablespoon dried Rhodiola Root, 2 cups hot water.

Preparation: Simmer Ginkgo and Rhodiola in hot water for 20 minutes. Strain and serve warm.

Suggested Usage: Drink 1 cup daily to reduce mental fatigue and promote energy.

Benefits: Ginkgo enhances blood circulation to the brain, while Rhodiola reduces mental fatigue and sharpens focus, making this elixir ideal for enhancing cognitive performance.

738. Lion's Mane and Reishi Stress-Resilience Capsules

Ingredients: 1 tablespoon Lion's Mane powder, 1 tablespoon Reishi Mushroom powder, empty gel capsules.

Preparation: Mix Lion's Mane and Reishi powders thoroughly. Fill empty capsules and seal.

Suggested Usage: Take 1 capsule daily to support brain health and resilience.

Benefits: Lion's Mane stimulates nerve regeneration, while Reishi supports cognitive function and reduces anxiety, making these capsules effective for promoting long-term brain health.

739. Gotu Kola and Sage Cognitive Health Capsules

Ingredients: 1 tablespoon Gotu Kola powder, 1 tablespoon Sage powder, empty gel capsules.

Preparation: Mix Gotu Kola and Sage powders thoroughly. Fill empty capsules and seal.

Suggested Usage: Take 1 capsule daily to enhance cognitive health and memory.

Benefits: Gotu Kola improves circulation and supports brain health, while Sage enhances memory and focus, making these capsules ideal for maintaining cognitive performance.

740. Bacopa and Ashwagandha Anti-Anxiety Tea

Ingredients: 1 tablespoon dried Bacopa, 1 tablespoon dried Ashwagandha, 2 cups hot water.

Preparation: Steep Bacopa and Ashwagandha in hot water for 15 minutes. Strain and serve warm.

Suggested Usage: Drink 1 cup up to twice daily to reduce anxiety and promote cognitive clarity.

Benefits: Bacopa enhances mental clarity, while Ashwagandha reduces stress and balances cortisol levels, making this tea effective for managing anxiety and supporting mental sharpness.

741. Holy Basil, Lemon Balm, and Chamomile Relaxation Tea

Ingredients: 1 tablespoon dried Holy Basil, 1 tablespoon dried Lemon Balm, 1 tablespoon dried Chamomile flowers, 2 cups hot water.

Preparation: Steep Holy Basil, Lemon Balm, and Chamomile in hot water for 15 minutes. Strain and serve warm.

Suggested Usage: Drink 1 cup daily to reduce stress and promote relaxation.

Benefits: Holy Basil, Lemon Balm, and Chamomile calm the nervous system, reduce anxiety, and promote emotional stability, making this tea ideal for maintaining mental clarity and focus.

Book 34: Natural Sleep Aids

Achieving restful and rejuvenating sleep is essential for overall health and well-being. The body and mind use sleep as a time for healing, regeneration, and maintaining balanced functions. Unfortunately, modern lifestyles, stress, and environmental factors can disrupt natural sleep patterns, leading to poor sleep quality or even insomnia. This chapter explores how herbs can be used to naturally promote sleep, restore circadian rhythms, and improve sleep quality, as well as how to integrate sleep-supporting herbal remedies into a healthy bedtime routine.

Herbs to Promote Restful Sleep

Herbs have been used for centuries to alleviate sleep disturbances, calm the nervous system, and promote relaxation. These herbs often work through gentle sedative properties, muscle relaxation, and mood-enhancing effects that prepare both the body and mind for a restful night's sleep.

One of the most widely used herbs for sleep is **Valerian Root**. Known for its natural sedative effects, Valerian Root has been shown to reduce the time it takes to fall asleep, improve sleep quality, and decrease nighttime awakenings. It works by increasing levels of gamma-aminobutyric acid (GABA) in the brain, a neurotransmitter that promotes relaxation. Valerian is most effective when taken consistently over a few weeks, making it ideal for those with chronic sleep difficulties.

Chamomile is another popular herb for sleep. Often consumed as a soothing tea, Chamomile contains apigenin, an antioxidant that binds to receptors in the brain, promoting relaxation and reducing anxiety. Chamomile tea is gentle enough to be used by children and the elderly, making it a versatile remedy for improving sleep quality and easing mild insomnia.

Lavender is not only known for its calming scent but also for its ability to enhance sleep. Lavender has been used in aromatherapy for its sedative and mood-stabilizing effects, making it beneficial for promoting restful sleep and reducing anxiety. Studies have shown that inhaling Lavender essential oil or using it in a bedtime massage can improve sleep quality, increase deep sleep, and reduce symptoms of insomnia.

Passionflower is a lesser-known but highly effective herb for promoting restful sleep. Like Valerian, Passionflower increases GABA levels in the brain, calming the nervous system and reducing racing thoughts that can disrupt sleep. Passionflower is particularly helpful for those who experience restlessness, anxiety, or an overactive mind at bedtime.

For those experiencing stress-induced insomnia, **Ashwagandha** can be a valuable addition to a sleep regimen. An adaptogen, Ashwagandha helps balance the body's stress response, lowering cortisol levels, and promoting a state of relaxation conducive to sleep. Regular use of Ashwagandha can help restore healthy sleep patterns, especially for individuals with high stress or anxiety.

Lemon Balm is another herb that has been traditionally used to ease tension and promote sleep. Known for its calming properties, Lemon Balm is often used in combination with other sleep-supporting herbs like Chamomile and Valerian. It helps reduce restlessness and supports a tranquil state of mind, making it ideal for those struggling with mild insomnia or stress-related sleep issues.

Hops, commonly used in beer brewing, is also an effective herbal sleep aid. Hops flowers contain a natural sedative compound that promotes deep, restful sleep. When combined with Valerian or Passionflower, Hops can be particularly effective in reducing the time it takes to fall asleep and improving overall sleep quality.

California Poppy is another powerful herb for promoting sleep and relaxation. It has mild sedative properties and is often used to ease tension and calm an overactive mind. California Poppy is especially useful for reducing sleep latency and encouraging a peaceful transition into sleep.

Skullcap, a lesser-known but highly effective herb, is used to calm an overactive mind and ease nervous tension. It is beneficial for those who experience racing thoughts or mental agitation before bedtime. Skullcap helps relax the body and mind, preparing you for a restful night's sleep.

St. John's Wort is another herb that, while primarily known for its mood-enhancing effects, can also promote restful sleep. By balancing serotonin levels and reducing anxiety, St. John's Wort can help regulate sleep patterns and support emotional well-being, making it an excellent option for individuals experiencing depression-related insomnia.

Sleep Hygiene Practices with Herbal Support

While herbal remedies can significantly improve sleep quality, incorporating them into a comprehensive sleep routine that supports healthy sleep hygiene is key for achieving long-term results. A few simple lifestyle adjustments, combined with the use of herbal sleep aids, can create an environment that promotes restorative sleep.

Creating a **calming bedtime routine** is one of the most effective ways to prepare the mind and body for sleep. Begin winding down at least an hour before bedtime by dimming the lights, turning off electronic devices, and engaging in relaxing activities such as reading or taking a warm bath. Incorporate herbs like Chamomile, Lemon Balm, or Lavender into this routine through teas, tinctures, or aromatherapy.

Establishing a **consistent sleep schedule** is also crucial. Going to bed and waking up at the same time each day helps regulate your internal clock, making it easier to fall asleep and wake up naturally. Herbal remedies such as Valerian and Hops can be used to support a healthy sleep cycle, especially if your sleep schedule has been disrupted.

Creating a **sleep-friendly environment** is equally important. Ensure that your bedroom is cool, dark, and quiet. Consider using herbal sachets filled with Lavender, Chamomile, and Hops, or essential oil diffusers with calming scents like Lavender and Cedarwood to enhance the atmosphere. Avoid stimulating activities or stressful conversations close to bedtime, and use herbal teas or tinctures to transition into a relaxed state.

Using **herbal teas** as part of your evening routine can help signal your body that it's time to unwind. For example, a cup of Chamomile and Lavender tea about an hour before bed can promote relaxation and help ease you into a restful sleep. Combining multiple herbs, such as Lemon Balm, Skullcap, and Passionflower, can provide a more potent calming effect, particularly for those who struggle with anxiety or an overactive mind.

Herbal **tinctures and elixirs** are also effective for those who prefer a more concentrated form of herbal support. Valerian, Passionflower, and California Poppy tinctures can be taken about 30 minutes before bedtime to induce sleep and reduce nighttime awakenings. Tinctures can be combined to address multiple sleep concerns, such as anxiety, restlessness, or difficulty falling asleep.

Incorporating **aromatherapy** into your bedtime routine can further enhance the sleep-promoting effects of herbs. Essential oils like Lavender, Cedarwood, and Roman Chamomile can be diffused in the bedroom, applied to pulse points, or added to a warm bath. Inhaling these calming scents signals the body to relax, helping to create a sleep-conducive environment.

Practicing **mindfulness and relaxation techniques** alongside herbal remedies can also be highly beneficial. Gentle yoga, deep breathing exercises, or meditation with calming herbs like Holy Basil or Lemon Balm can help reduce tension and promote a sense of peace before bedtime. Using herbal teas or tinctures that support relaxation can enhance the effectiveness of these practices.

By combining herbal remedies with healthy sleep hygiene practices, you can create a powerful, natural approach to achieving restorative and rejuvenating sleep. Implementing these strategies consistently will help regulate sleep patterns, reduce sleep disruptions, and improve overall sleep quality, leading to better physical and mental health.

Book 35: Mood-Boosting Herbal Remedies

Emotional health is an essential aspect of overall well-being, and herbs can play a powerful role in supporting a positive mood, alleviating symptoms of depression, and promoting a sense of happiness. By working to balance neurotransmitter levels, reduce stress, and support emotional stability, mood-enhancing herbs offer a natural alternative to conventional mood-altering medications. This chapter will explore various herbs known for their mood-boosting properties, their effects on the mind and body, and how to incorporate them into daily routines for enhanced emotional health. Additionally, it will provide recipes for teas, elixirs, and other herbal formulations that can provide an immediate mood boost and sustained emotional support.

Herbs to Elevate Mood and Happiness

There are many herbs traditionally used to promote happiness, reduce anxiety, and foster a sense of well-being. These herbs work by modulating neurotransmitters like serotonin, dopamine, and GABA, or by acting as adaptogens that balance the body's stress response. Here are some of the most effective herbs for elevating mood and promoting emotional health:

One of the best-known herbs for supporting a positive mood is **St. John's Wort**. This herb has been extensively studied for its antidepressant properties and is often used to alleviate mild to moderate depression. St. John's Wort works by inhibiting the reuptake of serotonin and dopamine, two neurotransmitters that regulate mood and happiness. This makes it an excellent choice for those experiencing low mood, sadness, or lack of motivation.

Another powerful herb for mood enhancement is **Saffron**. Often called "the sunshine spice," Saffron has been shown to increase serotonin levels and improve mood. Studies suggest that it may be as effective as some pharmaceutical antidepressants for alleviating symptoms of depression. Saffron's vibrant color and gentle effects on the nervous system make it ideal for adding to teas, elixirs, and culinary dishes to lift spirits and promote emotional well-being.

Rhodiola Rosea is an adaptogenic herb that enhances resilience to stress and promotes mental stamina. It works by balancing cortisol levels and supporting dopamine production, making it effective for reducing mental fatigue and uplifting mood. Rhodiola is particularly useful for individuals who experience burnout, lack of motivation, or emotional exhaustion.

Holy Basil, also known as Tulsi, is revered in Ayurveda for its ability to calm the mind, reduce stress, and enhance mood. Holy Basil works by modulating cortisol levels and supporting the body's natural stress response, making it an excellent choice for those dealing with anxiety, mood swings, or emotional instability.

Lemon Balm is another herb that gently lifts mood and promotes emotional balance. It works by increasing GABA levels in the brain, which helps to calm the nervous system and reduce anxiety. Lemon Balm is ideal for those experiencing restlessness, irritability, or low mood due to stress or anxiety.

Lavender is well-known for its calming and mood-enhancing properties. Its soothing scent can reduce anxiety and promote a sense of peace and well-being. Lavender can be used in teas, tinctures, or aromatherapy to reduce stress and create a calming environment.

Chamomile is a gentle herb that soothes the nervous system and promotes relaxation. Often used for its calming properties, Chamomile is ideal for reducing anxiety, easing tension, and promoting a positive outlook. It is particularly effective when used in teas or combined with other mood-enhancing herbs.

Ashwagandha is another adaptogen that supports emotional balance and reduces stress. By balancing cortisol levels and enhancing neurotransmitter function, Ashwagandha can improve mood, reduce anxiety, and promote a sense of calm. It is often used in capsules, teas, or tinctures for long-term support of emotional health.

Schisandra Berry is a lesser-known adaptogen that helps modulate stress, enhance energy, and uplift mood. It is particularly beneficial for those experiencing burnout or emotional fatigue, as it supports the adrenal system and enhances mental resilience.

Ginkgo Biloba, while primarily known for its cognitive-enhancing properties, also promotes a positive mood by improving circulation to the brain and supporting healthy neurotransmitter function. It can be used in teas or tinctures to boost mental clarity and foster emotional well-being.

Passionflower is a powerful nervine that promotes relaxation and reduces anxiety. It works by increasing GABA levels in the brain, making it effective for calming the mind and reducing overactivity that can contribute to anxiety or low mood.

Rose petals are not just beautiful but also emotionally uplifting. Rose is often used to open the heart, promote self-love, and enhance feelings of joy and happiness. Adding Rose petals to teas or using Rose water can create a sense of emotional well-being and peace.

Combining these herbs into blends and elixirs can provide a comprehensive approach to mood enhancement, supporting both immediate relief from low mood and long-term emotional health.

Recipes for Uplifting Elixirs

Creating herbal blends and elixirs that combine mood-enhancing herbs can offer powerful support for managing emotional health. These recipes are designed to be used during times of stress, low mood, or when a boost of happiness is needed.

For example, an **Uplifting Tea** that combines St. John's Wort, Lemon Balm, and Saffron can help elevate mood, reduce anxiety, and promote emotional resilience. This blend can be enjoyed daily to support overall emotional health or during times of increased stress.

A **Joyful Elixir** with Holy Basil, Rhodiola, and Lavender can reduce anxiety, enhance resilience to stress, and promote a sense of well-being. Adding a touch of honey can further enhance the soothing properties of the herbs, making it ideal for daily use or as a special treat when an emotional lift is needed.

For those experiencing emotional fatigue or burnout, a **Stress-Resilience Tonic** made with Ashwagandha, Schisandra, and Ginkgo Biloba can provide long-term support for energy and mood. This tonic can be taken in the morning to promote mental clarity and emotional balance throughout the day.

Creating **Mood-Boosting Capsules** with herbs like St. John's Wort, Rhodiola, and Saffron can provide a convenient way to support emotional health on a daily basis. Taking these capsules regularly can help stabilize mood, reduce anxiety, and promote a positive outlook.

For children or individuals who prefer a gentler approach, a **Gentle Mood Tea** with Chamomile, Lemon Balm, and Rose can provide relaxation and a sense of joy without causing drowsiness. This tea can be enjoyed any time of day to promote a calm, happy state of mind.

Incorporating **aromatherapy** with essential oils like Lavender, Lemon, and Bergamot can also enhance mood and reduce stress. Using these oils in a diffuser or creating a **Mood-Enhancing Spray** can create an uplifting environment and promote emotional well-being.

Whether using these herbs individually or in combination, mood-enhancing herbal remedies offer a natural way to support emotional health and promote a positive outlook. Regular use of these herbs, along with lifestyle practices such as mindfulness, exercise, and a balanced diet, can provide powerful support for emotional resilience and well-being.

Remedies for Mood Enhancement

742. St. John's Wort and Lemon Balm Mood-Lifting Tea

Ingredients: 1 tablespoon dried St. John's Wort, 1 tablespoon dried Lemon Balm, 2 cups hot water.
Preparation: Steep St. John's Wort and Lemon Balm in hot water for 15 minutes. Strain and serve warm.
Suggested Usage: Drink 1 cup daily to enhance mood and alleviate mild depression.
Benefits: St. John's Wort helps lift mood and reduce symptoms of depression, while Lemon Balm promotes calm and emotional stability, making this tea ideal for managing mood swings and promoting a positive mindset.

743. Holy Basil and Saffron Anti-Anxiety Capsules

Ingredients: 1 tablespoon Holy Basil powder, 1 teaspoon Saffron threads, empty gel capsules.
Preparation: Mix Holy Basil powder and Saffron threads thoroughly. Fill empty capsules and seal.
Suggested Usage: Take 1 capsule daily to reduce anxiety and promote emotional balance.
Benefits: Holy Basil calms the nervous system and lowers cortisol levels, while Saffron enhances mood and reduces anxiety, making these capsules effective for maintaining emotional well-being.

744. Chamomile and Lavender Calming Elixir

Ingredients: 1 tablespoon dried Chamomile flowers, 1 tablespoon dried Lavender flowers, 2 cups hot water.
Preparation: Steep Chamomile and Lavender in hot water for 15 minutes. Strain and serve warm.
Suggested Usage: Drink 1 cup in the evening to promote relaxation and reduce stress.
Benefits: Chamomile and Lavender calm the nervous system, promote relaxation, and enhance sleep quality, making this elixir ideal for winding down and reducing stress.

745. Lemon Balm and Skullcap Emotional Balance Tea

Ingredients: 1 tablespoon dried Lemon Balm, 1 tablespoon dried Skullcap, 2 cups hot water.
Preparation: Steep Lemon Balm and Skullcap in hot water for 15 minutes. Strain and serve warm.
Suggested Usage: Drink 1 cup daily to stabilize mood and promote emotional balance.
Benefits: Lemon Balm and Skullcap calm the mind, reduce anxiety, and support emotional stability, making this tea ideal for managing stress and promoting inner calm.

746. Rhodiola and Ashwagandha Stress-Relief Capsules

Ingredients: 1 tablespoon Rhodiola Root powder, 1 tablespoon Ashwagandha Root powder, empty gel capsules.
Preparation: Mix Rhodiola and Ashwagandha powders thoroughly. Fill empty capsules and seal.
Suggested Usage: Take 1 capsule daily to reduce stress and support resilience.
Benefits: Rhodiola enhances mental resilience and reduces fatigue, while Ashwagandha lowers cortisol levels and promotes calm, making these capsules effective for managing chronic stress.

747. Passionflower and Lemon Balm Nervous System Support Tincture

Ingredients: 1 tablespoon dried Passionflower, 1 tablespoon dried Lemon Balm, 1 cup vodka or brandy.
Preparation: Combine herbs and alcohol in a glass jar. Seal tightly and let steep for 4-6 weeks, shaking occasionally. Strain and store in a dark bottle.
Suggested Usage: Take ½ teaspoon up to twice daily to support the nervous system and reduce anxiety.
Benefits: Passionflower and Lemon Balm soothe the nervous system, reduce restlessness, and promote calm, making this tincture ideal for managing anxiety and stress.

748. Saffron and Holy Basil Antidepressant Tea

Ingredients: 1 teaspoon Saffron threads, 1 tablespoon dried Holy Basil, 2 cups hot water.
Preparation: Steep Saffron and Holy Basil in hot water for 15 minutes. Strain and serve warm.
Suggested Usage: Drink 1 cup daily to enhance mood and reduce depressive symptoms.
Benefits: Saffron elevates mood and reduces symptoms of depression, while Holy Basil promotes emotional stability and reduces anxiety, making this tea ideal for managing mood disorders.

749. Lavender and Lemon Balm Relaxation Tea

Ingredients: 1 tablespoon dried Lavender, 1 tablespoon dried Lemon Balm, 2 cups hot water.
Preparation: Steep Lavender and Lemon Balm in hot water for 15 minutes. Strain and serve warm.
Suggested Usage: Drink 1 cup in the evening to promote relaxation and reduce anxiety.
Benefits: Lavender and Lemon Balm calm the mind and body, promote a sense of peace, and support restful sleep, making this tea ideal for reducing stress and enhancing relaxation.

750. St. John's Wort and Skullcap Mood-Enhancing Capsules

Ingredients: 1 tablespoon St. John's Wort powder, 1 tablespoon Skullcap powder, empty gel capsules.
Preparation: Mix St. John's Wort and Skullcap powders thoroughly. Fill empty

capsules and seal.

Suggested Usage: Take 1 capsule daily to support mood and emotional stability.

Benefits: St. John's Wort lifts mood and reduces depressive symptoms, while Skullcap calms the nervous system, making these capsules effective for managing anxiety and promoting emotional well-being.

751. Chamomile, Lavender, and Lemon Balm Bedtime Tea

Ingredients: 1 tablespoon dried Chamomile flowers, 1 tablespoon dried Lavender flowers, 1 tablespoon dried Lemon Balm, 2 cups hot water.

Preparation: Steep Chamomile, Lavender, and Lemon Balm in hot water for 15 minutes. Strain and serve warm.

Suggested Usage: Drink 1 cup before bed to promote relaxation and restful sleep.

Benefits: Chamomile, Lavender, and Lemon Balm promote relaxation, reduce anxiety, and support restful sleep, making this tea ideal for calming the mind and preparing for a good night's sleep.

752. Gotu Kola and Rhodiola Stress-Relieving Capsules

Ingredients: 1 tablespoon Gotu Kola powder, 1 tablespoon Rhodiola Root powder, empty gel capsules.

Preparation: Mix Gotu Kola and Rhodiola powders thoroughly. Fill empty capsules and seal.

Suggested Usage: Take 1 capsule daily to reduce stress and enhance mental clarity.

Benefits: Gotu Kola improves circulation and cognitive function, while Rhodiola reduces stress and enhances focus, making

these capsules effective for promoting resilience and reducing anxiety.

753. Passionflower and Hops Sleep Support Tea

Ingredients: 1 tablespoon dried Passionflower, 1 tablespoon dried Hops flowers, 2 cups hot water.

Preparation: Steep Passionflower and Hops in hot water for 15 minutes. Strain and serve warm.

Suggested Usage: Drink 1 cup in the evening to promote restful sleep.

Benefits: Passionflower and Hops act as natural sedatives, promoting deep, restful sleep and reducing anxiety, making this tea ideal for managing insomnia and stress.

754. Lemon Balm and Valerian Calming Capsules

Ingredients: 1 tablespoon Lemon Balm powder, 1 tablespoon Valerian Root powder, empty gel capsules.

Preparation: Mix Lemon Balm and Valerian powders thoroughly. Fill empty capsules and seal.

Suggested Usage: Take 1 capsule up to twice daily to reduce anxiety and promote relaxation.

Benefits: Lemon Balm reduces nervous tension, while Valerian acts as a natural sedative, making these capsules effective for promoting calm and reducing anxiety.

755. Saffron and St. John's Wort Uplifting Tincture

Ingredients: 1 teaspoon Saffron threads, 1 tablespoon dried St. John's Wort, 1 cup vodka or brandy.

Preparation: Combine herbs and alcohol in a glass jar. Seal tightly and let steep for 4-6 weeks, shaking occasionally. Strain and store in a dark bottle.

Suggested Usage: Take ½ teaspoon up to twice daily to uplift mood and reduce depression.

Benefits: Saffron and St. John's Wort improve mood, reduce anxiety, and alleviate depressive symptoms, making this tincture ideal for managing mood disorders and enhancing emotional well-being.

756. Reishi and Schisandra Adaptogen Mood-Balancing Capsules

Ingredients: 1 tablespoon Reishi Mushroom powder, 1 tablespoon Schisandra Berry powder, empty gel capsules.

Preparation: Mix Reishi and Schisandra powders thoroughly. Fill empty capsules and seal.

Suggested Usage: Take 1 capsule daily to promote emotional balance and resilience.

Benefits: Reishi and Schisandra support adrenal health, balance mood, and promote mental clarity, making these capsules effective for managing stress and enhancing emotional well-being.

757. Lavender and Holy Basil Emotional Balance Tea

Ingredients: 1 tablespoon dried Lavender, 1 tablespoon dried Holy Basil, 2 cups hot water.

Preparation: Steep Lavender and Holy Basil in hot water for 15 minutes. Strain and serve warm.

Suggested Usage: Drink 1 cup daily to support emotional balance and reduce anxiety.

Benefits: Lavender calms the mind and body, while Holy Basil acts as an adaptogen to stabilize mood and reduce stress, making this tea effective for maintaining emotional well-being.

758. Chamomile and Skullcap Anti-Anxiety Capsules

Ingredients: 1 tablespoon Chamomile powder, 1 tablespoon Skullcap powder, empty gel capsules.

Preparation: Mix Chamomile and Skullcap powders thoroughly. Fill empty capsules and seal.

Suggested Usage: Take 1 capsule daily to reduce anxiety and promote calm.

Benefits: Chamomile soothes the nervous system, and Skullcap reduces anxiety and promotes relaxation, making these capsules ideal for managing stress and supporting a calm state of mind.

759. Lemon Balm and Holy Basil Mood-Stabilizing Elixir

Ingredients: 1 tablespoon dried Lemon Balm, 1 tablespoon dried Holy Basil, 2 cups hot water.

Preparation: Steep Lemon Balm and Holy Basil in hot water for 15 minutes. Strain and serve warm.

Suggested Usage: Drink 1 cup daily to stabilize mood and promote emotional resilience.

Benefits: Lemon Balm calms the nervous

system, while Holy Basil reduces cortisol levels and stabilizes mood, making this elixir ideal for promoting emotional balance.

760. Rhodiola and Ginseng Energy-Boosting Capsules

Ingredients: 1 tablespoon Rhodiola Root powder, 1 tablespoon Ginseng Root powder, empty gel capsules.
Preparation: Mix Rhodiola and Ginseng powders thoroughly. Fill empty capsules and seal.
Suggested Usage: Take 1 capsule daily to enhance energy levels and reduce mental fatigue.
Benefits: Rhodiola supports mental resilience, while Ginseng boosts energy and cognitive performance, making these capsules effective for reducing fatigue and maintaining focus.

761. Skullcap and Passionflower Nerve-Calming Tea

Ingredients: 1 tablespoon dried Skullcap, 1 tablespoon dried Passionflower, 2 cups hot water.
Preparation: Steep Skullcap and Passionflower in hot water for 15 minutes. Strain and serve warm.
Suggested Usage: Drink 1 cup in the evening to calm the nerves and promote relaxation.
Benefits: Skullcap and Passionflower soothe the nervous system, reduce anxiety, and promote relaxation, making this tea ideal for managing stress and calming an overactive mind.

762. Ashwagandha and Holy Basil Adrenal Support Capsules

Ingredients: 1 tablespoon Ashwagandha Root powder, 1 tablespoon Holy Basil powder, empty gel capsules.
Preparation: Mix Ashwagandha and Holy Basil powders thoroughly. Fill empty capsules and seal.
Suggested Usage: Take 1 capsule daily to support adrenal health and reduce stress.
Benefits: Ashwagandha balances cortisol levels and reduces anxiety, while Holy Basil acts as an adaptogen to support adrenal health, making these capsules effective for managing chronic stress.

763. Lemon Balm and Chamomile Emotional Soothing Tea

Ingredients: 1 tablespoon dried Lemon Balm, 1 tablespoon dried Chamomile, 2 cups hot water.
Preparation: Steep Lemon Balm and Chamomile in hot water for 15 minutes. Strain and serve warm.
Suggested Usage: Drink 1 cup daily to reduce anxiety and promote emotional calm.
Benefits: Lemon Balm and Chamomile soothe the nervous system, reduce restlessness, and promote a sense of peace, making this tea ideal for emotional soothing and managing stress.

764. Reishi and Ashwagandha Stress-Resilience Capsules

Ingredients: 1 tablespoon Reishi Mushroom powder, 1 tablespoon Ashwagandha Root powder, empty gel capsules.

Preparation: Mix Reishi and Ashwagandha powders thoroughly. Fill empty capsules and seal.

Suggested Usage: Take 1 capsule daily to enhance resilience and reduce stress.

Benefits: Reishi supports immune health and cognitive function, while Ashwagandha reduces cortisol levels and promotes calm, making these capsules ideal for managing chronic stress and enhancing resilience.

765. Saffron and Gotu Kola Emotional Balance Tea

Ingredients: 1 teaspoon Saffron threads, 1 tablespoon dried Gotu Kola, 2 cups hot water.

Preparation: Steep Saffron and Gotu Kola in hot water for 15 minutes. Strain and serve warm.

Suggested Usage: Drink 1 cup daily to promote emotional stability and reduce anxiety.

Benefits: Saffron elevates mood and reduces symptoms of depression, while Gotu Kola calms the mind and supports cognitive function, making this tea effective for promoting emotional balance.

766. St. John's Wort and Passionflower Mood-Stabilizing Capsules

Ingredients: 1 tablespoon St. John's Wort powder, 1 tablespoon Passionflower powder, empty gel capsules.

Preparation: Mix St. John's Wort and Passionflower powders thoroughly. Fill empty capsules and seal.

Suggested Usage: Take 1 capsule daily to support mood and reduce anxiety.

Benefits: St. John's Wort stabilizes mood and reduces depressive symptoms, while Passionflower calms the nervous system, making these capsules effective for managing mood disorders and promoting emotional stability.

767. Lemon Balm and Lavender Calm-Enhancing Capsules

Ingredients: 1 tablespoon Lemon Balm powder, 1 tablespoon Lavender powder, empty gel capsules.

Preparation: Mix Lemon Balm and Lavender powders thoroughly. Fill empty capsules and seal.

Suggested Usage: Take 1 capsule daily to reduce anxiety and promote calm.

Benefits: Lemon Balm and Lavender calm the mind, reduce stress, and support restful sleep, making these capsules ideal for maintaining emotional balance and promoting a sense of peace.

768. Holy Basil and Schisandra Adaptogen Tea

Ingredients: 1 tablespoon dried Holy Basil, 1 tablespoon dried Schisandra Berries, 2 cups hot water.

Preparation: Steep Holy Basil and Schisandra in hot water for 15 minutes. Strain and serve warm.

Suggested Usage: Drink 1 cup up to twice daily to promote resilience and support mental clarity.

Benefits: Holy Basil calms the mind and reduces cortisol levels, while Schisandra supports adrenal health and enhances cognitive performance, making this tea ideal for managing stress and promoting emotional resilience.

769. Chamomile and Lemon Balm Sleep-Enhancing Tea

Ingredients: 1 tablespoon dried Chamomile flowers, 1 tablespoon dried Lemon Balm leaves, 2 cups hot water.
Preparation: Steep Chamomile and Lemon Balm in hot water for 15 minutes. Strain and serve warm.
Suggested Usage: Drink 1 cup before bedtime to promote relaxation and enhance sleep quality.
Benefits: Chamomile soothes the nervous system, and Lemon Balm calms the mind, making this tea ideal for supporting restful sleep and reducing nighttime anxiety.

770. Skullcap and Lavender Nerve Support Capsules

Ingredients: 1 tablespoon Skullcap powder, 1 tablespoon Lavender powder, empty gel capsules.
Preparation: Mix Skullcap and Lavender powders thoroughly. Fill empty capsules and seal.
Suggested Usage: Take 1 capsule daily to calm the nerves and promote emotional stability.
Benefits: Skullcap reduces nervous tension, while Lavender supports emotional balance and promotes calm, making these capsules effective for managing stress and supporting the nervous system.

771. Rhodiola and Saffron Anti-Anxiety Elixir

Ingredients: 1 tablespoon dried Rhodiola Root, 1 teaspoon Saffron threads, 2 cups hot water.
Preparation: Steep Rhodiola and Saffron in hot water for 20 minutes. Strain and serve warm.
Suggested Usage: Drink 1 cup daily to reduce anxiety and promote mental resilience.
Benefits: Rhodiola enhances stress resilience and cognitive clarity, while Saffron improves mood and reduces anxiety, making this elixir effective for managing emotional stress and enhancing mental performance.

772. St. John's Wort and Rhodiola Stress-Balancing Capsules

Ingredients: 1 tablespoon St. John's Wort powder, 1 tablespoon Rhodiola Root powder, empty gel capsules.
Preparation: Mix St. John's Wort and Rhodiola powders thoroughly. Fill empty capsules and seal.
Suggested Usage: Take 1 capsule daily to support mood and reduce stress.
Benefits: St. John's Wort stabilizes mood and reduces depressive symptoms, while Rhodiola reduces mental fatigue and promotes resilience, making these capsules ideal for managing stress and supporting mental clarity.

773. Ashwagandha and Saffron Mood-Stabilizing Capsules

Ingredients: 1 tablespoon Ashwagandha Root powder, 1 teaspoon Saffron threads, empty gel capsules.
Preparation: Mix Ashwagandha and

Saffron thoroughly. Fill empty capsules and seal.

Suggested Usage: Take 1 capsule daily to stabilize mood and reduce anxiety.

Benefits: Ashwagandha reduces cortisol levels and balances stress, while Saffron elevates mood and reduces anxiety, making these capsules effective for managing mood swings and promoting emotional stability.

774. Skullcap and Passionflower Nervous System Calming Tea

Ingredients: 1 tablespoon dried Skullcap, 1 tablespoon dried Passionflower, 2 cups hot water.

Preparation: Steep Skullcap and Passionflower in hot water for 15 minutes. Strain and serve warm.

Suggested Usage: Drink 1 cup daily to calm the nervous system and reduce anxiety.

Benefits: Skullcap soothes the nerves, and Passionflower promotes relaxation, making this tea ideal for reducing mental tension and promoting a state of calm.

775. Lemon Balm, Lavender, and Holy Basil Relaxation Tea

Ingredients: 1 tablespoon dried Lemon Balm, 1 tablespoon dried Lavender, 1 tablespoon dried Holy Basil, 2 cups hot water.

Preparation: Steep Lemon Balm, Lavender, and Holy Basil in hot water for 15 minutes. Strain and serve warm.

Suggested Usage: Drink 1 cup in the evening to promote relaxation and reduce stress.

Benefits: Lemon Balm calms the mind, Lavender reduces tension, and Holy Basil stabilizes mood, making this tea effective for managing stress and promoting emotional balance.

776. Saffron and Chamomile Sleep Support Capsules

Ingredients: 1 teaspoon Saffron threads, 1 tablespoon Chamomile powder, empty gel capsules.

Preparation: Mix Saffron and Chamomile powders thoroughly. Fill empty capsules and seal.

Suggested Usage: Take 1 capsule daily before bedtime to promote restful sleep.

Benefits: Saffron reduces anxiety and improves mood, while Chamomile promotes relaxation and enhances sleep quality, making these capsules effective for managing insomnia and supporting restful sleep.

777. Reishi and Lemon Balm Emotional Balance Tea

Ingredients: 1 tablespoon dried Reishi Mushroom, 1 tablespoon dried Lemon Balm, 2 cups hot water.

Preparation: Simmer Reishi Mushroom and Lemon Balm in hot water for 20 minutes. Strain and serve warm.

Suggested Usage: Drink 1 cup daily to reduce anxiety and promote emotional stability.

Benefits: Reishi supports emotional balance and reduces stress, while Lemon Balm calms the mind, making this tea ideal for maintaining emotional well-being.

778. Gotu Kola and Holy Basil Stress-Reducing Capsules

Ingredients: 1 tablespoon Gotu Kola powder, 1 tablespoon Holy Basil powder, empty gel capsules.
Preparation: Mix Gotu Kola and Holy Basil powders thoroughly. Fill empty capsules and seal.
Suggested Usage: Take 1 capsule daily to reduce stress and support cognitive clarity.
Benefits: Gotu Kola enhances cognitive function, and Holy Basil reduces cortisol levels, making these capsules ideal for managing stress and supporting mental clarity.

779. Lavender, Chamomile, and Skullcap Sleep-Enhancing Tea

Ingredients: 1 tablespoon dried Lavender flowers, 1 tablespoon dried Chamomile flowers, 1 tablespoon dried Skullcap, 2 cups hot water.
Preparation: Steep Lavender, Chamomile, and Skullcap in hot water for 15 minutes. Strain and serve warm.
Suggested Usage: Drink 1 cup before bedtime to promote restful sleep.
Benefits: Lavender, Chamomile, and Skullcap calm the nervous system, reduce anxiety, and support deep, restful sleep, making this tea ideal for managing insomnia.

780. Saffron and Passionflower Anxiety-Reducing Elixir

Ingredients: 1 teaspoon Saffron threads, 1 tablespoon dried Passionflower, 2 cups hot water.
Preparation: Steep Saffron and Passionflower in hot water for 15 minutes. Strain and serve warm.
Suggested Usage: Drink 1 cup daily to reduce anxiety and support emotional stability.
Benefits: Saffron elevates mood and reduces anxiety, while Passionflower calms the mind and promotes relaxation, making this elixir effective for managing anxiety and supporting a calm state of mind.

781. Rhodiola and Schisandra Energy-Enhancing Capsules

Ingredients: 1 tablespoon Rhodiola Root powder, 1 tablespoon Schisandra Berry powder, empty gel capsules.
Preparation: Mix Rhodiola and Schisandra powders thoroughly. Fill empty capsules and seal.
Suggested Usage: Take 1 capsule daily to reduce fatigue and boost energy levels.
Benefits: Rhodiola enhances mental stamina and reduces stress, while Schisandra supports adrenal health and improves energy, making these capsules effective for reducing burnout and maintaining mental clarity.

782. Ashwagandha and Lemon Balm Stress Relief Tea

Ingredients: 1 tablespoon dried Ashwagandha Root, 1 tablespoon dried Lemon Balm, 2 cups hot water.
Preparation: Steep Ashwagandha and Lemon Balm in hot water for 15 minutes. Strain and serve warm.
Suggested Usage: Drink 1 cup up to twice daily to promote relaxation and reduce

anxiety.

Benefits: Ashwagandha reduces cortisol levels and balances stress, while Lemon Balm calms the nervous system, making this tea ideal for managing stress and promoting a state of calm.

783. St. John's Wort and Reishi Mood-Boosting Capsules

Ingredients: 1 tablespoon St. John's Wort powder, 1 tablespoon Reishi Mushroom powder, empty gel capsules.

Preparation: Mix St. John's Wort and Reishi powders thoroughly. Fill empty capsules and seal.

Suggested Usage: Take 1 capsule daily to enhance mood and reduce anxiety.

Benefits: St. John's Wort improves mood and reduces depressive symptoms, while Reishi supports emotional balance, making these capsules effective for maintaining a positive outlook.

784. Skullcap and Holy Basil Anti-Anxiety Tea

Ingredients: 1 tablespoon dried Skullcap, 1 tablespoon dried Holy Basil, 2 cups hot water.

Preparation: Steep Skullcap and Holy Basil in hot water for 15 minutes. Strain and serve warm.

Suggested Usage: Drink 1 cup up to twice daily to reduce anxiety and calm the nerves.

Benefits: Skullcap soothes nervous tension, and Holy Basil acts as an adaptogen to stabilize mood and reduce cortisol levels, making this tea ideal for managing anxiety and promoting emotional balance.

785. Lemon Balm and Passionflower Relaxation Tea

Ingredients: 1 tablespoon dried Lemon Balm, 1 tablespoon dried Passionflower, 2 cups hot water.

Preparation: Steep Lemon Balm and Passionflower in hot water for 15 minutes. Strain and serve warm.

Suggested Usage: Drink 1 cup in the evening to promote relaxation and reduce stress.

Benefits: Lemon Balm and Passionflower calm the mind and body, reduce anxiety, and promote relaxation, making this tea ideal for winding down in the evening.

786. Reishi and Rhodiola Immune-Boosting Capsules

Ingredients: 1 tablespoon Reishi Mushroom powder, 1 tablespoon Rhodiola Root powder, empty gel capsules.

Preparation: Mix Reishi and Rhodiola powders thoroughly. Fill empty capsules and seal.

Suggested Usage: Take 1 capsule daily to enhance immune health and reduce fatigue.

Benefits: Reishi supports immune function and cognitive health, while Rhodiola reduces stress and promotes mental clarity, making these capsules effective for maintaining resilience and immune balance.

787. Chamomile and Valerian Sleep-Inducing Tea

Ingredients: 1 tablespoon dried Chamomile flowers, 1 tablespoon dried

Valerian Root, 2 cups hot water.
Preparation: Steep Chamomile and Valerian in hot water for 15 minutes. Strain and serve warm.
Suggested Usage: Drink 1 cup 30 minutes before bed to promote restful sleep.
Benefits: Chamomile calms the mind and reduces anxiety, while Valerian acts as a natural sedative, making this tea ideal for supporting deep, restful sleep and reducing nighttime awakenings.

788. Holy Basil and Lemon Balm Adaptogenic Tea

Ingredients: 1 tablespoon dried Holy Basil, 1 tablespoon dried Lemon Balm, 2 cups hot water.
Preparation: Steep Holy Basil and Lemon Balm in hot water for 15 minutes. Strain and serve warm.
Suggested Usage: Drink 1 cup daily to promote emotional balance and reduce anxiety.
Benefits: Holy Basil balances cortisol levels and reduces stress, while Lemon Balm promotes relaxation and emotional stability, making this tea ideal for managing mood swings and enhancing resilience.

789. Ashwagandha and Gotu Kola Calm Focus Capsules

Ingredients: 1 tablespoon Ashwagandha Root powder, 1 tablespoon Gotu Kola powder, empty gel capsules.
Preparation: Mix Ashwagandha and Gotu Kola powders thoroughly. Fill empty capsules and seal.
Suggested Usage: Take 1 capsule daily to support focus and reduce stress.

Benefits: Ashwagandha lowers cortisol levels and reduces anxiety, while Gotu Kola enhances cognitive function and promotes mental clarity, making these capsules effective for maintaining calm focus under stress.

790. Skullcap, Lavender, and Lemon Balm Emotional Balance Tea

Ingredients: 1 tablespoon dried Skullcap, 1 tablespoon dried Lavender, 1 tablespoon dried Lemon Balm, 2 cups hot water.
Preparation: Steep Skullcap, Lavender, and Lemon Balm in hot water for 15 minutes. Strain and serve warm.
Suggested Usage: Drink 1 cup daily to reduce anxiety and promote emotional stability.
Benefits: Skullcap and Lavender calm the nervous system, and Lemon Balm reduces restlessness, making this tea effective for managing emotional turmoil and promoting inner peace.

791. Saffron and Lemon Balm Anti-Depressant Capsules

Ingredients: 1 teaspoon Saffron threads, 1 tablespoon Lemon Balm powder, empty gel capsules.
Preparation: Mix Saffron and Lemon Balm powders thoroughly. Fill empty capsules and seal.
Suggested Usage: Take 1 capsule daily to reduce depressive symptoms and promote emotional well-being.
Benefits: Saffron enhances mood and reduces symptoms of depression, while Lemon Balm calms the mind and promotes emotional stability, making

these capsules ideal for supporting mental health and reducing anxiety.

Book 36: Natural Remedies for ADHD

Attention Deficit Hyperactivity Disorder (ADHD) is a neurodevelopmental condition that affects both children and adults, characterized by symptoms such as inattention, impulsivity, and hyperactivity. While conventional treatments typically involve stimulant medications and behavioral therapy, many individuals seek natural remedies to support cognitive function and manage symptoms without the potential side effects associated with pharmaceuticals. This chapter explores various herbs known to enhance focus, attention, and mental clarity in individuals with ADHD, offering natural support to complement conventional treatments.

Herbal Support for Attention and Focus

Managing ADHD symptoms involves enhancing cognitive function, promoting calmness, and reducing stress and anxiety. Several herbs are recognized for their ability to support these aspects, improving focus and attention in a natural, balanced way.

One of the most effective herbs for supporting cognitive function in individuals with ADHD is **Bacopa Monnieri**. Known in Ayurvedic medicine as Brahmi, Bacopa has been traditionally used for enhancing memory, learning, and concentration. It works by modulating neurotransmitter activity, promoting synaptic communication, and protecting neurons from oxidative stress. Clinical studies suggest that Bacopa can reduce hyperactivity, improve attention, and support cognitive function, making it a cornerstone herb for ADHD protocols.

Ginkgo Biloba is another potent herb for supporting cognitive health and mental performance. It increases cerebral blood flow, enhancing the delivery of oxygen and nutrients to the brain, which can improve memory, attention, and processing speed. Its antioxidant properties protect neurons from damage, making it particularly effective for individuals with ADHD who struggle with attention and focus.

Gotu Kola is renowned in both Ayurvedic and Traditional Chinese Medicine for its ability to enhance memory, mental clarity, and focus. It works by improving circulation, strengthening blood vessels, and promoting neuroplasticity. These properties make Gotu Kola a powerful brain tonic for individuals seeking to improve cognitive function and sustain focus during tasks that require prolonged attention.

Rhodiola Rosea is an adaptogen that can benefit individuals with ADHD by reducing fatigue, enhancing focus, and supporting mental stamina. It works by balancing stress hormones and promoting the regulation of neurotransmitters like dopamine and serotonin, which are often implicated in ADHD. Rhodiola's ability to reduce mental burnout and increase resilience makes it particularly useful for managing ADHD-related cognitive fatigue.

Lion's Mane Mushroom is a nootropic and neuroprotective herb that supports the production of nerve growth factor (NGF), which is essential for the maintenance and regeneration of neurons. Lion's Mane enhances cognitive function, supports memory and focus, and promotes overall brain health. This mushroom is especially beneficial for individuals with ADHD who experience cognitive fog and lack of focus.

Passionflower and **Lemon Balm** are calming herbs that can help reduce hyperactivity and restlessness, common symptoms of ADHD. Passionflower increases GABA levels in the brain, which helps to promote relaxation and reduce excitability. Lemon Balm, on the other hand, alleviates anxiety and promotes a sense of calm, making it ideal for individuals who experience mood swings or irritability.

Ashwagandha, a renowned adaptogen in Ayurvedic medicine, helps balance cortisol levels and reduce stress, which can indirectly improve focus and reduce impulsivity in individuals with ADHD. It also promotes overall brain health and supports the nervous system, making it a valuable herb for long-term management of ADHD symptoms.

Skullcap is a nervine herb that helps calm an overactive mind, reduce nervous tension, and promote mental clarity. It can be particularly beneficial for managing the restlessness and agitation often associated with ADHD, allowing for improved focus and concentration.

Combining these herbs into herbal blends, teas, and capsules can provide a comprehensive approach to supporting cognitive health and managing ADHD symptoms naturally.

Recipes for Concentration-Enhancing Blends

Herbal remedies for ADHD can be used in various forms, including teas, tinctures, and capsules. Creating blends that combine multiple herbs with complementary effects can offer a more targeted approach to improving focus, reducing hyperactivity, and supporting emotional stability.

For example, a **Focus and Memory Tea** that combines Gotu Kola, Bacopa Monnieri, and Ginkgo Biloba can provide immediate and long-term support for cognitive function. This tea blend enhances memory, increases blood flow to the brain, and promotes synaptic communication, making it ideal for individuals who need sustained concentration for studying or work.

A **Calming Adaptogen Elixir** made with Rhodiola Rosea, Holy Basil, and Lemon Balm can reduce anxiety, stabilize mood, and support mental stamina. Adding a touch of honey can enhance the soothing properties of the herbs, making this elixir both effective and enjoyable to consume.

For children with ADHD, a **Gentle Nerve Tonic** with Skullcap, Chamomile, and Lemon Balm can provide relaxation and reduce restlessness without causing drowsiness. Adding a small amount of Licorice Root can improve the flavor and enhance the calming properties of the blend, making it more appealing for younger individuals.

Creating herbal capsules with **Lion's Mane Mushroom**, **Bacopa**, and **Gotu Kola** can provide long-term support for cognitive health. Taking these capsules regularly can help enhance focus, memory, and overall brain function, making them ideal for individuals who want a convenient, daily supplement for ADHD management.

For managing hyperactivity and impulsivity, a **Soothing Nervine Tea** made with Skullcap, Lemon Balm, and Passionflower can promote calmness and reduce excitability. This blend is particularly effective when used in the evening to promote relaxation and prepare the body for restful sleep.

A **Concentration-Enhancing Tincture** with Bacopa, Ginkgo Biloba, and Rhodiola can be taken during the day to boost focus and mental clarity. This tincture can be carried in a small bottle for use during times of intense cognitive demand, such as exams or important work projects.

For those who struggle with hyperactivity and impulsiveness, creating an **Adaptogen Tonic** that combines Ashwagandha, Reishi Mushroom, and Holy Basil can provide long-term support for emotional stability and focus. This blend balances stress hormones, supports adrenal health, and enhances overall cognitive function.

Incorporating **aromatherapy** can also be beneficial for supporting attention and focus in individuals with ADHD. Essential oils such as Rosemary, Peppermint, and Lemon have been shown to improve concentration and mental clarity. Creating a **Focus Aromatherapy Blend** with these essential oils can provide immediate support for attention and focus. Applying this blend to pulse points or using it in an inhaler can promote a calm, focused state of mind during challenging tasks.

By combining these herbs into effective formulations, individuals with ADHD can experience improved focus, reduced anxiety, and enhanced emotional stability. Using natural remedies alongside lifestyle modifications, dietary changes, and behavioral therapies can provide a holistic approach to managing ADHD and supporting cognitive health.

Remedies for ADHD

792. Rhodiola and Bacopa Focus Capsules

Ingredients: 1 tablespoon Rhodiola Root powder, 1 tablespoon Bacopa Monnieri powder, empty gel capsules.
Preparation: Mix Rhodiola and Bacopa

powders thoroughly. Fill empty capsules and seal.

Suggested Usage: Take 1 capsule in the morning to enhance focus and reduce mental fatigue.

Benefits: Rhodiola helps combat fatigue and increase stamina, while Bacopa improves memory and concentration, making this blend ideal for supporting mental clarity and cognitive function.

793. Lemon Balm and Passionflower Calm Tea

Ingredients: 1 tablespoon dried Lemon Balm, 1 tablespoon dried Passionflower, 2 cups hot water.

Preparation: Steep Lemon Balm and Passionflower in hot water for 10-15 minutes. Strain and serve warm.

Suggested Usage: Drink 1 cup up to twice daily to reduce anxiety and promote relaxation.

Benefits: Lemon Balm calms the nervous system and reduces anxiety, while Passionflower promotes relaxation and soothes restlessness, making this tea ideal for calming an overactive mind.

794. Ginkgo Biloba and Rosemary Concentration Capsules

Ingredients: 1 tablespoon Ginkgo Biloba powder, 1 tablespoon Rosemary powder, empty gel capsules.

Preparation: Mix Ginkgo Biloba and Rosemary powders thoroughly. Fill empty capsules and seal.

Suggested Usage: Take 1 capsule daily to support memory and mental sharpness.

Benefits: Ginkgo Biloba enhances circulation to the brain, improving memory and cognitive function, while Rosemary stimulates mental clarity and focus.

795. Holy Basil and Lavender Relaxation Capsules

Ingredients: 1 tablespoon Holy Basil powder, 1 tablespoon dried Lavender flowers, empty gel capsules.

Preparation: Grind Lavender flowers into a fine powder and mix with Holy Basil powder. Fill empty capsules and seal.

Suggested Usage: Take 1 capsule in the evening to promote relaxation and reduce stress.

Benefits: Holy Basil acts as an adaptogen to balance stress responses, while Lavender soothes the nervous system, making this blend ideal for relaxation and emotional balance.

796. Ashwagandha and Reishi Anti-Stress Tea

Ingredients: 1 tablespoon dried Ashwagandha Root, 1 tablespoon Reishi Mushroom powder, 2 cups hot water.

Preparation: Simmer Ashwagandha and Reishi in hot water for 15-20 minutes. Strain and serve warm.

Suggested Usage: Drink 1 cup daily to reduce stress and enhance resilience.

Benefits: Ashwagandha helps balance cortisol levels and reduce stress, while Reishi supports the immune system and promotes emotional stability, making this tea effective for managing daily stress.

797. Skullcap and Valerian Nerve Calming Capsules

Ingredients: 1 tablespoon Skullcap powder, 1 tablespoon Valerian Root powder, empty gel capsules.
Preparation: Mix Skullcap and Valerian powders thoroughly. Fill empty capsules and seal.
Suggested Usage: Take 1 capsule before bedtime to promote relaxation and support restful sleep.
Benefits: Skullcap calms the mind and reduces nervous tension, while Valerian acts as a natural sedative, promoting deep, restorative sleep.

798. Gotu Kola and Bacopa Memory Support Capsules

Ingredients: 1 tablespoon Gotu Kola powder, 1 tablespoon Bacopa Monnieri powder, empty gel capsules.
Preparation: Mix Gotu Kola and Bacopa powders thoroughly. Fill empty capsules and seal.
Suggested Usage: Take 1 capsule in the morning to enhance memory and mental clarity.
Benefits: Gotu Kola promotes mental alertness and reduces brain fog, while Bacopa supports cognitive function and improves memory.

799. Lion's Mane and Holy Basil Focus-Enhancing Tea

Ingredients: 1 tablespoon Lion's Mane Mushroom powder, 1 tablespoon dried Holy Basil, 2 cups hot water.
Preparation: Simmer Lion's Mane and Holy Basil in hot water for 15-20 minutes. Strain and serve warm.
Suggested Usage: Drink 1 cup in the morning to promote focus and mental clarity.
Benefits: Lion's Mane enhances cognitive function and supports nerve regeneration, while Holy Basil reduces stress and improves focus, making this tea effective for mental performance.

800. Peppermint and Lemon Balm Cognitive Clarity Tea

Ingredients: 1 tablespoon dried Peppermint, 1 tablespoon dried Lemon Balm, 2 cups hot water.
Preparation: Steep Peppermint and Lemon Balm in hot water for 10 minutes. Strain and serve warm.
Suggested Usage: Drink 1 cup up to twice daily to promote mental clarity and calm focus.
Benefits: Peppermint stimulates mental clarity and alertness, while Lemon Balm calms the mind and enhances concentration, making this blend ideal for staying focused during cognitive tasks.

801. Rhodiola and Saffron Mood-Balancing Capsules

Ingredients: 1 teaspoon Saffron threads, 1 tablespoon Rhodiola Root powder, empty gel capsules.
Preparation: Grind Saffron threads into a fine powder and mix with Rhodiola Root powder. Fill empty capsules and seal.
Suggested Usage: Take 1 capsule daily to enhance mood and reduce anxiety.
Benefits: Saffron improves mood and reduces symptoms of mild depression, while Rhodiola enhances resilience to stress and reduces mental fatigue.

802. Chamomile and Skullcap Nervous System Support Tea

Ingredients: 1 tablespoon dried Chamomile, 1 tablespoon Skullcap, 2 cups hot water.
Preparation: Steep Chamomile and Skullcap in hot water for 10-15 minutes. Strain and serve warm.
Suggested Usage: Drink 1 cup in the evening to promote relaxation and reduce anxiety.
Benefits: Chamomile calms the nervous system and promotes relaxation, while Skullcap soothes nervous tension, making this tea ideal for managing stress and supporting a balanced emotional state.

803. Ginkgo Biloba and Gotu Kola Brain Health Capsules

Ingredients: 1 tablespoon Ginkgo Biloba powder, 1 tablespoon Gotu Kola powder, empty gel capsules.
Preparation: Mix Ginkgo and Gotu Kola powders thoroughly. Fill empty capsules and seal.
Suggested Usage: Take 1 capsule daily to support brain health and cognitive function.
Benefits: Ginkgo Biloba improves cerebral circulation and enhances memory, while Gotu Kola supports mental clarity and reduces anxiety, making this combination ideal for long-term cognitive support.

804. Lavender and Passionflower Stress-Relieving Capsules

Ingredients: 1 tablespoon Lavender powder, 1 tablespoon Passionflower powder, empty gel capsules.
Preparation: Combine Lavender and Passionflower powders and fill capsules.
Suggested Usage: Take 1 capsule in the evening to reduce stress and promote relaxation.
Benefits: Lavender calms the mind and reduces tension, while Passionflower helps alleviate anxiety and soothes the nervous system, making this blend effective for managing stress and promoting emotional balance.

805. Reishi and Rhodiola Resilience Tea

Ingredients: 1 tablespoon Reishi Mushroom powder, 1 tablespoon dried Rhodiola Root, 2 cups hot water.
Preparation: Simmer Reishi and Rhodiola in hot water for 15-20 minutes. Strain and serve warm.
Suggested Usage: Drink 1 cup daily to enhance resilience and reduce mental fatigue.
Benefits: Reishi supports immune health and reduces stress, while Rhodiola boosts energy, stamina, and mental clarity, making this tea ideal for building resilience against daily stressors.

806. Lemon Balm, Holy Basil, and Ashwagandha Adaptogen Capsules

Ingredients: 1 tablespoon Lemon Balm powder, 1 tablespoon Holy Basil powder, 1 tablespoon Ashwagandha Root powder, empty gel capsules.
Preparation: Mix all three powders

thoroughly. Fill empty capsules and seal.

Suggested Usage: Take 1 capsule in the morning to balance stress and enhance cognitive function.

Benefits: Lemon Balm calms the nervous system, Holy Basil reduces cortisol levels, and Ashwagandha improves energy and focus, making this blend effective for stress management and mental performance.

807. St. John's Wort and Lavender Emotional Balance Capsules

Ingredients: 1 tablespoon St. John's Wort powder, 1 tablespoon Lavender powder, empty gel capsules.

Preparation: Mix the powders thoroughly and fill capsules.

Suggested Usage: Take 1 capsule in the morning to support mood stability and reduce anxiety.

Benefits: St. John's Wort acts as a natural antidepressant by balancing neurotransmitters, while Lavender provides calming effects, making this blend ideal for promoting emotional balance and reducing anxiety.

808. Lion's Mane and Ginseng Brain-Boosting Tea

Ingredients: 1 tablespoon Lion's Mane Mushroom powder, 1 tablespoon Ginseng Root powder, 2 cups hot water.

Preparation: Simmer Lion's Mane and Ginseng in hot water for 15-20 minutes. Strain and serve warm.

Suggested Usage: Drink 1 cup in the morning to enhance cognitive function and mental clarity.

Benefits: Lion's Mane supports nerve regeneration and improves cognitive health, while Ginseng boosts energy and mental focus, making this tea effective for mental performance and long-term brain support.

809. Holy Basil, Lemon Balm, and Skullcap Calm Capsules

Ingredients: 1 tablespoon Holy Basil powder, 1 tablespoon Lemon Balm powder, 1 tablespoon Skullcap powder, empty gel capsules.

Preparation: Mix the powders thoroughly and fill empty capsules.

Suggested Usage: Take 1 capsule in the evening to promote relaxation and reduce anxiety.

Benefits: Holy Basil balances stress hormones, Lemon Balm soothes the nervous system, and Skullcap calms the mind, making this blend effective for promoting calm and reducing overactivity.

810. Ginkgo, Peppermint, and Rosemary Focus Tea

Ingredients: 1 tablespoon Ginkgo Biloba, 1 tablespoon dried Peppermint, 1 tablespoon Rosemary, 2 cups hot water.

Preparation: Steep all herbs in hot water for 10-15 minutes. Strain and serve warm.

Suggested Usage: Drink 1 cup in the morning to enhance concentration and mental clarity.

Benefits: Ginkgo Biloba improves circulation and memory, Peppermint stimulates mental clarity, and Rosemary enhances focus, making this tea ideal for supporting cognitive performance.

811. Rhodiola and Gotu Kola Stress-Reduction Capsules

Ingredients: 1 tablespoon Rhodiola Root powder, 1 tablespoon Gotu Kola powder, empty gel capsules.
Preparation: Mix the powders thoroughly and fill empty capsules.
Suggested Usage: Take 1 capsule daily to reduce stress and improve mental stamina.
Benefits: Rhodiola reduces fatigue and enhances resilience, while Gotu Kola supports brain health and reduces anxiety, making this blend ideal for managing stress and promoting focus.

812. Ashwagandha and Reishi Brain Health Capsules

Ingredients: 1 tablespoon Ashwagandha Root powder, 1 tablespoon Reishi Mushroom powder, empty gel capsules.
Preparation: Mix the powders thoroughly and fill empty capsules.
Suggested Usage: Take 1 capsule daily to support brain health and reduce stress.
Benefits: Ashwagandha enhances cognitive function and reduces stress, while Reishi supports the immune system and promotes mental clarity.

813. Skullcap and Lemon Balm Emotional Soothing Tea

Ingredients: 1 tablespoon dried Skullcap, 1 tablespoon Lemon Balm, 2 cups hot water.
Preparation: Steep Skullcap and Lemon Balm in hot water for 10-15 minutes. Strain and serve warm.
Suggested Usage: Drink 1 cup in the evening to promote relaxation and support emotional balance.
Benefits: Skullcap calms the mind and reduces nervous tension, while Lemon Balm alleviates anxiety and promotes emotional stability, making this tea effective for soothing an overactive mind.

814. Bacopa and Lion's Mane Cognitive Function Capsules

Ingredients: 1 tablespoon Bacopa Monnieri powder, 1 tablespoon Lion's Mane Mushroom powder, empty gel capsules.
Preparation: Mix the powders thoroughly and fill empty capsules.
Suggested Usage: Take 1 capsule daily to enhance memory and support cognitive function.
Benefits: Bacopa improves memory retention and learning capacity, while Lion's Mane promotes nerve regeneration and enhances brain health.

815. Ginkgo and Holy Basil Brain-Enhancing Tea

Ingredients: 1 tablespoon Ginkgo Biloba, 1 tablespoon dried Holy Basil, 2 cups hot water.
Preparation: Steep Ginkgo and Holy Basil in hot water for 15 minutes. Strain and serve warm.
Suggested Usage: Drink 1 cup in the morning to improve focus and mental clarity.
Benefits: Ginkgo enhances cerebral circulation and cognitive function, while Holy Basil balances stress hormones and promotes emotional stability.

816. Reishi and Lavender Relaxation Capsules

Ingredients: 1 tablespoon Reishi Mushroom powder, 1 tablespoon Lavender powder, empty gel capsules.
Preparation: Mix the powders thoroughly and fill empty capsules.
Suggested Usage: Take 1 capsule in the evening to promote relaxation and reduce stress.
Benefits: Reishi soothes the nervous system and supports emotional stability, while Lavender calms the mind and reduces anxiety.

817. Rhodiola and Lemon Balm Focus Tea

Ingredients: 1 tablespoon Rhodiola Root, 1 tablespoon dried Lemon Balm, 2 cups hot water.
Preparation: Steep Rhodiola and Lemon Balm in hot water for 15 minutes. Strain and serve warm.
Suggested Usage: Drink 1 cup in the morning to enhance focus and reduce mental fatigue.
Benefits: Rhodiola boosts stamina and mental clarity, while Lemon Balm promotes calm focus and reduces anxiety.

818. Schisandra and Gotu Kola Memory-Enhancing Capsules

Ingredients: 1 tablespoon Schisandra powder, 1 tablespoon Gotu Kola powder, empty gel capsules.
Preparation: Mix the powders thoroughly and fill empty capsules.
Suggested Usage: Take 1 capsule daily to support memory and cognitive function.
Benefits: Schisandra enhances mental performance and reduces stress, while Gotu Kola supports brain health and improves memory.

819. Holy Basil and Passionflower Mood-Stabilizing Capsules

Ingredients: 1 tablespoon Holy Basil powder, 1 tablespoon Passionflower powder, empty gel capsules.
Preparation: Mix the powders thoroughly and fill empty capsules.
Suggested Usage: Take 1 capsule in the evening to promote emotional balance and reduce anxiety.
Benefits: Holy Basil balances stress hormones, while Passionflower calms the nervous system and promotes relaxation.

820. Chamomile and Lemon Balm Emotional Balance Capsules

Ingredients: 1 tablespoon Chamomile powder, 1 tablespoon Lemon Balm powder, empty gel capsules.
Preparation: Mix the powders thoroughly and fill empty capsules.
Suggested Usage: Take 1 capsule daily to support emotional balance and reduce stress.
Benefits: Chamomile soothes the nervous system, while Lemon Balm alleviates anxiety and promotes a calm mood.

821. Bacopa and Schisandra Mental Clarity Capsules

Ingredients: 1 tablespoon Bacopa Monnieri powder, 1 tablespoon Schisandra powder, empty gel capsules.
Preparation: Mix the powders thoroughly and fill empty capsules.
Suggested Usage: Take 1 capsule in the morning to enhance mental clarity and cognitive function.
Benefits: Bacopa improves memory and mental clarity, while Schisandra enhances resilience and supports mental performance.

822. Ashwagandha and Rhodiola Focus Tea

Ingredients: 1 tablespoon Ashwagandha Root, 1 tablespoon Rhodiola Root, 2 cups hot water.
Preparation: Simmer Ashwagandha and Rhodiola in hot water for 15 minutes. Strain and serve warm.
Suggested Usage: Drink 1 cup in the morning to enhance focus and reduce mental fatigue.
Benefits: Ashwagandha reduces stress and improves stamina, while Rhodiola enhances focus and resilience.

823. Ginkgo Biloba and Lion's Mane Brain Health Capsules

Ingredients: 1 tablespoon Ginkgo Biloba powder, 1 tablespoon Lion's Mane Mushroom powder, empty gel capsules.
Preparation: Mix the powders thoroughly and fill empty capsules.
Suggested Usage: Take 1 capsule daily to support brain health and cognitive function.
Benefits: Ginkgo enhances memory and mental performance, while Lion's Mane

supports nerve health and cognitive function.

824. Holy Basil and Lavender Emotional Soothing Tea

Ingredients: 1 tablespoon dried Holy Basil, 1 tablespoon dried Lavender, 2 cups hot water.
Preparation: Steep Holy Basil and Lavender in hot water for 15 minutes. Strain and serve warm.
Suggested Usage: Drink 1 cup in the evening to reduce stress and promote relaxation.
Benefits: Holy Basil balances the stress response, while Lavender calms the nervous system, making this tea effective for promoting emotional well-being.

825. Lemon Balm, Gotu Kola, and Skullcap Calm Capsules

Ingredients: 1 tablespoon Lemon Balm powder, 1 tablespoon Gotu Kola powder, 1 tablespoon Skullcap powder, empty gel capsules.
Preparation: Mix the powders thoroughly and fill empty capsules.
Suggested Usage: Take 1 capsule daily to reduce anxiety and promote relaxation.
Benefits: Lemon Balm calms the nervous system, Gotu Kola supports mental clarity, and Skullcap soothes nervous tension.

826. Rhodiola and Reishi Adaptogen Stress Relief Capsules

Ingredients: 1 tablespoon Rhodiola Root powder, 1 tablespoon Reishi Mushroom

powder, empty gel capsules.

Preparation: Mix the powders thoroughly and fill empty capsules.

Suggested Usage: Take 1 capsule daily to reduce stress and support emotional stability.

Benefits: Rhodiola enhances resilience and reduces fatigue, while Reishi calms the mind and promotes emotional stability.

827. Passionflower and Lemon Balm Nervous System Tea

Ingredients: 1 tablespoon dried Passionflower, 1 tablespoon dried Lemon Balm, 2 cups hot water.

Preparation: Steep Passionflower and Lemon Balm in hot water for 10-15 minutes. Strain and serve warm.

Suggested Usage: Drink 1 cup in the evening to calm the nervous system and reduce anxiety.

Benefits: Passionflower promotes relaxation and reduces nervous excitability, while Lemon Balm soothes the nervous system and helps alleviate anxiety.

828. Bacopa and Ginkgo Brain Function Capsules

Ingredients: 1 tablespoon Bacopa Monnieri powder, 1 tablespoon Ginkgo Biloba powder, empty gel capsules.

Preparation: Mix Bacopa and Ginkgo powders thoroughly. Fill empty capsules and seal.

Suggested Usage: Take 1 capsule daily to support memory and cognitive function.

Benefits: Bacopa enhances memory and learning ability, while Ginkgo improves blood flow to the brain, promoting focus and mental clarity.

829. Chamomile and Skullcap Relaxation Tea

Ingredients: 1 tablespoon dried Chamomile, 1 tablespoon Skullcap, 2 cups hot water.

Preparation: Steep Chamomile and Skullcap in hot water for 10-15 minutes. Strain and serve warm.

Suggested Usage: Drink 1 cup in the evening to promote relaxation and reduce anxiety.

Benefits: Chamomile calms the nervous system and promotes restful sleep, while Skullcap helps ease nervous tension and stress.

830. Gotu Kola and Ashwagandha Adaptogen Capsules

Ingredients: 1 tablespoon Gotu Kola powder, 1 tablespoon Ashwagandha Root powder, empty gel capsules.

Preparation: Mix the powders thoroughly and fill empty capsules.

Suggested Usage: Take 1 capsule in the morning to promote mental clarity and reduce stress.

Benefits: Gotu Kola supports brain health and reduces anxiety, while Ashwagandha balances cortisol levels and enhances stamina.

831. Ginseng and Holy Basil Stress-Reducing Tea

Ingredients: 1 tablespoon Ginseng Root, 1 tablespoon dried Holy Basil, 2 cups hot water.

Preparation: Steep Ginseng and Holy Basil in hot water for 15-20 minutes. Strain and serve warm.

Suggested Usage: Drink 1 cup in the morning to enhance mental clarity and reduce stress.

Benefits: Ginseng boosts energy and focus, while Holy Basil balances the stress response and promotes calm.

832. Lavender, Lemon Balm, and Skullcap Sleep Capsules

Ingredients: 1 tablespoon Lavender powder, 1 tablespoon Lemon Balm powder, 1 tablespoon Skullcap powder, empty gel capsules.

Preparation: Mix the powders thoroughly and fill empty capsules.

Suggested Usage: Take 1 capsule before bedtime to promote restful sleep and reduce anxiety.

Benefits: Lavender promotes relaxation, Lemon Balm calms the nervous system, and Skullcap eases nervous tension, making this blend ideal for sleep support.

833. Reishi and Schisandra Cognitive Function Capsules

Ingredients: 1 tablespoon Reishi Mushroom powder, 1 tablespoon Schisandra powder, empty gel capsules.

Preparation: Mix the powders thoroughly and fill empty capsules.

Suggested Usage: Take 1 capsule in the morning to enhance cognitive function and reduce stress.

Benefits: Reishi supports brain health and emotional balance, while Schisandra enhances memory and reduces mental fatigue.

834. St. John's Wort and Ashwagandha Emotional Balance Tea

Ingredients: 1 tablespoon dried St. John's Wort, 1 tablespoon dried Ashwagandha Root, 2 cups hot water.

Preparation: Steep St. John's Wort and Ashwagandha in hot water for 15-20 minutes. Strain and serve warm.

Suggested Usage: Drink 1 cup in the evening to promote emotional stability and reduce stress.

Benefits: St. John's Wort acts as a natural antidepressant, while Ashwagandha reduces stress and improves mood.

835. Rhodiola and Lemon Balm Nervine Tea

Ingredients: 1 tablespoon dried Rhodiola Root, 1 tablespoon Lemon Balm, 2 cups hot water.

Preparation: Steep Rhodiola and Lemon Balm in hot water for 15 minutes. Strain and serve warm.

Suggested Usage: Drink 1 cup in the morning to enhance focus and calm the nervous system.

Benefits: Rhodiola boosts mental clarity and stamina, while Lemon Balm soothes the nervous system and reduces anxiety.

836. Lion's Mane and Holy Basil Brain-Boosting Capsules

Ingredients: 1 tablespoon Lion's Mane Mushroom powder, 1 tablespoon Holy

Basil powder, empty gel capsules.
Preparation: Mix the powders thoroughly and fill empty capsules.
Suggested Usage: Take 1 capsule in the morning to enhance cognitive function and support brain health.
Benefits: Lion's Mane promotes nerve regeneration and cognitive health, while Holy Basil balances stress and supports mental clarity.

837. Bacopa, Lemon Balm, and Skullcap Focus Tea

Ingredients: 1 tablespoon Bacopa Monnieri, 1 tablespoon Lemon Balm, 1 tablespoon Skullcap, 2 cups hot water.
Preparation: Steep all herbs in hot water for 15 minutes. Strain and serve warm.
Suggested Usage: Drink 1 cup in the morning to enhance focus and mental clarity.
Benefits: Bacopa improves memory and cognitive function, Lemon Balm promotes calm, and Skullcap reduces anxiety.

838. Ginkgo Biloba and Schisandra Resilience Capsules

Ingredients: 1 tablespoon Ginkgo Biloba powder, 1 tablespoon Schisandra powder, empty gel capsules.
Preparation: Mix the powders thoroughly and fill empty capsules.
Suggested Usage: Take 1 capsule daily to enhance mental resilience and support cognitive health.

Benefits: Ginkgo improves circulation and cognitive performance, while Schisandra enhances memory and reduces fatigue.

839. Passionflower, Lavender, and Skullcap Calm-Enhancing Capsules

Ingredients: 1 tablespoon Passionflower powder, 1 tablespoon Lavender powder, 1 tablespoon Skullcap powder, empty gel capsules.
Preparation: Mix the powders thoroughly and fill empty capsules.
Suggested Usage: Take 1 capsule in the evening to reduce anxiety and promote relaxation.
Benefits: Passionflower calms the nervous system, Lavender promotes relaxation, and Skullcap eases nervous tension.

840. Lemon Balm and Ashwagandha Emotional Balance Capsules

Ingredients: 1 tablespoon Lemon Balm powder, 1 tablespoon Ashwagandha Root powder, empty gel capsules.
Preparation: Mix the powders thoroughly and fill empty capsules.
Suggested Usage: Take 1 capsule in the evening to support emotional balance and reduce stress.
Benefits: Lemon Balm soothes the nervous system, while Ashwagandha reduces anxiety and promotes emotional stability.

Book 37: Herbal Support for Cognitive Function

Enhancing Memory and Learning with Herbs

Memory and learning are complex cognitive processes influenced by various factors, including neurotransmitter levels, cerebral blood flow, and overall brain health. Herbs that enhance these processes work by supporting neurogenesis, improving blood circulation, reducing oxidative stress, and modulating neurotransmitters. Some of the most effective herbs for memory and learning include **Bacopa Monnieri, Ginkgo Biloba, Gotu Kola, Lion's Mane Mushroom**, and **Rosemary**.

Bacopa Monnieri, or Brahmi, is a well-known herb in Ayurvedic medicine traditionally used to improve cognitive function. It enhances memory retention and recall by increasing the levels of neurotransmitters such as acetylcholine. Studies show that Bacopa Monnieri also supports synaptic plasticity, which is crucial for learning.

Ginkgo Biloba is another powerful herb that works by improving blood flow to the brain. It enhances cerebral circulation, providing brain cells with more oxygen and nutrients, which is essential for optimal mental performance. Its potent antioxidant properties protect neurons from damage caused by free radicals, which is particularly beneficial for aging individuals experiencing memory decline.

Gotu Kola is often referred to as "food for the brain" due to its ability to promote the growth of new nerve cells and enhance communication between brain cells. It has a calming effect on the nervous system, making it ideal for improving memory and focus, especially in stressful situations.

Lion's Mane Mushroom is unique among medicinal mushrooms because it stimulates the production of Nerve Growth Factor (NGF), a protein that promotes the growth and maintenance of nerve cells. This property makes it beneficial for enhancing cognitive function, repairing nerve damage, and potentially slowing cognitive decline.

Rosemary is not just a culinary herb but also a potent memory enhancer. It contains compounds that increase acetylcholine levels, which are linked to memory and learning. The scent of rosemary alone has been shown to improve memory and cognitive performance, making it a versatile herb for cognitive support.

Recipes for Brain-Boosting Remedies

Herbal recipes designed to boost cognitive function are a combination of these powerful herbs, blended to create teas, tinctures, capsules, and even foods. The key is to combine herbs that work synergistically, enhancing each other's effects. For example, a **Bacopa and Ginkgo Biloba Tea** can provide a daily boost to memory and learning. Simply steep

1 teaspoon each of Bacopa and Ginkgo in hot water for 15 minutes. This tea can be taken in the morning to support mental sharpness throughout the day.

For a more potent formula, **Lion's Mane and Gotu Kola Capsules** can be created by blending equal parts of these powdered herbs and filling empty capsules. Take 1 capsule daily to support nerve regeneration and improve memory retention.

Another effective option is the **Ginkgo and Rosemary Focus Tea**. Steep 1 teaspoon of Ginkgo Biloba and 1 teaspoon of dried Rosemary in hot water for 15 minutes. This tea is ideal for individuals looking to enhance mental clarity and concentration during study or work.

Herbal tinctures are also a great way to consume these cognitive-supporting herbs. A **Gotu Kola and Bacopa Tincture** can be made by combining dried Gotu Kola and Bacopa in equal parts and soaking them in alcohol for 4-6 weeks. This tincture can be taken in small doses, about 1 dropperful, to promote mental clarity and reduce stress-induced cognitive impairment.

When making these formulations, it is important to source high-quality, organic herbs to ensure the efficacy and safety of the remedies. Additionally, these remedies should be taken consistently for several weeks to see noticeable improvements in memory, focus, and overall cognitive function.

Optimizing Cognitive Health Through Herbal Remedies

To fully benefit from these brain-boosting herbs, consider incorporating them into a broader lifestyle plan that includes a balanced diet, regular physical activity, and adequate sleep. A healthy lifestyle amplifies the effects of these herbs, creating an environment where the brain can thrive. Integrating these remedies into your daily routine, whether in the form of teas, capsules, or tinctures, can support long-term cognitive health and improve day-to-day mental performance. By harnessing the power of these herbs, it is possible to maintain sharp memory, improve learning, and enhance overall mental clarity.

Remedies for Cognitive Function

841. Bacopa and Gotu Kola Memory Support Capsules

Ingredients: 1 tablespoon Bacopa Monnieri powder, 1 tablespoon Gotu Kola powder, empty gel capsules.
Preparation: Mix Bacopa and Gotu Kola powders thoroughly. Fill empty capsules and seal.
Suggested Usage: Take 1 capsule daily to enhance memory retention and mental clarity.
Benefits: Bacopa enhances memory and learning, while Gotu Kola improves cerebral circulation and reduces anxiety,

making this blend effective for overall cognitive support.

842. Ginkgo and Rosemary Cognitive Clarity Tea

Ingredients: 1 tablespoon Ginkgo Biloba, 1 tablespoon dried Rosemary, 2 cups hot water.
Preparation: Steep Ginkgo and Rosemary in hot water for 10-15 minutes. Strain and serve warm.
Suggested Usage: Drink 1 cup daily to promote cognitive function and improve focus.
Benefits: Ginkgo supports blood flow to the brain, enhancing mental clarity, while Rosemary stimulates memory and concentration.

843. Lion's Mane and Ashwagandha Stress-Resilience Capsules

Ingredients: 1 tablespoon Lion's Mane Mushroom powder, 1 tablespoon Ashwagandha Root powder, empty gel capsules.
Preparation: Mix Lion's Mane and Ashwagandha powders thoroughly. Fill empty capsules and seal.
Suggested Usage: Take 1 capsule daily to reduce stress and support cognitive health.
Benefits: Lion's Mane promotes nerve health and cognitive function, while Ashwagandha balances cortisol levels, reducing the impact of stress.

844. Bacopa and Schisandra Mental Clarity Tea

Ingredients: 1 tablespoon Bacopa Monnieri, 1 tablespoon Schisandra Berries, 2 cups hot water.
Preparation: Steep Bacopa and Schisandra in hot water for 15 minutes. Strain and serve warm.
Suggested Usage: Drink 1 cup daily to enhance mental clarity and cognitive performance.
Benefits: Bacopa enhances memory and learning, while Schisandra reduces mental fatigue and promotes resilience.

845. Ginkgo and Lemon Balm Focus Tea

Ingredients: 1 tablespoon Ginkgo Biloba, 1 tablespoon Lemon Balm, 2 cups hot water.
Preparation: Steep Ginkgo and Lemon Balm in hot water for 10-15 minutes. Strain and serve warm.
Suggested Usage: Drink 1 cup in the morning to promote focus and calm mental clarity.
Benefits: Ginkgo improves blood flow to the brain, enhancing focus, while Lemon Balm calms the mind and reduces anxiety, making this blend ideal for balanced mental performance.

846. Gotu Kola and Rhodiola Brain Health Capsules

Ingredients: 1 tablespoon Gotu Kola powder, 1 tablespoon Rhodiola Root powder, empty gel capsules.
Preparation: Mix Gotu Kola and Rhodiola powders thoroughly. Fill empty capsules and seal.
Suggested Usage: Take 1 capsule daily to promote brain health and mental stamina.

Benefits: Gotu Kola supports cognitive health and mental clarity, while Rhodiola reduces stress and enhances focus.

847. Holy Basil and Rosemary Cognitive Enhancement Tea

Ingredients: 1 tablespoon Holy Basil, 1 tablespoon Rosemary, 2 cups hot water.
Preparation: Steep Holy Basil and Rosemary in hot water for 10-15 minutes. Strain and serve warm.
Suggested Usage: Drink 1 cup in the morning to enhance cognitive performance and reduce stress.
Benefits: Holy Basil balances stress hormones, while Rosemary enhances memory and concentration, making this tea ideal for cognitive enhancement.

848. Bacopa and Lion's Mane Concentration Capsules

Ingredients: 1 tablespoon Bacopa Monnieri powder, 1 tablespoon Lion's Mane Mushroom powder, empty gel capsules.
Preparation: Mix Bacopa and Lion's Mane powders thoroughly. Fill empty capsules and seal.
Suggested Usage: Take 1 capsule in the morning to promote concentration and cognitive health.
Benefits: Bacopa enhances learning and memory, while Lion's Mane supports nerve health and brain function.

849. Ginseng and Schisandra Vitality-Boosting Tea

Ingredients: 1 tablespoon Ginseng Root, 1 tablespoon dried Schisandra Berries, 2 cups hot water.
Preparation: Simmer Ginseng and Schisandra in hot water for 15-20 minutes. Strain and serve warm.
Suggested Usage: Drink 1 cup in the morning to boost vitality and mental clarity.
Benefits: Ginseng boosts energy and focus, while Schisandra reduces mental fatigue and supports cognitive performance.

850. Brahmi and Gotu Kola Memory Tea

Ingredients: 1 tablespoon Brahmi, 1 tablespoon Gotu Kola, 2 cups hot water.
Preparation: Steep Brahmi and Gotu Kola in hot water for 15 minutes. Strain and serve warm.
Suggested Usage: Drink 1 cup daily to promote memory and learning.
Benefits: Brahmi supports memory retention and mental clarity, while Gotu Kola enhances cognitive health and calms the mind.

851. Ginkgo Biloba and Peppermint Concentration Tea

Ingredients: 1 tablespoon Ginkgo Biloba, 1 tablespoon dried Peppermint, 2 cups hot water.
Preparation: Steep Ginkgo and Peppermint in hot water for 10 minutes. Strain and serve warm.
Suggested Usage: Drink 1 cup in the morning to promote concentration and cognitive function.
Benefits: Ginkgo enhances blood

circulation to the brain, while Peppermint stimulates mental clarity and focus.

852. Ashwagandha and Schisandra Brain-Boosting Capsules

Ingredients: 1 tablespoon Ashwagandha Root powder, 1 tablespoon Schisandra powder, empty gel capsules.
Preparation: Mix Ashwagandha and Schisandra powders thoroughly. Fill empty capsules and seal.
Suggested Usage: Take 1 capsule in the morning to support brain health and mental performance.
Benefits: Ashwagandha reduces stress and promotes mental stamina, while Schisandra enhances cognitive function and focus.

853. Lion's Mane and Bacopa Cognitive Health Capsules

Ingredients: 1 tablespoon Lion's Mane Mushroom powder, 1 tablespoon Bacopa Monnieri powder, empty gel capsules.
Preparation: Mix Lion's Mane and Bacopa powders thoroughly. Fill empty capsules and seal.
Suggested Usage: Take 1 capsule daily to enhance memory and support cognitive health.
Benefits: Lion's Mane supports nerve health and cognitive regeneration, while Bacopa promotes memory retention and learning capacity.

854. Rosemary and Lemon Balm Memory Support Tea

Ingredients: 1 tablespoon dried Rosemary, 1 tablespoon Lemon Balm, 2 cups hot water.
Preparation: Steep Rosemary and Lemon Balm in hot water for 15 minutes. Strain and serve warm.
Suggested Usage: Drink 1 cup in the morning to support memory retention and mental clarity.
Benefits: Rosemary enhances memory and concentration, while Lemon Balm calms the nervous system, promoting emotional balance and cognitive function.

855. Holy Basil and Ginkgo Focus Capsules

Ingredients: 1 tablespoon Holy Basil powder, 1 tablespoon Ginkgo Biloba powder, empty gel capsules.
Preparation: Mix Holy Basil and Ginkgo powders thoroughly. Fill empty capsules and seal.
Suggested Usage: Take 1 capsule in the morning to promote focus and mental clarity.
Benefits: Holy Basil balances stress hormones and improves mental stamina, while Ginkgo supports cerebral blood flow, enhancing concentration.

856. Lemon Balm and Lavender Calm Focus Tea

Ingredients: 1 tablespoon Lemon Balm, 1 tablespoon dried Lavender, 2 cups hot water.
Preparation: Steep Lemon Balm and Lavender in hot water for 10-15 minutes. Strain and serve warm.
Suggested Usage: Drink 1 cup in the afternoon to promote focus and calm.

Benefits: Lemon Balm calms the mind and supports mental clarity, while Lavender soothes the nervous system, reducing anxiety and promoting a focused state of mind.

857. Gotu Kola and Brahmi Cognitive Support Capsules

Ingredients: 1 tablespoon Gotu Kola powder, 1 tablespoon Brahmi powder, empty gel capsules.

Preparation: Mix Gotu Kola and Brahmi powders thoroughly. Fill empty capsules and seal.

Suggested Usage: Take 1 capsule daily to support cognitive function and memory.

Benefits: Gotu Kola promotes brain health and mental clarity, while Brahmi enhances memory retention and learning ability.

858. Ginseng and Rhodiola Mental Performance Capsules

Ingredients: 1 tablespoon Ginseng Root powder, 1 tablespoon Rhodiola Root powder, empty gel capsules.

Preparation: Mix Ginseng and Rhodiola powders thoroughly. Fill empty capsules and seal.

Suggested Usage: Take 1 capsule daily to enhance mental performance and stamina.

Benefits: Ginseng boosts energy and mental clarity, while Rhodiola improves cognitive function and reduces mental fatigue.

859. Schisandra and Lemon Peel Focus-Enhancing Tea

Ingredients: 1 tablespoon Schisandra Berries, 1 tablespoon dried Lemon Peel, 2 cups hot water.

Preparation: Steep Schisandra and Lemon Peel in hot water for 15 minutes. Strain and serve warm.

Suggested Usage: Drink 1 cup in the morning to boost focus and mental clarity.

Benefits: Schisandra enhances concentration and mental stamina, while Lemon Peel supports a clear and focused mind.

860. Rhodiola and Holy Basil Adaptogen Capsules

Ingredients: 1 tablespoon Rhodiola Root powder, 1 tablespoon Holy Basil powder, empty gel capsules.

Preparation: Mix Rhodiola and Holy Basil powders thoroughly. Fill empty capsules and seal.

Suggested Usage: Take 1 capsule in the morning to reduce stress and support cognitive health.

Benefits: Rhodiola improves resilience to stress and enhances focus, while Holy Basil promotes mental clarity and balances stress hormones.

861. Bacopa and Reishi Cognitive Function Capsules

Ingredients: 1 tablespoon Bacopa Monnieri powder, 1 tablespoon Reishi Mushroom powder, empty gel capsules.

Preparation: Mix Bacopa and Reishi powders thoroughly. Fill empty capsules and seal.

Suggested Usage: Take 1 capsule in the morning to support cognitive function and memory.

Benefits: Bacopa enhances memory and learning, while Reishi supports nerve health and reduces mental fatigue.

862. Lemon Balm and Skullcap Emotional Balance Tea

Ingredients: 1 tablespoon Lemon Balm, 1 tablespoon Skullcap, 2 cups hot water.
Preparation: Steep Lemon Balm and Skullcap in hot water for 15 minutes. Strain and serve warm.
Suggested Usage: Drink 1 cup in the evening to support emotional balance and reduce anxiety.
Benefits: Lemon Balm calms the nervous system, while Skullcap soothes nervous tension and promotes emotional stability.

863. Brahmi and Peppermint Clarity-Boosting Tea

Ingredients: 1 tablespoon Brahmi, 1 tablespoon dried Peppermint, 2 cups hot water.
Preparation: Steep Brahmi and Peppermint in hot water for 10-15 minutes. Strain and serve warm.
Suggested Usage: Drink 1 cup in the afternoon to promote mental clarity and focus.
Benefits: Brahmi supports cognitive function and memory, while Peppermint stimulates mental clarity and reduces fatigue.

864. Lion's Mane and Schisandra Stress-Relief Capsules

Ingredients: 1 tablespoon Lion's Mane Mushroom powder, 1 tablespoon Schisandra powder, empty gel capsules.
Preparation: Mix Lion's Mane and Schisandra powders thoroughly. Fill empty capsules and seal.
Suggested Usage: Take 1 capsule daily to reduce stress and support cognitive resilience.
Benefits: Lion's Mane promotes nerve health and cognitive function, while Schisandra enhances mental performance and reduces stress.

865. Holy Basil and Gotu Kola Brain Health Capsules

Ingredients: 1 tablespoon Holy Basil powder, 1 tablespoon Gotu Kola powder, empty gel capsules.
Preparation: Mix Holy Basil and Gotu Kola powders thoroughly. Fill empty capsules and seal.
Suggested Usage: Take 1 capsule in the morning to support brain health and reduce anxiety.
Benefits: Holy Basil balances stress hormones and promotes calm focus, while Gotu Kola enhances cognitive health and supports memory.

866. Ginkgo and Sage Focus Support Tea

Ingredients: 1 tablespoon Ginkgo Biloba, 1 tablespoon dried Sage, 2 cups hot water.
Preparation: Steep Ginkgo and Sage in hot water for 15 minutes. Strain and serve warm.
Suggested Usage: Drink 1 cup in the morning to promote focus and memory retention.

Benefits: Ginkgo supports blood flow to the brain, while Sage enhances concentration and cognitive clarity.

867. Bacopa and Brahmi Learning Support Capsules

Ingredients: 1 tablespoon Bacopa Monnieri powder, 1 tablespoon Brahmi powder, empty gel capsules.
Preparation: Mix Bacopa and Brahmi powders thoroughly. Fill empty capsules and seal.
Suggested Usage: Take 1 capsule in the morning to enhance learning and memory retention.
Benefits: Bacopa supports memory and learning, while Brahmi promotes mental clarity and reduces anxiety.

868. Reishi and Ginseng Cognitive Function Tea

Ingredients: 1 tablespoon Reishi Mushroom, 1 tablespoon Ginseng Root, 2 cups hot water.
Preparation: Steep Reishi and Ginseng in hot water for 15-20 minutes. Strain and serve warm.
Suggested Usage: Drink 1 cup in the morning to promote cognitive function and reduce mental fatigue.
Benefits: Reishi supports brain health and reduces stress, while Ginseng enhances energy and mental stamina.

869. Peppermint and Rosemary Memory-Enhancing Tea

Ingredients: 1 tablespoon dried Peppermint, 1 tablespoon Rosemary, 2 cups hot water.
Preparation: Steep Peppermint and Rosemary in hot water for 10-15 minutes. Strain and serve warm.
Suggested Usage: Drink 1 cup in the morning to improve memory and focus.
Benefits: Peppermint stimulates mental clarity, and Rosemary enhances memory retention and cognitive performance.

870. Lion's Mane and Holy Basil Brain Boost Capsules

Ingredients: 1 tablespoon Lion's Mane Mushroom powder, 1 tablespoon Holy Basil powder, empty gel capsules.
Preparation: Mix Lion's Mane and Holy Basil powders thoroughly. Fill empty capsules and seal.
Suggested Usage: Take 1 capsule daily to promote brain health and cognitive function.
Benefits: Lion's Mane supports nerve health and mental clarity, while Holy Basil balances stress hormones and enhances focus.

871. Schisandra and Rhodiola Anti-Fatigue Capsules

Ingredients: 1 tablespoon Schisandra powder, 1 tablespoon Rhodiola Root powder, empty gel capsules.
Preparation: Mix Schisandra and Rhodiola powders thoroughly. Fill empty capsules and seal.
Suggested Usage: Take 1 capsule in the morning to reduce fatigue and support mental performance.
Benefits: Schisandra reduces mental fatigue and supports resilience, while Rhodiola enhances focus and energy.

872. Ashwagandha and Peppermint Calm Focus Tea

Ingredients: 1 tablespoon Ashwagandha Root, 1 tablespoon dried Peppermint, 2 cups hot water.
Preparation: Steep Ashwagandha and Peppermint in hot water for 10-15 minutes. Strain and serve warm.
Suggested Usage: Drink 1 cup in the afternoon to promote calm focus and mental clarity.
Benefits: Ashwagandha balances cortisol levels, reducing stress, while Peppermint enhances focus and stimulates mental clarity.

873. Bacopa and Gotu Kola Brain Boost Tonic

Ingredients: 1 tablespoon Bacopa Monnieri, 1 tablespoon Gotu Kola, 2 cups hot water.
Preparation: Steep Bacopa and Gotu Kola in hot water for 15 minutes. Strain and serve warm.
Suggested Usage: Drink 1 cup in the morning to promote mental clarity and learning.
Benefits: Bacopa enhances learning and memory, while Gotu Kola supports brain health and reduces anxiety.

874. Ginkgo Biloba and Rosemary Focus Capsules

Ingredients: 1 tablespoon Ginkgo Biloba powder, 1 tablespoon Rosemary powder, empty gel capsules.
Preparation: Mix Ginkgo and Rosemary powders thoroughly. Fill empty capsules and seal.
Suggested Usage: Take 1 capsule daily to improve focus and cognitive function.
Benefits: Ginkgo enhances cerebral circulation and mental clarity, while Rosemary supports memory retention.

875. Schisandra and Lemon Balm Adaptogen Tea

Ingredients: 1 tablespoon Schisandra Berries, 1 tablespoon Lemon Balm, 2 cups hot water.
Preparation: Steep Schisandra and Lemon Balm in hot water for 15 minutes. Strain and serve warm.
Suggested Usage: Drink 1 cup in the afternoon to promote mental resilience and calm.
Benefits: Schisandra reduces mental fatigue and enhances cognitive performance, while Lemon Balm calms the nervous system.

876. Holy Basil and Rhodiola Mental Clarity Capsules

Ingredients: 1 tablespoon Holy Basil powder, 1 tablespoon Rhodiola Root powder, empty gel capsules.
Preparation: Mix Holy Basil and Rhodiola powders thoroughly. Fill empty capsules and seal.
Suggested Usage: Take 1 capsule daily to support mental clarity and reduce stress.
Benefits: Holy Basil balances stress hormones and improves cognitive function, while Rhodiola promotes resilience and focus.

877. Gotu Kola and Lemon Balm Nerve-Soothing Tea

Ingredients: 1 tablespoon Gotu Kola, 1 tablespoon Lemon Balm, 2 cups hot water.
Preparation: Steep Gotu Kola and Lemon Balm in hot water for 10-15 minutes. Strain and serve warm.
Suggested Usage: Drink 1 cup in the evening to soothe the nervous system and promote relaxation.
Benefits: Gotu Kola supports brain health and reduces anxiety, while Lemon Balm calms the mind and relieves stress.

878. Ginkgo and Lion's Mane Brain Health Capsules

Ingredients: 1 tablespoon Ginkgo Biloba powder, 1 tablespoon Lion's Mane Mushroom powder, empty gel capsules.
Preparation: Mix Ginkgo and Lion's Mane powders thoroughly. Fill empty capsules and seal.
Suggested Usage: Take 1 capsule in the morning to promote brain health and cognitive clarity.
Benefits: Ginkgo enhances cerebral circulation and focus, while Lion's Mane promotes nerve health and cognitive function.

879. Rhodiola and Ginseng Energy-Enhancing Capsules

Ingredients: 1 tablespoon Rhodiola Root powder, 1 tablespoon Ginseng Root powder, empty gel capsules.
Preparation: Mix Rhodiola and Ginseng powders thoroughly. Fill empty capsules and seal.
Suggested Usage: Take 1 capsule daily to boost energy and mental performance.
Benefits: Rhodiola reduces mental fatigue and promotes focus, while Ginseng enhances energy and cognitive function.

880. Brahmi and Ashwagandha Cognitive Support Capsules

Ingredients: 1 tablespoon Brahmi powder, 1 tablespoon Ashwagandha Root powder, empty gel capsules.
Preparation: Mix Brahmi and Ashwagandha powders thoroughly. Fill empty capsules and seal.
Suggested Usage: Take 1 capsule in the morning to support memory and reduce stress.
Benefits: Brahmi enhances memory retention, while Ashwagandha balances cortisol and supports cognitive health.

881. Peppermint and Rosemary Mental Clarity Capsules

Ingredients: 1 tablespoon dried Peppermint powder, 1 tablespoon Rosemary powder, empty gel capsules.
Preparation: Mix Peppermint and Rosemary powders thoroughly. Fill empty capsules and seal.
Suggested Usage: Take 1 capsule in the morning to support mental clarity and concentration.
Benefits: Peppermint stimulates cognitive function and alertness, while Rosemary enhances memory and focus.

882. Bacopa and Lemon Balm Memory-Enhancing Tea

Ingredients: 1 tablespoon Bacopa Monnieri, 1 tablespoon Lemon Balm, 2 cups hot water.
Preparation: Steep Bacopa and Lemon Balm in hot water for 15 minutes. Strain and serve warm.
Suggested Usage: Drink 1 cup daily to promote memory and cognitive function.
Benefits: Bacopa supports memory retention and learning, while Lemon Balm soothes the nervous system, enhancing mental clarity.

883. Schisandra and Reishi Adaptogen Brain Boost Capsules

Ingredients: 1 tablespoon Schisandra powder, 1 tablespoon Reishi Mushroom powder, empty gel capsules.
Preparation: Mix Schisandra and Reishi powders thoroughly. Fill empty capsules and seal.
Suggested Usage: Take 1 capsule in the morning to promote resilience and cognitive health.
Benefits: Schisandra enhances mental performance and reduces fatigue, while Reishi supports brain health and reduces stress.

884. Lemon Balm and Rhodiola Stress-Relief Tea

Ingredients: 1 tablespoon Lemon Balm, 1 tablespoon Rhodiola Root, 2 cups hot water.
Preparation: Steep Lemon Balm and Rhodiola in hot water for 10-15 minutes. Strain and serve warm.
Suggested Usage: Drink 1 cup in the afternoon to promote mental clarity and reduce stress.

Benefits: Lemon Balm calms the mind and reduces anxiety, while Rhodiola enhances resilience and cognitive performance.

885. Holy Basil and Ginseng Brain Health Capsules

Ingredients: 1 tablespoon Holy Basil powder, 1 tablespoon Ginseng Root powder, empty gel capsules.
Preparation: Mix Holy Basil and Ginseng powders thoroughly. Fill empty capsules and seal.
Suggested Usage: Take 1 capsule in the morning to support brain health and energy levels.
Benefits: Holy Basil reduces stress and supports cognitive function, while Ginseng enhances energy and mental clarity.

886. Lion's Mane and Ginkgo Cognitive Clarity Capsules

Ingredients: 1 tablespoon Lion's Mane Mushroom powder, 1 tablespoon Ginkgo Biloba powder, empty gel capsules.
Preparation: Mix Lion's Mane and Ginkgo powders thoroughly. Fill empty capsules and seal.
Suggested Usage: Take 1 capsule daily to enhance cognitive function and mental clarity.
Benefits: Lion's Mane supports nerve health and brain function, while Ginkgo improves blood flow to the brain, enhancing focus and memory.

887. Gotu Kola and Bacopa Mental Clarity Tea

Ingredients: 1 tablespoon Gotu Kola, 1 tablespoon Bacopa Monnieri, 2 cups hot water.
Preparation: Steep Gotu Kola and Bacopa in hot water for 15 minutes. Strain and serve warm.
Suggested Usage: Drink 1 cup in the morning to support mental clarity and memory.
Benefits: Gotu Kola enhances cerebral circulation and mental focus, while Bacopa promotes memory retention and cognitive health.

888. Rhodiola and Schisandra Cognitive Health Capsules

Ingredients: 1 tablespoon Rhodiola Root powder, 1 tablespoon Schisandra powder, empty gel capsules.
Preparation: Mix Rhodiola and Schisandra powders thoroughly. Fill empty capsules and seal.
Suggested Usage: Take 1 capsule in the morning to support cognitive function and reduce fatigue.
Benefits: Rhodiola improves resilience to stress and enhances focus, while Schisandra reduces mental fatigue and promotes cognitive performance.

889. Ginkgo, Gotu Kola, and Rosemary Focus Tea

Ingredients: 1 tablespoon Ginkgo Biloba, 1 tablespoon Gotu Kola, 1 tablespoon dried Rosemary, 2 cups hot water.
Preparation: Steep Ginkgo, Gotu Kola, and Rosemary in hot water for 15 minutes. Strain and serve warm.
Suggested Usage: Drink 1 cup daily to support focus and concentration.
Benefits: Ginkgo enhances cerebral circulation, Gotu Kola supports brain health, and Rosemary promotes memory retention and mental clarity.

890. Lion's Mane and Brahmi Nerve-Support Capsules

Ingredients: 1 tablespoon Lion's Mane Mushroom powder, 1 tablespoon Brahmi powder, empty gel capsules.
Preparation: Mix Lion's Mane and Brahmi powders thoroughly. Fill empty capsules and seal.
Suggested Usage: Take 1 capsule daily to support nerve health and enhance cognitive function.
Benefits: Lion's Mane promotes nerve regeneration and cognitive clarity, while Brahmi enhances memory and learning.

Book 38: Mindfulness and Herbal Integration

Combining Mindfulness Practices with Herbal Remedies

Mindfulness practices, such as meditation, yoga, and breathwork, are essential tools for promoting mental clarity, emotional balance, and overall well-being. Integrating herbal remedies into these practices can further enhance their effectiveness by preparing the mind and body for deeper states of relaxation and awareness. Certain herbs, known for their calming and centering properties, can help to quiet the mind, reduce stress, and support the body's natural rhythms, making them ideal companions for mindfulness.

Herbs like **Holy Basil** (Tulsi), **Ashwagandha**, and **Lemon Balm** are particularly effective for reducing anxiety and promoting a sense of calm focus, which is essential for a productive meditation or mindfulness session. Adaptogenic herbs like **Rhodiola** and **Reishi Mushroom** help regulate the body's stress response, making it easier to achieve a state of mental equilibrium. Additionally, herbs such as **Lavender** and **Chamomile** can be used to create a tranquil environment, either through teas or aromatic preparations, enhancing the sensory experience of mindfulness practices.

Incorporating herbal teas, tinctures, or elixirs into a pre-meditation routine can prepare the body and mind for stillness. For instance, sipping a warm cup of **Holy Basil and Lemon Balm Tea** before meditation can set a peaceful tone, while **Lavender and Skullcap Tea** can be consumed after an intense yoga session to support relaxation and muscle recovery. Each herb has its own unique properties that align with various mindfulness practices, making it easy to customize herbal support based on the specific needs of the individual.

To maximize the benefits of combining herbs with mindfulness, it's important to use high-quality, organic herbs and to prepare them mindfully, paying attention to the sensory experience of making and consuming herbal teas or tinctures. This process itself can become a meditative practice, deepening the connection between body and mind.

Recipes for Meditative Elixirs

Herbal elixirs can be a wonderful addition to any mindfulness routine, offering nourishment for both body and soul. These blends often incorporate herbs that promote relaxation, enhance focus, or support emotional balance. A **Chamomile, Lavender, and Lemon Balm Elixir**, for instance, can be sipped slowly before bedtime to transition into a restful night's sleep. For those looking to deepen their meditation practice, a **Holy Basil and Gotu Kola Adaptogen Elixir** can enhance mental clarity and sustain energy levels without overstimulation.

Other blends, such as **Ashwagandha and Reishi Mushroom Stress-Relief Tonic**, can help to ground the body and mind, promoting resilience and calm during times of stress. Preparing these elixirs with intention—selecting each herb thoughtfully, measuring, and brewing them with care—creates a ritual that enhances the practice of mindfulness itself.

The sensory experience of herbal elixirs can also be amplified by incorporating spices like **Cinnamon**, **Cardamom**, or **Ginger**, which add warmth and complexity to the blend, making the experience of sipping an herbal tea or tonic a sensory delight that engages the taste, smell, and touch.

By mindfully integrating herbs into meditation, yoga, and relaxation routines, individuals can cultivate a more holistic approach to wellness, aligning the body's physical needs with the mental and emotional benefits of mindfulness practices.

Remedies for Mindfulness

891. Holy Basil and Lemon Balm Calm Focus Tea

Ingredients: 1 tablespoon Holy Basil, 1 tablespoon Lemon Balm, 2 cups hot water.
Preparation: Steep Holy Basil and Lemon Balm in hot water for 10-15 minutes. Strain and serve warm.
Suggested Usage: Drink 1 cup in the afternoon to promote calm focus and mental clarity.
Benefits: Holy Basil helps balance stress hormones and enhances mental stamina, while Lemon Balm soothes the nervous system, promoting a clear and focused state of mind.

892. Ashwagandha and Reishi Mushroom Grounding Tonic

Ingredients: 1 tablespoon Ashwagandha Root powder, 1 tablespoon Reishi Mushroom powder, 2 cups hot water.
Preparation: Simmer Ashwagandha and Reishi Mushroom powders in hot water for 15-20 minutes. Strain and serve warm.
Suggested Usage: Drink 1 cup in the evening to promote grounding and relaxation.
Benefits: Ashwagandha reduces stress and promotes mental calm, while Reishi enhances emotional resilience and supports overall well-being.

893. Lavender and Skullcap Relaxation Tea

Ingredients: 1 tablespoon dried Lavender flowers, 1 tablespoon Skullcap, 2 cups hot water.
Preparation: Steep Lavender and Skullcap in hot water for 10-15 minutes. Strain and serve warm.
Suggested Usage: Drink 1 cup in the evening to support relaxation and mental calm.
Benefits: Lavender promotes relaxation and reduces anxiety, while Skullcap soothes nervous tension, making this tea ideal for stress relief.

894. Gotu Kola and Holy Basil Meditation Capsules

Ingredients: 1 tablespoon Gotu Kola powder, 1 tablespoon Holy Basil powder, empty gel capsules.
Preparation: Mix Gotu Kola and Holy Basil powders thoroughly. Fill empty capsules and seal.
Suggested Usage: Take 1 capsule before meditation to enhance focus and emotional stability.
Benefits: Gotu Kola improves mental clarity and focus, while Holy Basil calms the mind and reduces anxiety, making these capsules ideal for deepening meditation practices.

895. Chamomile and Passionflower Sleep-Inducing Tea

Ingredients: 1 tablespoon dried Chamomile flowers, 1 tablespoon Passionflower, 2 cups hot water.
Preparation: Steep Chamomile and Passionflower in hot water for 10-15 minutes. Strain and serve warm.
Suggested Usage: Drink 1 cup 30 minutes before bedtime to promote restful sleep.
Benefits: Chamomile relaxes the mind and body, while Passionflower helps alleviate insomnia and calm the nervous system, promoting a deeper and more restful sleep.

896. Rhodiola and Schisandra Adaptogen Elixir

Ingredients: 1 tablespoon Rhodiola Root powder, 1 tablespoon Schisandra Berry powder, 2 cups hot water.
Preparation: Simmer Rhodiola and Schisandra in hot water for 15-20 minutes. Strain and serve warm.

Suggested Usage: Drink 1 cup in the morning to enhance focus and reduce stress.
Benefits: Rhodiola improves resilience to stress and enhances mental stamina, while Schisandra reduces mental fatigue and supports cognitive function.

897. Lemon Balm, Lavender, and Rose Calming Tea

Ingredients: 1 tablespoon Lemon Balm, 1 tablespoon dried Lavender, 1 teaspoon dried Rose petals, 2 cups hot water.
Preparation: Steep Lemon Balm, Lavender, and Rose in hot water for 10-15 minutes. Strain and serve warm.
Suggested Usage: Drink 1 cup in the evening to promote calm and emotional balance.
Benefits: Lemon Balm soothes the nervous system, Lavender calms the mind, and Rose petals uplift the mood, creating a harmonizing tea for emotional well-being.

898. Tulsi and Peppermint Mind-Soothing Tea

Ingredients: 1 tablespoon Tulsi (Holy Basil), 1 tablespoon dried Peppermint, 2 cups hot water.
Preparation: Steep Tulsi and Peppermint in hot water for 10-15 minutes. Strain and serve warm.
Suggested Usage: Drink 1 cup in the afternoon to promote calm and mental clarity.
Benefits: Tulsi balances stress hormones and enhances mental clarity, while Peppermint stimulates the mind and soothes digestive tension, making this blend ideal for overall well-being.

899. Skullcap and Oatstraw Nervine Support Tincture

Ingredients: 1 tablespoon Skullcap, 1 tablespoon dried Oatstraw, 1 cup vodka or brandy.
Preparation: Combine Skullcap and Oatstraw in a glass jar and cover with alcohol. Seal tightly and let sit for 4-6 weeks, shaking daily. Strain and store in a dark glass bottle.
Suggested Usage: Take 1 teaspoon in the evening to calm the nervous system and support relaxation.
Benefits: Skullcap soothes nervous tension and promotes relaxation, while Oatstraw nourishes the nervous system and helps alleviate stress.

900. Reishi Mushroom and Ashwagandha Stress-Relief Capsules

Ingredients: 1 tablespoon Reishi Mushroom powder, 1 tablespoon Ashwagandha Root powder, empty gel capsules.
Preparation: Mix Reishi and Ashwagandha powders thoroughly. Fill empty capsules and seal.
Suggested Usage: Take 1 capsule daily to promote resilience and reduce stress.
Benefits: Reishi supports emotional resilience and reduces stress, while Ashwagandha balances cortisol levels, making this blend ideal for stress management.

901. Lemon Balm, Chamomile, and Holy Basil Relaxation Capsules

Ingredients: 1 tablespoon Lemon Balm powder, 1 tablespoon Chamomile powder, 1 tablespoon Holy Basil powder, empty gel capsules.
Preparation: Mix Lemon Balm, Chamomile, and Holy Basil powders thoroughly. Fill empty capsules and seal.
Suggested Usage: Take 1 capsule in the evening to promote relaxation and reduce anxiety.
Benefits: Lemon Balm calms the nervous system, Chamomile relaxes the mind and body, and Holy Basil balances stress hormones, making this blend effective for relaxation and emotional balance.

902. Ginkgo and Rosemary Cognitive Clarity Tea

Ingredients: 1 tablespoon Ginkgo Biloba, 1 tablespoon dried Rosemary, 2 cups hot water.
Preparation: Steep Ginkgo and Rosemary in hot water for 15 minutes. Strain and serve warm.
Suggested Usage: Drink 1 cup in the morning to enhance memory retention and mental clarity.
Benefits: Ginkgo promotes cerebral circulation, while Rosemary stimulates memory and concentration, making this tea ideal for cognitive support.

903. Bacopa and Gotu Kola Memory-Enhancing Tincture

Ingredients: 1 tablespoon Bacopa Monnieri, 1 tablespoon Gotu Kola, 1 cup vodka or brandy.
Preparation: Combine Bacopa and Gotu Kola in a glass jar, cover with alcohol, and seal. Let sit for 4-6 weeks, shaking daily.

Strain and store in a dark glass bottle.
Suggested Usage: Take 1 teaspoon twice daily to support memory and cognitive function.
Benefits: Bacopa enhances learning and memory, while Gotu Kola improves mental clarity and reduces anxiety, making this tincture effective for memory enhancement.

904. Holy Basil and Rhodiola Focus-Enhancing Capsules

Ingredients: 1 tablespoon Holy Basil powder, 1 tablespoon Rhodiola Root powder, empty gel capsules.
Preparation: Mix Holy Basil and Rhodiola powders thoroughly. Fill empty capsules and seal.
Suggested Usage: Take 1 capsule daily to promote mental focus and reduce stress.
Benefits: Holy Basil balances stress hormones and improves mental clarity, while Rhodiola reduces mental fatigue and enhances concentration.

905. Passionflower and Lemon Balm Sleep Support Elixir

Ingredients: 1 tablespoon Passionflower, 1 tablespoon Lemon Balm, 1 cup water, 1 cup honey.
Preparation: Simmer Passionflower and Lemon Balm in water for 15 minutes. Strain and combine the liquid with honey. Store in a glass jar.
Suggested Usage: Take 1 tablespoon 30 minutes before bedtime to promote restful sleep.
Benefits: Passionflower calms the nervous system and reduces anxiety, while Lemon Balm promotes relaxation and helps alleviate insomnia.

906. Lavender and Chamomile Bedtime Tea

Ingredients: 1 tablespoon dried Lavender, 1 tablespoon dried Chamomile, 2 cups hot water.
Preparation: Steep Lavender and Chamomile in hot water for 10-15 minutes. Strain and serve warm.
Suggested Usage: Drink 1 cup 30 minutes before bedtime to support relaxation and sleep.
Benefits: Lavender reduces anxiety and promotes relaxation, while Chamomile soothes the mind and body, creating the perfect blend for restful sleep.

907. Lemon Balm and Skullcap Nervous System Support Tea

Ingredients: 1 tablespoon Lemon Balm, 1 tablespoon Skullcap, 2 cups hot water.
Preparation: Steep Lemon Balm and Skullcap in hot water for 15 minutes. Strain and serve warm.
Suggested Usage: Drink 1 cup in the evening to support the nervous system and reduce stress.
Benefits: Lemon Balm calms the nervous system, while Skullcap soothes nervous tension and promotes emotional stability.

908. Peppermint and Rosemary Mental Clarity Capsules

Ingredients: 1 tablespoon dried Peppermint powder, 1 tablespoon Rosemary powder, empty gel capsules.

Preparation: Mix Peppermint and Rosemary powders thoroughly. Fill empty capsules and seal.

Suggested Usage: Take 1 capsule in the morning to support mental clarity and focus.

Benefits: Peppermint stimulates cognitive function and alertness, while Rosemary enhances memory and concentration, making this blend ideal for mental clarity.

909. Lemon Balm and Valerian Root Emotional Balance Tea

Ingredients: 1 tablespoon Lemon Balm, 1 tablespoon Valerian Root, 2 cups hot water.

Preparation: Steep Lemon Balm and Valerian Root in hot water for 15-20 minutes. Strain and serve warm.

Suggested Usage: Drink 1 cup in the evening to promote emotional balance and reduce anxiety.

Benefits: Lemon Balm calms the nervous system, while Valerian Root reduces stress and supports emotional well-being, making this tea effective for emotional stability.

910. Gotu Kola and Ginkgo Biloba Cognitive Function Capsules

Ingredients: 1 tablespoon Gotu Kola powder, 1 tablespoon Ginkgo Biloba powder, empty gel capsules.

Preparation: Mix Gotu Kola and Ginkgo powders thoroughly. Fill empty capsules and seal.

Suggested Usage: Take 1 capsule daily to support cognitive function and enhance memory.

Benefits: Gotu Kola enhances cerebral circulation and mental focus, while Ginkgo improves memory retention and cognitive clarity.

Book 39: Herbal Support for Emotional Balance

Managing Emotions with Herbal Remedies

Emotional balance is a key component of overall well-being, influencing how we handle stress, relationships, and daily challenges. Herbs have been used for centuries to help regulate and stabilize emotions, acting as natural allies in managing mood swings, anxiety, and even mild depression. By targeting the nervous system and supporting the adrenal and endocrine systems, herbs can help the body achieve a state of emotional equilibrium. For those experiencing stress-induced mood disorders, herbs such as **Ashwagandha** and **Holy Basil** work to lower cortisol levels and support the body's natural stress response, making them ideal adaptogens for emotional stability.

For regulating anxiety and promoting calm, herbs like **Lemon Balm**, **Skullcap**, and **Passionflower** are highly effective. These herbs act on the nervous system to reduce excitability and anxiety, fostering a sense of tranquility and mental clarity. **Chamomile** is another well-known herb for its gentle yet effective calming properties, making it useful for those who experience irritability or nervousness. Additionally, **St. John's Wort** and **Saffron** have shown promise in supporting mood stability and alleviating symptoms of mild depression by modulating neurotransmitters like serotonin and dopamine.

For emotional upheavals caused by hormonal fluctuations, herbs such as **Vitex** (Chaste Tree Berry) and **Dong Quai** are particularly effective for women experiencing mood swings related to PMS or menopause. By balancing hormonal levels, these herbs can help smooth emotional transitions and promote a more stable mood. **Schisandra** and **Rhodiola**, known for their adaptogenic properties, can also be used to balance emotional highs and lows by supporting the adrenal system and promoting mental resilience.

The key to using herbs for emotional balance lies in understanding their unique properties and how they interact with the body's systems. Selecting the right herb based on individual needs and emotional patterns can make a significant difference in achieving and maintaining emotional harmony. It's also important to incorporate these herbs consistently, as emotional health is deeply tied to the body's overall state of balance and rhythm.

Recipes for Calming and Balancing Elixirs

Herbal elixirs are an excellent way to incorporate the benefits of emotional-supporting herbs into a daily routine. These blends often combine herbs that support the nervous system, soothe the adrenal glands, and promote mental clarity, creating a holistic approach to emotional balance. For example, a **Chamomile, Lemon Balm, and Lavender Tea** can be sipped in the evening to ease stress and prepare for restful sleep.

Alternatively, an **Ashwagandha and Reishi Adaptogen Tonic** can be taken in the morning to build emotional resilience and reduce the impact of daily stressors.

Another effective blend is the **Holy Basil and Rhodiola Uplifting Tea**, which combines two powerful adaptogens to support emotional stability and energy levels without overstimulation. For mood swings related to hormonal changes, a **Vitex and Dong Quai Hormonal Balance Elixir** can be highly beneficial, helping to smooth out emotional fluctuations by regulating hormonal activity.

Creating herbal elixirs can also become a mindfulness practice, allowing for a moment of calm as you brew, blend, and sip with intention. This mindful approach to herbal medicine can deepen the effects of the remedies, helping to foster a stronger connection between mind and body. By carefully selecting and preparing these blends, you can create a repertoire of herbal allies that support your emotional well-being throughout life's ups and downs.

Remedies for Emotional Balance

911. Holy Basil and Lemon Balm Calm Tea

Ingredients: 1 tablespoon Holy Basil, 1 tablespoon Lemon Balm, 2 cups hot water.
Preparation: Steep Holy Basil and Lemon Balm in hot water for 10-15 minutes. Strain and serve warm.
Suggested Usage: Drink 1 cup in the morning to promote calm and emotional clarity.
Benefits: Holy Basil supports stress management and emotional resilience, while Lemon Balm soothes the nervous system, promoting calmness and reducing anxiety.

912. Ashwagandha and Reishi Mushroom Adaptogen Tonic

Ingredients: 1 tablespoon Ashwagandha Root, 1 tablespoon Reishi Mushroom, 2 cups hot water.
Preparation: Simmer Ashwagandha and Reishi in hot water for 15-20 minutes. Strain and serve warm.
Suggested Usage: Drink 1 cup daily to promote emotional stability and reduce stress.
Benefits: Ashwagandha balances cortisol levels and enhances emotional balance, while Reishi supports mental resilience and calm.

913. Chamomile, Lemon Balm, and Lavender Stress Relief Tea

Ingredients: 1 tablespoon Chamomile, 1 tablespoon Lemon Balm, 1 teaspoon dried Lavender flowers, 2 cups hot water.
Preparation: Steep Chamomile, Lemon Balm, and Lavender in hot water for 10-15 minutes. Strain and serve warm.
Suggested Usage: Drink 1 cup in the evening to promote relaxation and reduce irritability.
Benefits: Chamomile relaxes the mind and body, Lemon Balm calms the nerves, and Lavender uplifts the mood, making this tea ideal for stress relief.

914. St. John's Wort and Saffron Uplifting Capsules

Ingredients: 1 tablespoon St. John's Wort powder, 1 teaspoon Saffron threads, empty gel capsules.
Preparation: Mix St. John's Wort and Saffron powders thoroughly. Fill empty capsules and seal.
Suggested Usage: Take 1 capsule daily to promote a positive mood and reduce mild depression.
Benefits: St. John's Wort modulates neurotransmitters to support mood stability, while Saffron enhances emotional well-being and reduces anxiety.

915. Passionflower and Skullcap Anti-Anxiety Tincture

Ingredients: 1 tablespoon Passionflower, 1 tablespoon Skullcap, 1 cup vodka or brandy.
Preparation: Combine Passionflower and Skullcap in a glass jar, cover with alcohol, and seal. Let sit for 4-6 weeks, shaking daily. Strain and store in a dark glass bottle.
Suggested Usage: Take 1 teaspoon in the evening to reduce anxiety and promote calm.
Benefits: Passionflower reduces anxiety and calms the mind, while Skullcap soothes nervous tension, making this tincture ideal for managing stress and anxiety.

916. Rhodiola and Schisandra Adaptogen Capsules

Ingredients: 1 tablespoon Rhodiola Root powder, 1 tablespoon Schisandra Berry powder, empty gel capsules.
Preparation: Mix Rhodiola and Schisandra powders thoroughly. Fill empty capsules and seal.
Suggested Usage: Take 1 capsule in the morning to reduce fatigue and support emotional stability.
Benefits: Rhodiola enhances mental resilience and reduces stress, while Schisandra balances emotions and promotes cognitive clarity.

917. Lavender, Lemon Balm, and Skullcap Bedtime Elixir

Ingredients: 1 tablespoon dried Lavender, 1 tablespoon Lemon Balm, 1 tablespoon Skullcap, 2 cups hot water, 1 cup honey.
Preparation: Simmer Lavender, Lemon Balm, and Skullcap in water for 15 minutes. Strain and combine with honey. Store in a glass jar.
Suggested Usage: Take 1 tablespoon 30 minutes before bed to promote restful sleep and emotional calm.
Benefits: Lavender reduces anxiety and promotes relaxation, Lemon Balm calms the nervous system, and Skullcap soothes tension, making this blend perfect for emotional stability.

918. Ashwagandha and Holy Basil Stress-Reducing Capsules

Ingredients: 1 tablespoon Ashwagandha Root powder, 1 tablespoon Holy Basil powder, empty gel capsules.
Preparation: Mix Ashwagandha and Holy Basil powders thoroughly. Fill empty capsules and seal.

Suggested Usage: Take 1 capsule in the morning to promote resilience and emotional balance.
Benefits: Ashwagandha reduces cortisol levels and promotes emotional stability, while Holy Basil enhances mental clarity and calm.

919. Lemon Balm and Chamomile Emotional Balance Tea

Ingredients: 1 tablespoon Lemon Balm, 1 tablespoon dried Chamomile flowers, 2 cups hot water.
Preparation: Steep Lemon Balm and Chamomile in hot water for 10-15 minutes. Strain and serve warm.
Suggested Usage: Drink 1 cup in the evening to promote calm and reduce emotional turbulence.
Benefits: Lemon Balm calms the mind, while Chamomile soothes irritability and promotes relaxation, making this tea ideal for emotional stability.

920. Holy Basil and Rhodiola Focus-Enhancing Capsules

Ingredients: 1 tablespoon Holy Basil powder, 1 tablespoon Rhodiola Root powder, empty gel capsules.
Preparation: Mix Holy Basil and Rhodiola powders thoroughly. Fill empty capsules and seal.
Suggested Usage: Take 1 capsule in the morning to enhance focus and emotional clarity.
Benefits: Holy Basil reduces anxiety and balances emotional states, while Rhodiola enhances resilience and focus.

921. Lavender and Passionflower Calming Tea

Ingredients: 1 tablespoon dried Lavender, 1 tablespoon Passionflower, 2 cups hot water.
Preparation: Steep Lavender and Passionflower in hot water for 10-15 minutes. Strain and serve warm.
Suggested Usage: Drink 1 cup in the evening to promote calm and reduce anxiety.
Benefits: Lavender relaxes the mind, while Passionflower alleviates anxiety, making this tea ideal for calming the nervous system.

922. Lemon Balm and Skullcap Emotional Soothing Tincture

Ingredients: 1 tablespoon Lemon Balm, 1 tablespoon Skullcap, 1 cup vodka or brandy.
Preparation: Combine Lemon Balm and Skullcap in a glass jar, cover with alcohol, and seal. Let sit for 4-6 weeks, shaking daily. Strain and store in a dark glass bottle.
Suggested Usage: Take 1 teaspoon in the evening to reduce stress and promote emotional stability.
Benefits: Lemon Balm calms the nervous system, while Skullcap soothes emotional tension, promoting relaxation and mental clarity.

923. Chamomile and Lavender Emotional Balance Capsules

Ingredients: 1 tablespoon Chamomile powder, 1 tablespoon dried Lavender

powder, empty gel capsules.

Preparation: Mix Chamomile and Lavender powders thoroughly. Fill empty capsules and seal.

Suggested Usage: Take 1 capsule in the evening to promote calm and emotional balance.

Benefits: Chamomile soothes the mind and body, while Lavender promotes relaxation, making this blend ideal for stress relief and emotional stability.

924. Gotu Kola and Holy Basil Mood-Stabilizing Tea

Ingredients: 1 tablespoon Gotu Kola, 1 tablespoon Holy Basil, 2 cups hot water.

Preparation: Steep Gotu Kola and Holy Basil in hot water for 15 minutes. Strain and serve warm.

Suggested Usage: Drink 1 cup in the morning to promote mood stability and mental clarity.

Benefits: Gotu Kola supports cognitive function and mental balance, while Holy Basil reduces anxiety and enhances emotional well-being.

925. Passionflower and Valerian Anti-Anxiety Tincture

Ingredients: 1 tablespoon Passionflower, 1 tablespoon Valerian Root, 1 cup vodka or brandy.

Preparation: Combine Passionflower and Valerian in a glass jar, cover with alcohol, and seal. Let sit for 4-6 weeks, shaking daily. Strain and store in a dark glass bottle.

Suggested Usage: Take 1 teaspoon before bed to alleviate anxiety and promote restful sleep.

Benefits: Passionflower reduces anxiety, while Valerian calms the nervous system and promotes relaxation, making this tincture ideal for emotional balance and sleep support.

926. Rhodiola and Lemon Balm Emotional Resilience Capsules

Ingredients: 1 tablespoon Rhodiola Root powder, 1 tablespoon Lemon Balm powder, empty gel capsules.

Preparation: Mix Rhodiola and Lemon Balm powders thoroughly. Fill empty capsules and seal.

Suggested Usage: Take 1 capsule in the morning to reduce stress and promote emotional stability.

Benefits: Rhodiola enhances mental stamina and resilience to stress, while Lemon Balm calms the mind and stabilizes emotions.

927. Schisandra and Ashwagandha Stress-Relief Capsules

Ingredients: 1 tablespoon Schisandra Berry powder, 1 tablespoon Ashwagandha Root powder, empty gel capsules.

Preparation: Mix Schisandra and Ashwagandha powders thoroughly. Fill empty capsules and seal.

Suggested Usage: Take 1 capsule daily to reduce stress and enhance emotional balance.

Benefits: Schisandra promotes emotional stability and reduces fatigue, while Ashwagandha enhances resilience to stress, making this blend effective for stress management.

928. Lemon Balm and Chamomile Mood-Calming Tea

Ingredients: 1 tablespoon Lemon Balm, 1 tablespoon dried Chamomile, 2 cups hot water.
Preparation: Steep Lemon Balm and Chamomile in hot water for 10-15 minutes. Strain and serve warm.
Suggested Usage: Drink 1 cup in the evening to reduce anxiety and promote relaxation.
Benefits: Lemon Balm soothes the nervous system, while Chamomile reduces irritability and promotes a calm state of mind.

929. St. John's Wort and Schisandra Emotional Balance Capsules

Ingredients: 1 tablespoon St. John's Wort powder, 1 tablespoon Schisandra Berry powder, empty gel capsules.
Preparation: Mix St. John's Wort and Schisandra powders thoroughly. Fill empty capsules and seal.
Suggested Usage: Take 1 capsule daily to promote emotional stability and alleviate mild depression.
Benefits: St. John's Wort stabilizes mood by modulating neurotransmitter levels, while Schisandra enhances resilience and emotional balance.

930. Lavender and Skullcap Relaxation Tea

Ingredients: 1 tablespoon dried Lavender, 1 tablespoon Skullcap, 2 cups hot water.
Preparation: Steep Lavender and Skullcap in hot water for 10-15 minutes. Strain and serve warm.
Suggested Usage: Drink 1 cup before bed to promote relaxation and emotional stability.
Benefits: Lavender reduces anxiety and tension, while Skullcap calms the nervous system and promotes restful sleep.

931. Holy Basil and Gotu Kola Emotional Balance Capsules

Ingredients: 1 tablespoon Holy Basil powder, 1 tablespoon Gotu Kola powder, empty gel capsules.
Preparation: Mix Holy Basil and Gotu Kola powders thoroughly. Fill empty capsules and seal.
Suggested Usage: Take 1 capsule in the morning to promote emotional stability and mental clarity.
Benefits: Holy Basil balances emotional states and reduces stress, while Gotu Kola enhances mental focus and emotional resilience.

932. Lemon Balm and Skullcap Anti-Anxiety Elixir

Ingredients: 1 tablespoon Lemon Balm, 1 tablespoon Skullcap, 1 cup honey, 1 cup water.
Preparation: Simmer Lemon Balm and Skullcap in water for 15 minutes. Strain and combine with honey. Store in a glass jar.
Suggested Usage: Take 1 tablespoon in the evening to reduce anxiety and promote emotional calm.
Benefits: Lemon Balm calms the nervous system, while Skullcap reduces emotional tension and promotes relaxation.

933. Rhodiola and Schisandra Adaptogen Mood-Balancing Capsules

Ingredients: 1 tablespoon Rhodiola Root powder, 1 tablespoon Schisandra Berry powder, empty gel capsules.
Preparation: Mix Rhodiola and Schisandra powders thoroughly. Fill empty capsules and seal.
Suggested Usage: Take 1 capsule daily to support mood stability and reduce fatigue.
Benefits: Rhodiola enhances mental stamina and resilience, while Schisandra reduces emotional fatigue and supports overall emotional well-being.

934. Lavender and Passionflower Bedtime Tea

Ingredients: 1 tablespoon dried Lavender, 1 tablespoon Passionflower, 2 cups hot water.
Preparation: Steep Lavender and Passionflower in hot water for 10-15 minutes. Strain and serve warm.
Suggested Usage: Drink 1 cup 30 minutes before bed to promote restful sleep and reduce anxiety.
Benefits: Lavender promotes relaxation and reduces anxiety, while Passionflower soothes the nervous system and promotes a sense of tranquility.

935. Bacopa and Gotu Kola Emotional Clarity Tincture

Ingredients: 1 tablespoon Bacopa Monnieri, 1 tablespoon Gotu Kola, 1 cup vodka or brandy.
Preparation: Combine Bacopa and Gotu Kola in a glass jar, cover with alcohol, and seal. Let sit for 4-6 weeks, shaking daily. Strain and store in a dark glass bottle.
Suggested Usage: Take 1 teaspoon in the morning to support mental clarity and emotional stability.
Benefits: Bacopa enhances cognitive clarity and emotional stability, while Gotu Kola reduces anxiety and improves focus.

936. Holy Basil and Ashwagandha Adaptogen Tea

Ingredients: 1 tablespoon Holy Basil, 1 tablespoon Ashwagandha Root, 2 cups hot water.
Preparation: Simmer Holy Basil and Ashwagandha in hot water for 10-15 minutes. Strain and serve warm.
Suggested Usage: Drink 1 cup in the morning to promote emotional balance and reduce stress.
Benefits: Holy Basil supports stress management and mental clarity, while Ashwagandha enhances resilience and emotional stability.

Book 40: Natural Remedies for Memory Enhancement

Herbs to Improve Memory and Recall

Memory and cognitive recall are vital components of mental function, significantly affecting learning, problem-solving, and daily activities. Certain herbs, known for their neuroprotective properties, have been used traditionally to enhance memory retention, sharpen cognitive abilities, and support overall brain health. The primary mechanism by which these herbs work is by increasing cerebral blood flow, protecting neurons from oxidative damage, and modulating neurotransmitter activity, thus supporting long-term cognitive health.

One of the most renowned memory-enhancing herbs is **Ginkgo Biloba**, which has been extensively studied for its ability to increase blood flow to the brain, enhance synaptic plasticity, and protect against age-related cognitive decline. **Gotu Kola** is another powerful herb that has been used in Ayurvedic medicine for centuries to improve mental clarity, memory, and concentration. It works by supporting microcirculation and promoting the health of the brain's blood vessels.

Another effective herb is **Bacopa Monnieri**, also known as Brahmi. Bacopa is widely used in Ayurvedic traditions to enhance learning and memory. Its active compounds, called bacosides, have been shown to support cognitive processing, reduce anxiety, and improve the retention of new information. **Rosemary**, with its fragrant aroma, is believed to stimulate memory and concentration, making it a versatile herb for both culinary and therapeutic purposes. The use of **Lion's Mane Mushroom** has gained popularity for its potential to stimulate nerve growth factor (NGF), which supports the health and regeneration of neurons, making it a valuable herb for maintaining cognitive health and memory.

For optimal results, these herbs can be used individually or in combination, depending on the desired effects. When creating herbal blends for memory enhancement, it is important to consider the unique properties of each herb and how they can complement one another. For instance, combining **Ginkgo Biloba** with **Rosemary** can amplify the cognitive benefits, while blending **Bacopa** and **Gotu Kola** can create a powerful formula for enhancing learning and recall.

Recipes for Memory-Boosting Teas

Memory-boosting teas and tinctures are a simple and effective way to incorporate these cognitive-supporting herbs into a daily routine. Herbal teas such as **Ginkgo and Rosemary Memory Tea** can be sipped in the morning to enhance focus and clarity, while a **Gotu Kola and Bacopa Cognitive Support Tea** can be enjoyed during study sessions to support concentration and memory retention.

For a more potent formula, tinctures like **Bacopa and Lion's Mane Memory Elixir** can be taken daily to support long-term cognitive health. These herbal preparations can be made by combining herbs with complementary actions, such as using adaptogens like **Ashwagandha** or **Rhodiola** to reduce stress and promote mental stamina alongside memory-enhancing herbs. Including aromatic herbs like **Rosemary** and **Peppermint** in tea blends can also stimulate mental alertness and clarity, adding an invigorating sensory experience to the memory-boosting effects.

Creating a routine around these herbal remedies can enhance their benefits. Pairing memory-enhancing teas with mental exercises such as puzzles, reading, or mindfulness practices can create a synergistic effect, supporting both short-term and long-term cognitive health. By incorporating these herbs into a comprehensive approach to mental wellness, it is possible to maintain and even improve memory and recall abilities over time, supporting a sharper and more resilient mind.

Remedies for Memory Enhancement

937. Ginkgo Biloba and Gotu Kola Memory Boost Tea

Ingredients: 1 tablespoon Ginkgo Biloba, 1 tablespoon Gotu Kola, 2 cups hot water.
Preparation: Steep Ginkgo Biloba and Gotu Kola in hot water for 15 minutes. Strain and serve warm.
Suggested Usage: Drink 1 cup daily to support memory and cognitive health.
Benefits: Ginkgo enhances cerebral circulation, while Gotu Kola supports cognitive clarity and reduces mental fatigue.

938. Bacopa and Lion's Mane Cognitive Clarity Capsules

Ingredients: 1 tablespoon Bacopa powder, 1 tablespoon Lion's Mane powder, empty gel capsules.
Preparation: Mix Bacopa and Lion's Mane powders thoroughly. Fill empty capsules and seal.
Suggested Usage: Take 1 capsule daily to enhance learning and memory retention.
Benefits: Bacopa improves memory recall and cognitive function, while Lion's Mane promotes nerve regeneration and mental clarity.

939. Rosemary and Peppermint Focus Tea

Ingredients: 1 tablespoon dried Rosemary, 1 tablespoon Peppermint, 2 cups hot water.
Preparation: Steep Rosemary and Peppermint in hot water for 10-15 minutes. Strain and serve warm.
Suggested Usage: Drink 1 cup in the morning to promote alertness and focus.
Benefits: Rosemary stimulates memory and concentration, while Peppermint invigorates the mind and enhances clarity.

940. Gotu Kola and Ashwagandha Brain Health Elixir

Ingredients: 1 tablespoon Gotu Kola, 1 tablespoon Ashwagandha Root, 1 cup water, 1 cup honey.

Preparation: Simmer Gotu Kola and Ashwagandha in water for 15 minutes. Strain and combine with honey. Store in a glass jar.

Suggested Usage: Take 1 tablespoon daily to promote cognitive function and reduce stress.

Benefits: Gotu Kola enhances memory and focus, while Ashwagandha reduces stress and supports mental resilience.

941. Ginseng and Rhodiola Adaptogen Capsules

Ingredients: 1 tablespoon Ginseng powder, 1 tablespoon Rhodiola Root powder, empty gel capsules.

Preparation: Mix Ginseng and Rhodiola powders thoroughly. Fill empty capsules and seal.

Suggested Usage: Take 1 capsule in the morning to enhance energy and mental stamina.

Benefits: Ginseng boosts energy and mental clarity, while Rhodiola reduces mental fatigue and enhances cognitive resilience.

942. Ginkgo and Brahmi Memory-Enhancing Tincture

Ingredients: 1 tablespoon Ginkgo Biloba, 1 tablespoon Brahmi, 1 cup vodka or brandy.

Preparation: Combine Ginkgo and Brahmi in a glass jar, cover with alcohol, and seal. Let sit for 4-6 weeks, shaking daily. Strain and store in a dark glass bottle.

Suggested Usage: Take 1 teaspoon twice daily to support memory and learning.

Benefits: Ginkgo improves blood flow to the brain, while Brahmi enhances memory and cognitive clarity.

943. Lion's Mane and Schisandra Brain Support Capsules

Ingredients: 1 tablespoon Lion's Mane powder, 1 tablespoon Schisandra Berry powder, empty gel capsules.

Preparation: Mix Lion's Mane and Schisandra powders thoroughly. Fill empty capsules and seal.

Suggested Usage: Take 1 capsule daily to support cognitive health and mental resilience.

Benefits: Lion's Mane supports nerve regeneration and brain function, while Schisandra reduces mental fatigue and enhances clarity.

944. Gotu Kola and Bacopa Memory Tonic

Ingredients: 1 tablespoon Gotu Kola, 1 tablespoon Bacopa, 2 cups hot water.

Preparation: Steep Gotu Kola and Bacopa in hot water for 15 minutes. Strain and serve warm.

Suggested Usage: Drink 1 cup daily to promote learning and memory retention.

Benefits: Gotu Kola enhances mental clarity, while Bacopa supports memory retention and cognitive function.

945. Ginkgo Biloba and Rosemary Cognitive Health Tea

Ingredients: 1 tablespoon Ginkgo Biloba, 1 tablespoon Rosemary, 2 cups hot water.

Preparation: Steep Ginkgo and Rosemary in hot water for 15 minutes. Strain and serve warm.

Suggested Usage: Drink 1 cup in the morning to promote memory and concentration.

Benefits: Ginkgo increases cerebral circulation, while Rosemary improves memory and focus.

946. Ashwagandha and Holy Basil Adaptogen Capsules

Ingredients: 1 tablespoon Ashwagandha Root powder, 1 tablespoon Holy Basil powder, empty gel capsules.

Preparation: Mix Ashwagandha and Holy Basil powders thoroughly. Fill empty capsules and seal.

Suggested Usage: Take 1 capsule daily to support emotional and cognitive resilience.

Benefits: Ashwagandha reduces stress and enhances mental stamina, while Holy Basil supports emotional stability and cognitive function.

947. Peppermint and Lemon Balm Focus Tea

Ingredients: 1 tablespoon Peppermint, 1 tablespoon Lemon Balm, 2 cups hot water.

Preparation: Steep Peppermint and Lemon Balm in hot water for 10-15 minutes. Strain and serve warm.

Suggested Usage: Drink 1 cup in the afternoon to promote mental clarity and reduce anxiety.

Benefits: Peppermint stimulates cognitive function and enhances alertness, while Lemon Balm soothes anxiety and promotes calm focus.

948. Rhodiola and Schisandra Cognitive Support Elixir

Ingredients: 1 tablespoon Rhodiola Root, 1 tablespoon Schisandra Berry, 1 cup honey, 1 cup water.

Preparation: Simmer Rhodiola and Schisandra in water for 15 minutes. Strain and combine with honey. Store in a glass jar.

Suggested Usage: Take 1 tablespoon in the morning to support mental stamina and reduce stress.

Benefits: Rhodiola enhances cognitive resilience and mental clarity, while Schisandra supports emotional balance and memory function.

949. Lemon Balm and Lavender Relaxation Capsules

Ingredients: 1 tablespoon Lemon Balm powder, 1 tablespoon Lavender powder, empty gel capsules.

Preparation: Mix Lemon Balm and Lavender powders thoroughly. Fill empty capsules and seal.

Suggested Usage: Take 1 capsule in the evening to reduce stress and promote relaxation.

Benefits: Lemon Balm calms the nervous system, while Lavender reduces anxiety and supports emotional stability.

950. Gotu Kola and Rosemary Focus Capsules

Ingredients: 1 tablespoon Gotu Kola powder, 1 tablespoon Rosemary powder, empty gel capsules.

Preparation: Mix Gotu Kola and

Rosemary powders thoroughly. Fill empty capsules and seal.

Suggested Usage: Take 1 capsule daily to promote focus and mental clarity.

Benefits: Gotu Kola supports cognitive clarity and mental stamina, while Rosemary enhances concentration and memory.

951. Brahmi and Ginkgo Memory-Enhancing Capsules

Ingredients: 1 tablespoon Brahmi powder, 1 tablespoon Ginkgo Biloba powder, empty gel capsules.

Preparation: Mix Brahmi and Ginkgo powders thoroughly. Fill empty capsules and seal.

Suggested Usage: Take 1 capsule daily to support memory retention and cognitive health.

Benefits: Brahmi enhances learning and cognitive clarity, while Ginkgo improves blood flow to the brain and supports memory function.

952. Lion's Mane and Peppermint Brain-Boosting Tea

Ingredients: 1 tablespoon dried Lion's Mane, 1 tablespoon dried Peppermint, 2 cups hot water.

Preparation: Steep Lion's Mane and Peppermint in hot water for 15 minutes. Strain and serve warm.

Suggested Usage: Drink 1 cup in the morning to promote mental clarity and focus.

Benefits: Lion's Mane supports cognitive function and nerve health, while Peppermint invigorates the mind and enhances alertness.

953. Bacopa and Ashwagandha Cognitive Support Capsules

Ingredients: 1 tablespoon Bacopa powder, 1 tablespoon Ashwagandha Root powder, empty gel capsules.

Preparation: Mix Bacopa and Ashwagandha powders thoroughly. Fill empty capsules and seal.

Suggested Usage: Take 1 capsule daily to reduce mental fatigue and enhance cognitive function.

Benefits: Bacopa supports memory and learning, while Ashwagandha enhances resilience to stress and promotes mental clarity.

954. Rosemary and Lemon Peel Mental Clarity Tea

Ingredients: 1 tablespoon dried Rosemary, 1 tablespoon Lemon Peel, 2 cups hot water.

Preparation: Steep Rosemary and Lemon Peel in hot water for 10-15 minutes. Strain and serve warm.

Suggested Usage: Drink 1 cup in the morning to promote mental clarity and concentration.

Benefits: Rosemary enhances memory and focus, while Lemon Peel supports digestion and cognitive health.

955. Ginseng and Brahmi Concentration Tonic

Ingredients: 1 tablespoon Ginseng Root, 1 tablespoon Brahmi, 2 cups hot water, 1 cup honey.

Preparation: Simmer Ginseng and Brahmi in water for 15 minutes. Strain and

combine with honey. Store in a glass jar.
Suggested Usage: Take 1 tablespoon in the morning to enhance concentration and reduce mental fatigue.
Benefits: Ginseng boosts mental energy and resilience, while Brahmi improves memory and cognitive function.

956. Gotu Kola and Peppermint Brain-Boosting Capsules

Ingredients: 1 tablespoon Gotu Kola powder, 1 tablespoon Peppermint powder, empty gel capsules.
Preparation: Mix Gotu Kola and Peppermint powders thoroughly. Fill empty capsules and seal.
Suggested Usage: Take 1 capsule in the morning to promote mental clarity and alertness.
Benefits: Gotu Kola supports cognitive clarity and focus, while Peppermint enhances concentration and mental performance.

957. Ginkgo and Schisandra Stress-Relief Capsules

Ingredients: 1 tablespoon Ginkgo Biloba powder, 1 tablespoon Schisandra Berry powder, empty gel capsules.
Preparation: Mix Ginkgo and Schisandra powders thoroughly. Fill empty capsules and seal.
Suggested Usage: Take 1 capsule daily to promote cognitive health and reduce stress.
Benefits: Ginkgo enhances cerebral circulation and memory function, while Schisandra supports emotional balance and mental resilience.

958. Holy Basil and Ashwagandha Brain-Calming Tea

Ingredients: 1 tablespoon Holy Basil, 1 tablespoon Ashwagandha Root, 2 cups hot water.
Preparation: Steep Holy Basil and Ashwagandha in hot water for 15 minutes. Strain and serve warm.
Suggested Usage: Drink 1 cup in the evening to reduce stress and promote mental calm.
Benefits: Holy Basil supports mental clarity and reduces anxiety, while Ashwagandha enhances stress resilience and cognitive function.

959. Peppermint and Lemon Balm Focus Capsules

Ingredients: 1 tablespoon Peppermint powder, 1 tablespoon Lemon Balm powder, empty gel capsules.
Preparation: Mix Peppermint and Lemon Balm powders thoroughly. Fill empty capsules and seal.
Suggested Usage: Take 1 capsule in the afternoon to promote focus and reduce stress.
Benefits: Peppermint stimulates mental alertness, while Lemon Balm calms the mind and promotes emotional balance.

960. Ginkgo Biloba and Gotu Kola Concentration Elixir

Ingredients: 1 tablespoon Ginkgo Biloba, 1 tablespoon Gotu Kola, 1 cup water, 1 cup honey.
Preparation: Simmer Ginkgo and Gotu Kola in water for 15 minutes. Strain and

combine with honey. Store in a glass jar.

Suggested Usage: Take 1 tablespoon daily to support concentration and mental clarity.

Benefits: Ginkgo enhances memory and cerebral circulation, while Gotu Kola promotes cognitive clarity and reduces mental fatigue.

961. Lion's Mane and Ginkgo Brain-Boosting Capsules

Ingredients: 1 tablespoon Lion's Mane powder, 1 tablespoon Ginkgo Biloba powder, empty gel capsules.

Preparation: Mix Lion's Mane and Ginkgo powders thoroughly. Fill empty capsules and seal.

Suggested Usage: Take 1 capsule daily to support cognitive function and nerve health.

Benefits: Lion's Mane stimulates nerve regeneration and supports cognitive health, while Ginkgo enhances memory and mental clarity.

962. Gotu Kola and Schisandra Emotional Balance Capsules

Ingredients: 1 tablespoon Gotu Kola powder, 1 tablespoon Schisandra Berry powder, empty gel capsules.

Preparation: Mix Gotu Kola and Schisandra powders thoroughly. Fill empty capsules and seal.

Suggested Usage: Take 1 capsule daily to promote emotional stability and mental focus.

Benefits: Gotu Kola supports cognitive clarity and mental stamina, while Schisandra reduces stress and supports emotional balance.

963. Bacopa and Peppermint Clarity Tea

Ingredients: 1 tablespoon Bacopa Monnieri, 1 tablespoon Peppermint, 2 cups hot water.

Preparation: Steep Bacopa and Peppermint in hot water for 15 minutes. Strain and serve warm.

Suggested Usage: Drink 1 cup in the morning to promote mental clarity and enhance learning.

Benefits: Bacopa supports memory retention and cognitive processing, while Peppermint enhances focus and mental clarity.

964. Ginkgo and Lemon Balm Cognitive Health Capsules

Ingredients: 1 tablespoon Ginkgo Biloba powder, 1 tablespoon Lemon Balm powder, empty gel capsules.

Preparation: Mix Ginkgo and Lemon Balm powders thoroughly. Fill empty capsules and seal.

Suggested Usage: Take 1 capsule daily to support cognitive health and emotional balance.

Benefits: Ginkgo enhances cerebral circulation and memory function, while Lemon Balm promotes emotional stability and cognitive clarity.

Section IV: Physical Health and Vitality

Book 41: Natural Pain Relief

Herbal Analgesics for Chronic and Acute Pain

Pain management is a critical aspect of physical health, affecting the quality of life and overall well-being. Conventional pain relief methods often come with potential side effects, leading many individuals to seek out natural alternatives. Herbal analgesics provide a gentle yet effective option for managing both chronic and acute pain, targeting the underlying causes and offering relief without the harsh effects of synthetic medications. Herbs like **Willow Bark**, **Turmeric**, and **Devil's Claw** have been used for centuries to reduce inflammation and alleviate pain, making them essential components of a natural pain relief regimen.

Willow Bark, often referred to as "nature's aspirin," contains salicin, a compound similar to acetylsalicylic acid (the active ingredient in aspirin). It is particularly effective for joint pain, headaches, and muscle soreness. Similarly, **Turmeric**, with its active compound curcumin, is a powerful anti-inflammatory agent that can help reduce pain associated with arthritis and other inflammatory conditions. It works by modulating inflammatory pathways in the body, offering long-term relief without the gastrointestinal side effects commonly associated with NSAIDs.

For those experiencing nerve pain or sciatica, **St. John's Wort** has been shown to be beneficial due to its nervine properties, which support the health of the nervous system. **California Poppy** and **Valerian** are also effective for relieving tension and promoting relaxation, making them ideal for pain related to muscle spasms or tension headaches. **Ginger** and **Cayenne Pepper** are known for their warming properties, which stimulate circulation and provide relief from localized pain when used topically. Cayenne contains capsaicin, which depletes substance P—a neurotransmitter involved in pain signaling—resulting in pain reduction over time.

Chronic pain, such as that caused by arthritis, fibromyalgia, or lower back issues, often requires a multifaceted approach. **Devil's Claw**, a herb traditionally used in African medicine, has shown promise in reducing inflammation and pain in individuals with osteoarthritis. It is often paired with other anti-inflammatory herbs like **Boswellia** and **Turmeric** to create a comprehensive approach to managing chronic conditions. For acute pain, such as muscle strains or sprains, **Arnica** is commonly used as a topical remedy due to its anti-inflammatory and analgesic properties. It can reduce swelling and speed up the healing process, making it a go-to herb for sports injuries or acute muscle pain.

By integrating these herbs into a pain management routine, individuals can experience effective relief while supporting overall health and reducing reliance on conventional pain medications. However, it is important to consider the underlying causes of pain and address them with a combination of herbal, dietary, and lifestyle interventions for long-term management.

Recipes for Pain-Relieving Salves and Tinctures

Creating herbal formulations for pain relief allows for targeted applications and a personalized approach to managing discomfort. Salves, tinctures, and oils can be tailored to address specific types of pain, whether it's joint pain, muscle soreness, or nerve pain. A **Willow Bark and St. John's Wort Tincture** can be taken internally to reduce nerve pain and inflammation, while a **Cayenne and Ginger Warming Salve** can be applied topically to alleviate muscle stiffness and soreness.

For chronic pain conditions like arthritis, a **Turmeric and Boswellia Anti-Inflammatory Oil** can be massaged into the affected areas to reduce inflammation and promote joint mobility. An **Arnica and Comfrey Healing Salve** is excellent for acute injuries, as it reduces swelling and accelerates tissue repair. These remedies can be incorporated into a daily routine or used as needed for pain flare-ups, providing a natural, effective means of managing discomfort.

The combination of internal and topical herbal remedies can create a synergistic effect, enhancing the overall efficacy of pain relief protocols. For example, using a **Turmeric and Devil's Claw Tincture** internally along with a **Cayenne and Arnica Pain Relief Salve** externally can address both systemic inflammation and localized pain, providing comprehensive support for pain management.

Creating a pain-relief regimen that includes herbal remedies, dietary modifications, and physical therapies such as yoga or gentle stretching can significantly improve quality of life for individuals dealing with chronic pain. Herbal pain relief is not just about symptom management; it is about promoting healing, reducing inflammation, and supporting the body's natural pain response for long-term wellness and vitality.

Remedies for Pain Relief

965. Willow Bark and Turmeric Anti-Inflammatory Capsules

Ingredients: 1 tablespoon Willow Bark powder, 1 tablespoon Turmeric powder, empty gel capsules.
Preparation: Mix Willow Bark and Turmeric powders thoroughly. Fill empty capsules and seal.
Suggested Usage: Take 1 capsule twice daily to reduce inflammation and manage chronic pain.
Benefits: Willow Bark provides natural pain relief similar to aspirin, while

Turmeric reduces inflammation and supports joint health.

966. St. John's Wort and Skullcap Nerve Pain Tincture

Ingredients: 1 tablespoon St. John's Wort, 1 tablespoon Skullcap, 1 cup vodka or brandy.
Preparation: Combine St. John's Wort and Skullcap in a glass jar, cover with alcohol, and seal. Let sit for 4-6 weeks, shaking daily. Strain and store in a dark glass bottle.
Suggested Usage: Take 1 teaspoon twice daily to alleviate nerve pain and calm the nervous system.
Benefits: St. John's Wort soothes nerve pain, while Skullcap calms the nervous system and reduces tension.

967. Arnica and Comfrey Healing Salve

Ingredients: 1 tablespoon Arnica flowers, 1 tablespoon Comfrey Root, 1 cup olive oil, 1/4 cup beeswax.
Preparation: Simmer Arnica and Comfrey in olive oil for 30 minutes. Strain and melt in beeswax. Pour into a container and let cool.
Suggested Usage: Apply to bruises, sprains, and sore muscles to reduce pain and inflammation.
Benefits: Arnica reduces swelling and pain, while Comfrey accelerates tissue repair and healing.

968. Turmeric and Ginger Anti-Inflammatory Tonic

Ingredients: 1 tablespoon Turmeric powder, 1 tablespoon Ginger Root, 1 cup warm water, 1 tablespoon honey.
Preparation: Combine all ingredients in a cup and stir well. Serve warm.
Suggested Usage: Drink 1 cup daily to reduce systemic inflammation and alleviate pain.
Benefits: Turmeric and Ginger work together to reduce inflammation and promote circulation, easing muscle and joint pain.

969. Devil's Claw and Boswellia Joint Relief Capsules

Ingredients: 1 tablespoon Devil's Claw powder, 1 tablespoon Boswellia powder, empty gel capsules.
Preparation: Mix Devil's Claw and Boswellia powders thoroughly. Fill empty capsules and seal.
Suggested Usage: Take 1 capsule twice daily to alleviate joint pain and stiffness.
Benefits: Devil's Claw reduces inflammation and pain, while Boswellia supports joint health and mobility.

970. Cayenne and Ginger Warming Salve

Ingredients: 1 tablespoon Cayenne powder, 1 tablespoon Ginger Root, 1 cup coconut oil, 1/4 cup beeswax.
Preparation: Simmer Cayenne and Ginger in coconut oil for 30 minutes. Strain and melt in beeswax. Pour into a container and let cool.
Suggested Usage: Apply to sore muscles and joints to increase circulation and alleviate pain.
Benefits: Cayenne contains capsaicin,

which reduces pain signaling, while Ginger provides additional warming and anti-inflammatory effects.

971. Turmeric and Black Pepper Pain-Relief Capsules

Ingredients: 1 tablespoon Turmeric powder, 1 teaspoon Black Pepper, empty gel capsules.
Preparation: Mix Turmeric and Black Pepper powders thoroughly. Fill empty capsules and seal.
Suggested Usage: Take 1 capsule daily to reduce inflammation and manage chronic pain.
Benefits: Turmeric reduces inflammation and Black Pepper enhances curcumin absorption for more effective pain relief.

972. California Poppy and Valerian Sleep Support Tincture

Ingredients: 1 tablespoon California Poppy, 1 tablespoon Valerian Root, 1 cup vodka or brandy.
Preparation: Combine California Poppy and Valerian in a glass jar, cover with alcohol, and seal. Let sit for 4-6 weeks, shaking daily. Strain and store in a dark glass bottle.
Suggested Usage: Take 1 teaspoon before bed to reduce pain-related insomnia and promote restful sleep.
Benefits: California Poppy reduces pain and promotes relaxation, while Valerian supports deep, restorative sleep.

973. Ginger and Turmeric Anti-Spasm Tea

Ingredients: 1 tablespoon Ginger Root, 1 tablespoon Turmeric, 2 cups hot water.
Preparation: Steep Ginger and Turmeric in hot water for 10-15 minutes. Strain and serve warm.
Suggested Usage: Drink 1 cup to alleviate muscle spasms and reduce tension.
Benefits: Ginger and Turmeric reduce muscle pain and promote relaxation through their anti-inflammatory and warming properties.

974. White Willow Bark and Meadowsweet Pain Relief Tea

Ingredients: 1 tablespoon Willow Bark, 1 tablespoon Meadowsweet, 2 cups hot water.
Preparation: Steep Willow Bark and Meadowsweet in hot water for 15 minutes. Strain and serve warm.
Suggested Usage: Drink 1 cup as needed to relieve headaches, joint pain, and muscle soreness.
Benefits: Willow Bark provides natural pain relief similar to aspirin, while Meadowsweet soothes inflammation and promotes joint health.

975. Ginger and Cayenne Circulation Tonic

Ingredients: 1 tablespoon Ginger Root, 1 teaspoon Cayenne Pepper, 1 cup warm water, 1 tablespoon honey.
Preparation: Combine all ingredients in a cup and stir well. Serve warm.
Suggested Usage: Drink 1 cup daily to stimulate circulation and alleviate pain.
Benefits: Ginger and Cayenne work together to promote blood flow and reduce pain in stiff or sore muscles.

976. Chamomile and Lavender Tension Relief Tea

Ingredients: 1 tablespoon Chamomile, 1 tablespoon Lavender, 2 cups hot water.
Preparation: Steep Chamomile and Lavender in hot water for 10-15 minutes. Strain and serve warm.
Suggested Usage: Drink 1 cup to reduce tension headaches and promote relaxation.
Benefits: Chamomile and Lavender work together to relax the nervous system and alleviate tension.

977. Peppermint and Rosemary Muscle Pain-Relief Oil

Ingredients: 1 tablespoon dried Peppermint, 1 tablespoon Rosemary, 1 cup olive oil, 1/4 cup beeswax.
Preparation: Simmer Peppermint and Rosemary in olive oil for 30 minutes. Strain and melt in beeswax. Pour into a container and let cool.
Suggested Usage: Apply to sore muscles and joints to reduce pain and inflammation.
Benefits: Peppermint provides a cooling sensation, while Rosemary enhances circulation and reduces pain.

978. Clove and Cinnamon Toothache Relief Oil

Ingredients: 1 tablespoon Clove powder, 1 tablespoon Cinnamon, 1/2 cup coconut oil.
Preparation: Simmer Clove and Cinnamon in coconut oil for 30 minutes. Strain and store in a glass jar.
Suggested Usage: Apply a small amount to the affected area to relieve toothache pain.
Benefits: Clove and Cinnamon have natural analgesic properties, providing pain relief and reducing inflammation.

979. Boswellia and Turmeric Inflammation Relief Capsules

Ingredients: 1 tablespoon Boswellia powder, 1 tablespoon Turmeric powder, empty gel capsules.
Preparation: Mix Boswellia and Turmeric powders thoroughly. Fill empty capsules and seal.
Suggested Usage: Take 1 capsule twice daily to reduce chronic pain and inflammation.
Benefits: Boswellia supports joint health and reduces inflammation, while Turmeric provides systemic anti-inflammatory benefits.

980. Eucalyptus and Peppermint Tension-Relief Balm

Ingredients: 1 tablespoon Eucalyptus, 1 tablespoon Peppermint, 1 cup coconut oil, 1/4 cup beeswax.
Preparation: Simmer Eucalyptus and Peppermint in coconut oil for 30 minutes. Strain and melt in beeswax. Pour into a container and let cool.
Suggested Usage: Apply to temples and neck to reduce tension headaches and promote relaxation.
Benefits: Eucalyptus and Peppermint provide cooling relief and reduce tension, making this balm ideal for headaches and muscle pain.

981. Devil's Claw and Turmeric Joint Pain Capsules

Ingredients: 1 tablespoon Devil's Claw powder, 1 tablespoon Turmeric powder, empty gel capsules.
Preparation: Mix Devil's Claw and Turmeric powders thoroughly. Fill empty capsules and seal.
Suggested Usage: Take 1 capsule twice daily to alleviate joint pain and stiffness.
Benefits: Devil's Claw reduces inflammation and pain, while Turmeric supports joint health and mobility.

982. Valerian and Passionflower Muscle Relaxation Tea

Ingredients: 1 tablespoon Valerian Root, 1 tablespoon Passionflower, 2 cups hot water.
Preparation: Steep Valerian and Passionflower in hot water for 15 minutes. Strain and serve warm.
Suggested Usage: Drink 1 cup before bed to reduce muscle tension and promote restful sleep.
Benefits: Valerian promotes deep relaxation, while Passionflower soothes the nervous system and reduces muscle spasms.

983. Arnica and Calendula Bruise-Soothing Salve

Ingredients: 1 tablespoon Arnica, 1 tablespoon Calendula, 1 cup olive oil, 1/4 cup beeswax.
Preparation: Simmer Arnica and Calendula in olive oil for 30 minutes. Strain and melt in beeswax. Pour into a container and let cool.
Suggested Usage: Apply to bruises and sprains to reduce pain, inflammation, and discoloration.
Benefits: Arnica reduces bruising and swelling, while Calendula accelerates skin healing and reduces inflammation.

984. Ginger and Cinnamon Warming Tea

Ingredients: 1 tablespoon Ginger Root, 1 tablespoon Cinnamon, 2 cups hot water.
Preparation: Steep Ginger and Cinnamon in hot water for 15 minutes. Strain and serve warm.
Suggested Usage: Drink 1 cup in the morning to alleviate joint pain and promote circulation.
Benefits: Ginger and Cinnamon provide warming and anti-inflammatory effects, making this tea ideal for cold, achy joints.

985. Peppermint and Clove Tension Relief Tincture

Ingredients: 1 tablespoon Peppermint, 1 tablespoon Clove, 1 cup vodka or brandy.
Preparation: Combine Peppermint and Clove in a glass jar, cover with alcohol, and seal. Let sit for 4-6 weeks, shaking daily. Strain and store in a dark glass bottle.
Suggested Usage: Take 1 teaspoon as needed to relieve tension headaches and muscle pain.
Benefits: Peppermint provides a cooling, relaxing sensation, while Clove reduces pain and inflammation.

986. White Willow Bark and Boswellia Pain Relief Capsules

Ingredients: 1 tablespoon Willow Bark powder, 1 tablespoon Boswellia powder, empty gel capsules.
Preparation: Mix Willow Bark and Boswellia powders thoroughly. Fill empty capsules and seal.
Suggested Usage: Take 1 capsule twice daily to reduce pain and support joint health.
Benefits: Willow Bark offers natural pain relief similar to aspirin, while Boswellia supports joint health and reduces inflammation.

987. Cayenne and St. John's Wort Nerve Pain Salve

Ingredients: 1 tablespoon Cayenne powder, 1 tablespoon St. John's Wort, 1 cup olive oil, 1/4 cup beeswax.
Preparation: Simmer Cayenne and St. John's Wort in olive oil for 30 minutes. Strain and melt in beeswax. Pour into a container and let cool.
Suggested Usage: Apply to affected areas to reduce nerve pain and promote circulation.
Benefits: Cayenne depletes substance P, a pain-signaling neurotransmitter, while St. John's Wort soothes nerve pain and supports the nervous system.

988. Chamomile and Lavender Anti-Spasm Capsules

Ingredients: 1 tablespoon Chamomile powder, 1 tablespoon Lavender powder, empty gel capsules.
Preparation: Mix Chamomile and Lavender powders thoroughly. Fill empty capsules and seal.
Suggested Usage: Take 1 capsule twice daily to reduce muscle spasms and promote relaxation.
Benefits: Chamomile relaxes muscle tension, while Lavender calms the nervous system and reduces pain.

989. Turmeric and Black Pepper Anti-Inflammatory Salve

Ingredients: 1 tablespoon Turmeric, 1 teaspoon Black Pepper, 1 cup coconut oil, 1/4 cup beeswax.
Preparation: Simmer Turmeric and Black Pepper in coconut oil for 30 minutes. Strain and melt in beeswax. Pour into a container and let cool.
Suggested Usage: Apply to inflamed joints and muscles to reduce pain and promote circulation.
Benefits: Turmeric reduces inflammation, and Black Pepper enhances curcumin absorption, increasing the effectiveness of the salve.

990. Ginger and Peppermint Headache Relief Tea

Ingredients: 1 tablespoon Ginger Root, 1 tablespoon Peppermint, 2 cups hot water.
Preparation: Steep Ginger and Peppermint in hot water for 10-15 minutes. Strain and serve warm.
Suggested Usage: Drink 1 cup as needed to relieve headaches and reduce nausea.
Benefits: Ginger alleviates pain and nausea, while Peppermint provides cooling relief and reduces tension.

991. Turmeric and Willow Bark Anti-Inflammatory Capsules

Ingredients: 1 tablespoon Turmeric powder, 1 tablespoon Willow Bark powder, empty gel capsules.
Preparation: Mix Turmeric and Willow Bark powders thoroughly. Fill empty capsules and seal.
Suggested Usage: Take 1 capsule twice daily to manage chronic pain and reduce inflammation.
Benefits: Turmeric and Willow Bark work together to provide natural pain relief and reduce inflammation.

992. Calendula and Comfrey Muscle-Repair Salve

Ingredients: 1 tablespoon Calendula, 1 tablespoon Comfrey Root, 1 cup olive oil, 1/4 cup beeswax.
Preparation: Simmer Calendula and Comfrey in olive oil for 30 minutes. Strain and melt in beeswax. Pour into a container and let cool.
Suggested Usage: Apply to sore muscles and bruises to reduce pain and promote tissue repair.
Benefits: Calendula reduces inflammation and supports skin healing, while Comfrey promotes the repair of muscle and connective tissue.

993. Lemon Balm and Skullcap Tension Relief Capsules

Ingredients: 1 tablespoon Lemon Balm powder, 1 tablespoon Skullcap powder, empty gel capsules.
Preparation: Mix Lemon Balm and Skullcap powders thoroughly. Fill empty capsules and seal.
Suggested Usage: Take 1 capsule in the evening to reduce tension and promote relaxation.
Benefits: Lemon Balm calms the nervous system, while Skullcap reduces anxiety and tension headaches.

994. Eucalyptus and Peppermint Pain Relief Massage Oil

Ingredients: 1 tablespoon Eucalyptus, 1 tablespoon Peppermint, 1 cup olive oil.
Preparation: Combine Eucalyptus and Peppermint in olive oil and let infuse for 2 weeks. Strain and store in a dark glass bottle.
Suggested Usage: Massage into sore muscles and joints to reduce pain and tension.
Benefits: Eucalyptus and Peppermint provide cooling relief, reduce inflammation, and promote relaxation of tense muscles.

995. White Willow Bark and Devil's Claw Pain Relief Tincture

Ingredients: 1 tablespoon Willow Bark, 1 tablespoon Devil's Claw, 1 cup vodka or brandy.
Preparation: Combine Willow Bark and Devil's Claw in a glass jar, cover with alcohol, and seal. Let sit for 4-6 weeks, shaking daily. Strain and store in a dark glass bottle.
Suggested Usage: Take 1 teaspoon twice daily to reduce inflammation and manage chronic pain.

Benefits: Willow Bark provides natural pain relief, while Devil's Claw supports joint health and reduces inflammation.

Book 42: Herbal Remedies for Joint Health

Supporting Joint Function with Herbs

Maintaining joint health is crucial for mobility and overall physical well-being, especially as one ages or experiences conditions like arthritis or joint injuries. Joint health is often compromised due to inflammation, wear and tear, or autoimmune conditions that affect the connective tissues. Herbs can play a significant role in supporting joint health, reducing inflammation, promoting flexibility, and slowing down degenerative processes. By incorporating herbal remedies into daily routines, it is possible to improve joint function and alleviate discomfort naturally.

Several herbs have been traditionally used to support joint health. **Turmeric**, with its active compound curcumin, is a well-known anti-inflammatory agent that can significantly reduce joint inflammation and pain. Curcumin works by blocking inflammatory pathways in the body, making it highly effective for managing conditions like arthritis and general joint soreness. **Boswellia**, also known as Indian frankincense, is another potent anti-inflammatory herb that inhibits enzymes responsible for the production of inflammatory molecules, helping reduce stiffness and improve mobility in people suffering from osteoarthritis or rheumatoid arthritis.

For long-term joint support, **Devil's Claw** and **Willow Bark** are excellent choices. Devil's Claw has been used traditionally in African medicine to treat inflammation and joint pain, while Willow Bark is considered "nature's aspirin" due to its salicin content, which is metabolized into salicylic acid in the body. These herbs can be particularly effective for managing chronic joint conditions, providing pain relief without the adverse side effects of synthetic medications.

Other beneficial herbs for joint health include **Ginger** and **Nettle Leaf**. Ginger's warming properties and anti-inflammatory effects help soothe sore joints and increase circulation, making it an ideal remedy for people suffering from stiffness and limited mobility. Nettle Leaf, on the other hand, is rich in minerals such as silica and magnesium, which support joint and connective tissue health. When combined, these herbs create a powerful synergy that not only alleviates joint pain but also nourishes and strengthens the joints.

Recipes for Anti-Inflammatory Blends

Herbal formulations for joint health can be prepared as teas, tinctures, or topical applications, depending on the specific needs of the individual. For internal use, a **Turmeric and Boswellia Anti-Inflammatory Tea** can be consumed daily to reduce inflammation and support joint flexibility. To prepare, simply simmer 1 tablespoon of

Turmeric powder and 1 teaspoon of Boswellia powder in 2 cups of water for 10-15 minutes. Add honey to taste, and drink twice daily for best results.

For those who prefer topical applications, a **Ginger and Cayenne Pain-Relieving Salve** can be made by simmering 1 tablespoon of dried Ginger and 1 tablespoon of Cayenne powder in 1 cup of olive oil. After straining, melt in 1/4 cup of beeswax and pour into a container to cool. This salve can be applied to sore joints to promote circulation, reduce inflammation, and provide localized pain relief.

Another effective remedy for joint health is a **Devil's Claw and Willow Bark Tincture**, which combines the pain-relieving properties of Willow Bark with the anti-inflammatory effects of Devil's Claw. To make this tincture, combine 1 tablespoon of each herb in a glass jar, cover with 1 cup of vodka or brandy, and seal. Let the mixture sit for 4-6 weeks, shaking daily. Strain and store in a dark glass bottle. Take 1 teaspoon twice daily to alleviate chronic joint pain and inflammation.

Incorporating these herbal blends into a holistic joint health regimen, along with a balanced diet and regular exercise, can significantly improve joint mobility, reduce pain, and enhance overall quality of life. These natural remedies provide a safe and effective alternative to conventional treatments, allowing for long-term support of joint function and comfort.

Remedies for Joint Health

996. Turmeric and Boswellia Joint Support Capsules

Ingredients: 1 tablespoon Turmeric powder, 1 tablespoon Boswellia powder, empty gel capsules.
Preparation: Mix Turmeric and Boswellia powders thoroughly. Fill empty capsules and seal.
Suggested Usage: Take 1 capsule twice daily to reduce joint inflammation and support flexibility.
Benefits: Turmeric reduces inflammation, while Boswellia inhibits enzymes that contribute to joint pain and stiffness.

997. Devil's Claw and Willow Bark Pain-Relief Tea

Ingredients: 1 tablespoon Devil's Claw, 1 tablespoon Willow Bark, 2 cups hot water.
Preparation: Steep Devil's Claw and Willow Bark in hot water for 15 minutes. Strain and serve warm.
Suggested Usage: Drink 1 cup in the morning to alleviate joint pain and reduce stiffness.
Benefits: Devil's Claw and Willow Bark provide natural pain relief and reduce joint inflammation.

998. Ginger and Cayenne Warming Salve

Ingredients: 1 tablespoon Ginger Root, 1 tablespoon Cayenne Pepper, 1 cup coconut oil, 1/4 cup beeswax.
Preparation: Simmer Ginger and

Cayenne in coconut oil for 30 minutes. Strain and melt in beeswax. Pour into a container and let cool.

Suggested Usage: Apply to sore joints and muscles to increase circulation and reduce pain.

Benefits: Ginger and Cayenne stimulate blood flow, reduce stiffness, and provide a warming sensation that alleviates pain.

999. Nettle and Horsetail Mineral-Rich Infusion

Ingredients: 1 tablespoon dried Nettle, 1 tablespoon dried Horsetail, 2 cups hot water.

Preparation: Steep Nettle and Horsetail in hot water for 20 minutes. Strain and serve warm.

Suggested Usage: Drink 1 cup daily to nourish joints and connective tissues.

Benefits: Nettle and Horsetail are rich in silica and magnesium, which support joint strength and flexibility.

1000. Turmeric and Ginger Anti-Inflammatory Tonic

Ingredients: 1 tablespoon Turmeric powder, 1 tablespoon Ginger Root, 1 cup warm water, 1 tablespoon honey.

Preparation: Combine all ingredients in a cup and stir well. Serve warm.

Suggested Usage: Drink 1 cup daily to reduce joint pain and promote mobility.

Benefits: Turmeric and Ginger work synergistically to reduce inflammation and enhance circulation.

1001. Boswellia and Ashwagandha Joint Health Capsules

Ingredients: 1 tablespoon Boswellia powder, 1 tablespoon Ashwagandha powder, empty gel capsules.

Preparation: Mix Boswellia and Ashwagandha powders thoroughly. Fill empty capsules and seal.

Suggested Usage: Take 1 capsule twice daily to support joint health and reduce stress-related pain.

Benefits: Boswellia reduces inflammation, while Ashwagandha promotes overall joint resilience and stress reduction.

1002. Turmeric and Black Pepper Golden Milk

Ingredients: 1 tablespoon Turmeric powder, 1/4 teaspoon Black Pepper, 1 cup warm milk (or dairy-free alternative), 1 teaspoon honey.

Preparation: Mix Turmeric and Black Pepper in warm milk. Stir well and add honey to taste.

Suggested Usage: Drink 1 cup daily to reduce joint inflammation and promote relaxation.

Benefits: Turmeric reduces inflammation, and Black Pepper enhances curcumin absorption for more effective pain relief.

1003. White Willow Bark and Ginger Joint Pain Tea

Ingredients: 1 tablespoon White Willow Bark, 1 tablespoon Ginger Root, 2 cups hot water.

Preparation: Steep White Willow Bark and Ginger in hot water for 15 minutes. Strain and serve warm.

Suggested Usage: Drink 1 cup in the evening to relieve joint pain and reduce

inflammation.

Benefits: White Willow Bark provides natural pain relief, and Ginger enhances circulation and reduces joint stiffness.

1004. Arnica and Calendula Joint-Soothing Oil

Ingredients: 1 tablespoon Arnica flowers, 1 tablespoon Calendula, 1 cup olive oil, 1/4 cup beeswax.

Preparation: Simmer Arnica and Calendula in olive oil for 30 minutes. Strain and melt in beeswax. Pour into a container and let cool.

Suggested Usage: Apply to swollen or painful joints to reduce pain and promote healing.

Benefits: Arnica and Calendula reduce inflammation, soothe joint pain, and accelerate healing.

1005. Ginger and Peppermint Muscle Relief Tea

Ingredients: 1 tablespoon Ginger Root, 1 tablespoon Peppermint, 2 cups hot water.

Preparation: Steep Ginger and Peppermint in hot water for 10-15 minutes. Strain and serve warm.

Suggested Usage: Drink 1 cup to reduce muscle stiffness and promote relaxation.

Benefits: Ginger and Peppermint enhance circulation and reduce tension in sore muscles and joints.

1006. Devil's Claw and Boswellia Pain-Relief Capsules

Ingredients: 1 tablespoon Devil's Claw powder, 1 tablespoon Boswellia powder, empty gel capsules.

Preparation: Mix Devil's Claw and Boswellia powders thoroughly. Fill empty capsules and seal.

Suggested Usage: Take 1 capsule twice daily to reduce joint pain and support mobility.

Benefits: Devil's Claw reduces pain and inflammation, while Boswellia supports joint health and flexibility.

1007. Turmeric and Cinnamon Anti-Inflammatory Tea

Ingredients: 1 tablespoon Turmeric, 1 tablespoon Cinnamon, 2 cups hot water.

Preparation: Steep Turmeric and Cinnamon in hot water for 15 minutes. Strain and serve warm.

Suggested Usage: Drink 1 cup daily to reduce inflammation and promote joint health.

Benefits: Turmeric and Cinnamon provide anti-inflammatory benefits, supporting joint flexibility and reducing pain.

1008. Comfrey and Arnica Joint Repair Salve

Ingredients: 1 tablespoon Comfrey Root, 1 tablespoon Arnica flowers, 1 cup olive oil, 1/4 cup beeswax.

Preparation: Simmer Comfrey and Arnica in olive oil for 30 minutes. Strain and melt in beeswax. Pour into a container and let cool.

Suggested Usage: Apply to painful joints to reduce inflammation and support healing.

Benefits: Comfrey supports tissue repair, while Arnica reduces swelling and pain.

1009. Cayenne and Ginger Joint-Soothing Oil

Ingredients: 1 tablespoon Cayenne powder, 1 tablespoon Ginger Root, 1 cup olive oil.
Preparation: Simmer Cayenne and Ginger in olive oil for 30 minutes. Strain and store in a glass bottle.
Suggested Usage: Massage into painful joints to increase circulation and reduce stiffness.
Benefits: Cayenne and Ginger stimulate blood flow and reduce pain in sore joints.

1010. Ashwagandha and Licorice Joint Support Capsules

Ingredients: 1 tablespoon Ashwagandha powder, 1 tablespoon Licorice Root powder, empty gel capsules.
Preparation: Mix Ashwagandha and Licorice powders thoroughly. Fill empty capsules and seal.
Suggested Usage: Take 1 capsule daily to support joint health and reduce stress-related pain.
Benefits: Ashwagandha supports joint strength, while Licorice reduces inflammation and supports adrenal health.

1011. Devil's Claw and Nettle Leaf Joint Flexibility Tea

Ingredients: 1 tablespoon Devil's Claw, 1 tablespoon Nettle Leaf, 2 cups hot water.
Preparation: Steep Devil's Claw and Nettle in hot water for 15 minutes. Strain and serve warm.
Suggested Usage: Drink 1 cup daily to support joint flexibility and reduce inflammation.
Benefits: Devil's Claw and Nettle reduce joint stiffness and inflammation while supporting overall joint health.

1012. Ginger and Turmeric Joint-Soothing Tea

Ingredients: 1 tablespoon Ginger Root, 1 tablespoon Turmeric powder, 2 cups hot water.
Preparation: Steep Ginger and Turmeric in hot water for 15 minutes. Strain and serve warm.
Suggested Usage: Drink 1 cup daily to alleviate joint pain and improve circulation.
Benefits: Ginger and Turmeric reduce inflammation and promote blood flow, helping to ease joint stiffness and pain.

1013. Boswellia and Ginger Joint Flexibility Capsules

Ingredients: 1 tablespoon Boswellia powder, 1 tablespoon Ginger powder, empty gel capsules.
Preparation: Mix Boswellia and Ginger powders thoroughly. Fill empty capsules and seal.
Suggested Usage: Take 1 capsule twice daily to reduce inflammation and enhance joint mobility.
Benefits: Boswellia reduces joint pain and swelling, while Ginger enhances circulation and flexibility.

1014. Nettle and Turmeric Anti-Inflammatory Capsules

Ingredients: 1 tablespoon Nettle powder, 1 tablespoon Turmeric powder, empty gel capsules.

Preparation: Mix Nettle and Turmeric powders thoroughly. Fill empty capsules and seal.

Suggested Usage: Take 1 capsule daily to reduce joint inflammation and support joint health.

Benefits: Nettle provides minerals for bone and joint health, while Turmeric reduces systemic inflammation.

1015. Licorice and Marshmallow Joint-Soothing Tea

Ingredients: 1 tablespoon Licorice Root, 1 tablespoon Marshmallow Root, 2 cups hot water.

Preparation: Steep Licorice and Marshmallow in hot water for 15 minutes. Strain and serve warm.

Suggested Usage: Drink 1 cup as needed to soothe sore joints and reduce pain.

Benefits: Licorice and Marshmallow soothe inflammation, reduce pain, and support joint health.

1016. Ginger, Cinnamon, and Turmeric Joint-Strengthening Tea

Ingredients: 1 tablespoon Ginger Root, 1 tablespoon Turmeric, 1 teaspoon Cinnamon, 2 cups hot water.

Preparation: Steep Ginger, Turmeric, and Cinnamon in hot water for 15 minutes. Strain and serve warm.

Suggested Usage: Drink 1 cup in the morning to support joint strength and reduce inflammation.

Benefits: Ginger, Turmeric, and Cinnamon work together to reduce inflammation, enhance circulation, and promote joint flexibility.

1017. Ashwagandha and Holy Basil Joint Support Capsules

Ingredients: 1 tablespoon Ashwagandha powder, 1 tablespoon Holy Basil powder, empty gel capsules.

Preparation: Mix Ashwagandha and Holy Basil powders thoroughly. Fill empty capsules and seal.

Suggested Usage: Take 1 capsule twice daily to reduce joint inflammation and support overall resilience.

Benefits: Ashwagandha and Holy Basil support stress management and reduce inflammation, promoting joint health.

1018. Devil's Claw and Ginger Anti-Inflammatory Tincture

Ingredients: 1 tablespoon Devil's Claw, 1 tablespoon Ginger Root, 1 cup vodka or brandy.

Preparation: Combine Devil's Claw and Ginger in a glass jar, cover with alcohol, and seal. Let sit for 4-6 weeks, shaking daily. Strain and store in a dark glass bottle.

Suggested Usage: Take 1 teaspoon twice daily to alleviate chronic joint pain and reduce inflammation.

Benefits: Devil's Claw and Ginger provide anti-inflammatory benefits and support joint health.

1019. Boswellia and Turmeric Pain-Relief Oil

Ingredients: 1 tablespoon Boswellia powder, 1 tablespoon Turmeric powder, 1 cup olive oil, 1/4 cup beeswax.
Preparation: Simmer Boswellia and Turmeric in olive oil for 30 minutes. Strain and melt in beeswax. Pour into a container and let cool.
Suggested Usage: Apply to painful joints to reduce inflammation and alleviate pain.
Benefits: Boswellia and Turmeric support joint mobility, reduce pain, and promote healing.

1020. Reishi and Schisandra Anti-Inflammatory Capsules

Ingredients: 1 tablespoon Reishi powder, 1 tablespoon Schisandra powder, empty gel capsules.
Preparation: Mix Reishi and Schisandra powders thoroughly. Fill empty capsules and seal.
Suggested Usage: Take 1 capsule daily to reduce joint inflammation and promote flexibility.
Benefits: Reishi and Schisandra provide adaptogenic and anti-inflammatory benefits, supporting joint resilience and reducing pain.

1021. Turmeric and Boswellia Anti-Inflammatory Tincture

Ingredients: 1 tablespoon Turmeric, 1 tablespoon Boswellia, 1 cup vodka or brandy.
Preparation: Combine Turmeric and Boswellia in a glass jar, cover with alcohol, and seal. Let sit for 4-6 weeks, shaking daily. Strain and store in a dark glass bottle.
Suggested Usage: Take 1 teaspoon twice daily to reduce inflammation and alleviate joint pain.
Benefits: Turmeric and Boswellia work synergistically to reduce inflammation and promote joint health.

1022. White Willow Bark and Devil's Claw Joint Relief Capsules

Ingredients: 1 tablespoon Willow Bark powder, 1 tablespoon Devil's Claw powder, empty gel capsules.
Preparation: Mix Willow Bark and Devil's Claw powders thoroughly. Fill empty capsules and seal.
Suggested Usage: Take 1 capsule twice daily to reduce joint pain and inflammation.
Benefits: Willow Bark provides natural pain relief, while Devil's Claw reduces inflammation and supports joint flexibility.

1023. Turmeric, Ginger, and Cinnamon Joint Health Tea

Ingredients: 1 tablespoon Turmeric, 1 tablespoon Ginger, 1 teaspoon Cinnamon, 2 cups hot water.
Preparation: Steep Turmeric, Ginger, and Cinnamon in hot water for 15 minutes. Strain and serve warm.
Suggested Usage: Drink 1 cup in the evening to support joint health and reduce stiffness.
Benefits: Turmeric, Ginger, and Cinnamon provide anti-inflammatory and warming benefits, promoting flexibility and joint comfort.

1024. Nettle and Horsetail Joint Health Capsules

Ingredients: 1 tablespoon Nettle powder, 1 tablespoon Horsetail powder, empty gel capsules.

Preparation: Mix Nettle and Horsetail powders thoroughly. Fill empty capsules and seal.

Suggested Usage: Take 1 capsule twice daily to nourish joints and connective tissues.

Benefits: Nettle and Horsetail are rich in minerals that support joint health, reduce inflammation, and promote flexibility.

1025. Ginger and Cayenne Circulation-Boosting Tonic

Ingredients: 1 tablespoon Ginger Root, 1/4 teaspoon Cayenne Pepper, 1 cup warm water, 1 tablespoon honey.

Preparation: Combine all ingredients in a cup and stir well. Serve warm.

Suggested Usage: Drink 1 cup daily to increase circulation and reduce joint stiffness.

Benefits: Ginger and Cayenne stimulate blood flow, reduce stiffness, and provide warming relief for sore joints.

Book 43: Supporting Heart Health Naturally

Herbs to Promote Cardiovascular Health

Maintaining a healthy heart is essential for overall well-being and longevity. Cardiovascular health involves not only the heart but also the entire network of blood vessels that support the body's circulation. Various factors such as high blood pressure, elevated cholesterol levels, and poor circulation can impact heart health. Herbs can be powerful allies in supporting cardiovascular function, improving circulation, and promoting healthy blood pressure levels. By incorporating specific heart-supporting herbs into daily routines, individuals can naturally promote heart health and reduce the risk of cardiovascular issues.

Some of the most beneficial herbs for heart health include **Hawthorn**, **Garlic**, and **Ginkgo Biloba**. **Hawthorn**, often referred to as the "heart herb," has been used traditionally to strengthen the heart muscle, enhance blood flow, and regulate blood pressure. Its bioflavonoids and procyanidins help dilate blood vessels, reducing resistance and improving circulation. This makes Hawthorn an excellent herb for individuals dealing with hypertension or early-stage heart disease.

Garlic is another potent herb for cardiovascular support. Its active compound, allicin, helps reduce blood pressure, lower cholesterol levels, and prevent plaque buildup in the arteries. Regular consumption of Garlic can decrease the risk of atherosclerosis and other cardiovascular complications. It can be incorporated into daily meals or taken as a supplement for a more targeted approach.

Ginkgo Biloba is known for its ability to enhance circulation, particularly in the brain and extremities. By improving blood flow, Ginkgo can help reduce the risk of blood clots and support healthy arterial function. Additionally, Ginkgo's antioxidant properties protect the cardiovascular system from oxidative stress, which can lead to damage in the blood vessels and contribute to heart disease over time.

Other beneficial herbs for heart health include **Motherwort**, **Cayenne Pepper**, and **Linden Blossom**. **Motherwort** is a calming herb that helps reduce anxiety and stress, which are common contributors to heart issues. It has mild sedative properties that can help stabilize heart rhythm and reduce palpitations. **Cayenne Pepper**, known for its hot and spicy nature, is a circulatory stimulant that improves blood flow and strengthens the heart. It can also help clear arterial blockages and reduce cholesterol levels. **Linden Blossom** is a gentle heart tonic that relaxes the blood vessels, lowers blood pressure, and supports overall cardiovascular health.

Recipes for Heart-Healthy Elixirs

Heart-healthy herbal formulations can be prepared in a variety of forms, including teas, tinctures, and capsules. A **Hawthorn and Hibiscus Heart Tonic Tea** is an excellent choice for daily heart support. To prepare, combine 1 tablespoon of dried Hawthorn berries and 1 tablespoon of dried Hibiscus flowers in 2 cups of hot water. Steep for 15 minutes, strain, and drink 1 cup twice daily to support heart function and regulate blood pressure.

For those looking for a stronger cardiovascular boost, a **Garlic and Ginger Circulation Tonic** can be effective. Combine 2 cloves of crushed Garlic, 1 tablespoon of freshly grated Ginger, and 1 tablespoon of honey in 1 cup of warm water. Drink this tonic once daily to promote healthy blood flow and reduce the risk of arterial plaque buildup.

A **Motherwort and Lemon Balm Calming Tea** is perfect for individuals dealing with stress-related heart concerns. Simply combine 1 tablespoon of dried Motherwort and 1 tablespoon of dried Lemon Balm in 2 cups of hot water. Steep for 10-15 minutes, strain, and enjoy before bedtime to reduce anxiety and support heart rhythm.

For those interested in improving circulation and strengthening the heart, a **Cayenne and Hawthorn Berry Tincture** can be prepared. Combine 1 tablespoon of Cayenne powder and 1 tablespoon of crushed Hawthorn berries in a glass jar, cover with 1 cup of vodka or brandy, and seal. Let sit for 4-6 weeks, shaking daily. Strain and store in a dark glass bottle. Take 1/2 teaspoon twice daily to enhance circulation, support heart function, and reduce blood pressure.

By incorporating these herbs and elixirs into a daily health regimen, individuals can support their cardiovascular health naturally, promoting longevity and overall well-being. Regular use of heart-healthy herbs, combined with a balanced diet and regular physical activity, can significantly improve heart function, regulate blood pressure, and protect against cardiovascular disease.

Remedies for Heart Health

1026. Hawthorn Berry and Hibiscus Heart Tonic

Ingredients: 1 tablespoon Hawthorn berries, 1 tablespoon Hibiscus flowers, 2 cups hot water.
Preparation: Steep Hawthorn and Hibiscus in hot water for 15 minutes. Strain and serve warm.

Suggested Usage: Drink 1 cup twice daily to support heart function and regulate blood pressure.
Benefits: Hawthorn strengthens the heart muscle and improves circulation, while Hibiscus helps lower blood pressure.

1027. Garlic and Ginger Circulation Boosting Tea

Ingredients: 2 cloves of crushed Garlic, 1 tablespoon grated Ginger, 1 tablespoon honey, 1 cup hot water.

Preparation: Steep Garlic and Ginger in hot water for 10 minutes. Strain, add honey, and serve warm.

Suggested Usage: Drink once daily to promote circulation and reduce arterial plaque buildup.

Benefits: Garlic and Ginger enhance blood flow and lower cholesterol, supporting overall cardiovascular health.

1028. Hawthorn and Lemon Balm Relaxation Tea

Ingredients: 1 tablespoon Hawthorn berries, 1 tablespoon Lemon Balm, 2 cups hot water.

Preparation: Steep Hawthorn and Lemon Balm in hot water for 15 minutes. Strain and serve warm.

Suggested Usage: Drink 1 cup in the evening to reduce anxiety and support heart rhythm.

Benefits: Hawthorn and Lemon Balm work together to reduce stress-related heart issues and promote a calm cardiovascular system.

1029. Motherwort and Linden Blossom Heart-Calming Tea

Ingredients: 1 tablespoon Motherwort, 1 tablespoon Linden Blossom, 2 cups hot water.

Preparation: Steep Motherwort and Linden Blossom in hot water for 10-15 minutes. Strain and serve warm.

Suggested Usage: Drink 1 cup before bedtime to reduce heart palpitations and promote relaxation.

Benefits: Motherwort stabilizes heart rhythm, while Linden Blossom helps lower blood pressure.

1030. Cayenne and Hawthorn Berry Heart Health Tincture

Ingredients: 1 tablespoon Cayenne powder, 1 tablespoon crushed Hawthorn berries, 1 cup vodka or brandy.

Preparation: Combine Cayenne and Hawthorn in a glass jar, cover with alcohol, and seal. Let sit for 4-6 weeks, shaking daily. Strain and store in a dark glass bottle.

Suggested Usage: Take 1/2 teaspoon twice daily to enhance circulation and reduce blood pressure.

Benefits: Cayenne stimulates circulation, while Hawthorn supports heart function and arterial health.

1031. Garlic and Turmeric Cholesterol-Reducing Capsules

Ingredients: 1 tablespoon Garlic powder, 1 tablespoon Turmeric powder, empty gel capsules.

Preparation: Mix Garlic and Turmeric powders thoroughly. Fill empty capsules and seal.

Suggested Usage: Take 1 capsule twice daily to lower cholesterol and reduce inflammation.

Benefits: Garlic lowers cholesterol, while Turmeric reduces arterial inflammation, supporting heart health.

1032. Ginger and Cinnamon Heart-Warming Tea

Ingredients: 1 tablespoon Ginger Root, 1 tablespoon Cinnamon, 2 cups hot water.
Preparation: Steep Ginger and Cinnamon in hot water for 15 minutes. Strain and serve warm.
Suggested Usage: Drink 1 cup daily to improve circulation and reduce inflammation.
Benefits: Ginger and Cinnamon promote blood flow, reduce inflammation, and support heart function.

1033. Hawthorn and Reishi Mushroom Heart Tonic Capsules

Ingredients: 1 tablespoon Hawthorn powder, 1 tablespoon Reishi Mushroom powder, empty gel capsules.
Preparation: Mix Hawthorn and Reishi powders thoroughly. Fill empty capsules and seal.
Suggested Usage: Take 1 capsule twice daily to strengthen heart function and enhance circulation.
Benefits: Hawthorn strengthens the heart, while Reishi provides adaptogenic support to reduce stress and inflammation.

1034. Lemon Balm and Skullcap Nerve-Calming Tea

Ingredients: 1 tablespoon Lemon Balm, 1 tablespoon Skullcap, 2 cups hot water.
Preparation: Steep Lemon Balm and Skullcap in hot water for 15 minutes. Strain and serve warm.
Suggested Usage: Drink 1 cup daily to reduce stress and support cardiovascular health.
Benefits: Lemon Balm calms the nervous system, while Skullcap supports a steady heart rhythm.

1035. Garlic, Ginger, and Turmeric Cholesterol Support Tea

Ingredients: 2 cloves crushed Garlic, 1 tablespoon grated Ginger, 1 teaspoon Turmeric, 2 cups hot water.
Preparation: Steep Garlic, Ginger, and Turmeric in hot water for 10 minutes. Strain and serve warm.
Suggested Usage: Drink once daily to reduce cholesterol and support arterial health.
Benefits: Garlic, Ginger, and Turmeric lower cholesterol, reduce inflammation, and promote circulation.

1036. Holy Basil and Linden Blossom Heart Relaxation Tea

Ingredients: 1 tablespoon Holy Basil, 1 tablespoon Linden Blossom, 2 cups hot water.
Preparation: Steep Holy Basil and Linden in hot water for 10-15 minutes. Strain and serve warm.
Suggested Usage: Drink 1 cup in the evening to reduce anxiety and promote a calm cardiovascular system.
Benefits: Holy Basil and Linden calm the heart, reduce stress, and lower blood pressure.

1037. Ginkgo Biloba and Gotu Kola Circulation Capsules

Ingredients: 1 tablespoon Ginkgo Biloba powder, 1 tablespoon Gotu Kola powder, empty gel capsules.
Preparation: Mix Ginkgo and Gotu Kola powders thoroughly. Fill empty capsules

and seal.

Suggested Usage: Take 1 capsule twice daily to enhance blood circulation and support cognitive and heart health.

Benefits: Ginkgo enhances circulation, while Gotu Kola strengthens blood vessels and improves overall heart health.

1038. Hawthorn and Garlic Blood Pressure Support Capsules

Ingredients: 1 tablespoon Hawthorn powder, 1 tablespoon Garlic powder, empty gel capsules.

Preparation: Mix Hawthorn and Garlic powders thoroughly. Fill empty capsules and seal.

Suggested Usage: Take 1 capsule twice daily to lower blood pressure and support cardiovascular health.

Benefits: Hawthorn reduces blood pressure and strengthens the heart, while Garlic lowers cholesterol and supports arterial health.

1039. Reishi Mushroom and Holy Basil Heart Health Tincture

Ingredients: 1 tablespoon Reishi powder, 1 tablespoon Holy Basil, 1 cup vodka or brandy.

Preparation: Combine Reishi and Holy Basil in a glass jar, cover with alcohol, and seal. Let sit for 4-6 weeks, shaking daily. Strain and store in a dark glass bottle.

Suggested Usage: Take 1/2 teaspoon twice daily to reduce stress and support heart function.

Benefits: Reishi and Holy Basil reduce inflammation and strengthen heart function.

1040. Ginger, Garlic, and Lemon Arterial Cleanse

Ingredients: 1 tablespoon grated Ginger, 2 cloves crushed Garlic, 1 tablespoon fresh Lemon juice, 1 cup warm water.

Preparation: Mix all ingredients in warm water and stir well. Serve immediately.

Suggested Usage: Drink once daily to cleanse the arteries and promote cardiovascular health.

Benefits: Ginger, Garlic, and Lemon promote arterial health, reduce cholesterol, and enhance circulation.

Book 44: Herbal Solutions for Weight Management

Natural Weight Loss Remedies

Achieving and maintaining a healthy weight is not only essential for physical appearance but also for overall health and longevity. Weight management can be a complex process influenced by diet, lifestyle, metabolism, and even stress levels. While a balanced diet and regular exercise are fundamental to effective weight management, certain herbs can play a supportive role in enhancing metabolic function, curbing appetite, and promoting fat breakdown. By using these herbs as part of a comprehensive health regimen, individuals can achieve their weight loss goals more effectively and sustainably.

One of the most popular herbs for weight management is **Green Tea**, known for its high levels of catechins, which stimulate thermogenesis and enhance fat oxidation. The presence of caffeine in Green Tea also helps increase energy levels, making it easier to engage in physical activity. Drinking Green Tea regularly has been shown to promote weight loss by boosting metabolism and reducing overall body fat.

Another powerful herb is **Cinnamon**, which helps regulate blood sugar levels, reducing cravings and preventing energy crashes that can lead to overeating. Cinnamon's ability to improve insulin sensitivity also makes it beneficial for those struggling with weight gain due to insulin resistance or metabolic syndrome. Adding Cinnamon to meals or consuming it in tea form can help balance blood sugar and curb appetite.

Garcinia Cambogia, a tropical fruit, has gained popularity as a natural weight loss aid due to its high content of hydroxycitric acid (HCA). HCA is known to inhibit an enzyme called citrate lyase, which the body uses to produce fat. By blocking this enzyme, Garcinia Cambogia can reduce fat accumulation and promote a feeling of fullness, helping to prevent overeating.

Gymnema Sylvestre, known as the "sugar destroyer," is another beneficial herb for weight management. It works by reducing the ability of the taste buds to detect sweetness, thereby decreasing the desire for sugary foods. Additionally, Gymnema has been shown to support blood sugar regulation, making it particularly useful for those with sugar cravings or who struggle with maintaining a healthy diet.

Dandelion Root is often used in weight loss protocols due to its diuretic properties, which help reduce water retention and promote detoxification. By flushing out excess fluids and toxins, Dandelion Root supports the liver in metabolizing fats more effectively, aiding in overall weight management.

Recipes for Metabolism-Boosting Teas

Herbal teas can be a delightful and effective way to support weight management. They are easy to prepare, enjoyable to consume, and can deliver potent health benefits when used consistently. For example, a **Green Tea and Ginger Metabolism-Boosting Tea** can be made by combining 1 tablespoon of Green Tea leaves with 1 tablespoon of freshly grated Ginger Root in 2 cups of hot water. Steep for 10-15 minutes, strain, and enjoy twice daily. This blend not only boosts metabolic rate but also helps reduce inflammation and support digestion.

For appetite control, a **Cinnamon and Gymnema Appetite-Suppressing Tea** can be prepared by steeping 1 tablespoon of Cinnamon sticks and 1 tablespoon of dried Gymnema leaves in 2 cups of hot water for 15 minutes. Strain and drink 1 cup before meals to curb sugar cravings and prevent overeating.

Another effective weight management formula is a **Garcinia Cambogia and Lemon Fat-Burning Elixir**, which can be made by mixing 1 tablespoon of Garcinia Cambogia extract with 1 tablespoon of fresh Lemon juice in 1 cup of warm water. Drink this elixir 30 minutes before meals to reduce fat production and promote a sense of fullness.

A **Dandelion Root and Fennel Digestive Tea** is excellent for reducing bloating and water retention. To prepare, simmer 1 tablespoon of Dandelion Root and 1 tablespoon of Fennel seeds in 2 cups of water for 15 minutes. Strain and enjoy before bedtime to support digestion and detoxification.

By incorporating these herbal teas and remedies into daily routines, individuals can naturally support their weight management efforts, boost metabolism, and reduce cravings in a healthy and sustainable manner. Regular use of these herbs, combined with mindful eating and physical activity, provides a holistic approach to achieving and maintaining a healthy weight.

Remedies for Weight Management

1041. Green Tea and Ginger Metabolism-Boosting Tea

Ingredients: 1 tablespoon Green Tea leaves, 1 tablespoon freshly grated Ginger Root, 2 cups hot water.
Preparation: Steep Green Tea and Ginger in hot water for 10-15 minutes. Strain and serve warm.
Suggested Usage: Drink 1 cup twice daily to increase metabolism and support fat burning.
Benefits: Green Tea boosts metabolic rate, while Ginger enhances digestion and reduces inflammation.

1042. Cinnamon and Gymnema Appetite-Suppressing Tea

392

Ingredients: 1 tablespoon Cinnamon sticks, 1 tablespoon dried Gymnema leaves, 2 cups hot water.
Preparation: Steep Cinnamon and Gymnema in hot water for 15 minutes. Strain and serve warm.
Suggested Usage: Drink 1 cup before meals to reduce sugar cravings and control appetite.
Benefits: Cinnamon balances blood sugar, and Gymnema reduces the desire for sugary foods.

1043. Garcinia Cambogia and Lemon Fat-Burning Elixir

Ingredients: 1 tablespoon Garcinia Cambogia extract, 1 tablespoon fresh Lemon juice, 1 cup warm water.
Preparation: Mix all ingredients thoroughly and serve warm.
Suggested Usage: Drink 30 minutes before meals to inhibit fat production and promote satiety.
Benefits: Garcinia Cambogia blocks fat formation, and Lemon enhances digestion and detoxification.

1044. Dandelion Root and Fennel Digestive Tea

Ingredients: 1 tablespoon Dandelion Root, 1 tablespoon Fennel seeds, 2 cups water.
Preparation: Simmer Dandelion and Fennel in water for 15 minutes. Strain and serve warm.
Suggested Usage: Drink once daily before bedtime to reduce bloating and support liver health.
Benefits: Dandelion acts as a diuretic, while Fennel reduces water retention and improves digestion.

1045. Yerba Mate and Ginseng Energy Tea

Ingredients: 1 tablespoon Yerba Mate, 1 tablespoon Ginseng Root, 2 cups hot water.
Preparation: Steep Yerba Mate and Ginseng in hot water for 10 minutes. Strain and serve warm.
Suggested Usage: Drink once daily to boost energy and increase metabolic rate.
Benefits: Yerba Mate stimulates metabolism, and Ginseng provides sustained energy without jitters.

1046. Cayenne and Ginger Thermogenic Capsules

Ingredients: 1 tablespoon Cayenne powder, 1 tablespoon Ginger powder, empty gel capsules.
Preparation: Mix Cayenne and Ginger powders thoroughly. Fill empty capsules and seal.
Suggested Usage: Take 1 capsule twice daily to enhance metabolism and promote fat burning.
Benefits: Cayenne and Ginger boost thermogenesis, increasing calorie burn and supporting weight loss.

1047. Holy Basil and Lemon Balm Stress-Reducing Tea

Ingredients: 1 tablespoon Holy Basil, 1 tablespoon Lemon Balm, 2 cups hot water.
Preparation: Steep Holy Basil and Lemon Balm in hot water for 15 minutes.

Strain and serve warm.

Suggested Usage: Drink 1 cup in the evening to reduce stress-related cravings and support relaxation.

Benefits: Holy Basil and Lemon Balm reduce cortisol levels, helping to prevent stress-related weight gain.

1048. Ginseng and Green Tea Energy Capsules

Ingredients: 1 tablespoon Ginseng powder, 1 tablespoon Green Tea powder, empty gel capsules.

Preparation: Mix Ginseng and Green Tea powders thoroughly. Fill empty capsules and seal.

Suggested Usage: Take 1 capsule twice daily to boost energy and enhance fat metabolism.

Benefits: Ginseng supports energy levels, and Green Tea enhances metabolic rate for weight loss.

1049. Ginger and Lemon Digestive Tonic

Ingredients: 1 tablespoon grated Ginger, 1 tablespoon fresh Lemon juice, 1 cup warm water.

Preparation: Mix all ingredients in warm water and stir well. Serve immediately.

Suggested Usage: Drink before meals to enhance digestion and reduce bloating.

Benefits: Ginger and Lemon stimulate digestive enzymes, improving nutrient absorption and reducing bloating.

1050. Turmeric and Black Pepper Anti-Inflammatory Tea

Ingredients: 1 tablespoon Turmeric, 1/4 teaspoon Black Pepper, 2 cups hot water.

Preparation: Steep Turmeric and Black Pepper in hot water for 10 minutes. Strain and serve warm.

Suggested Usage: Drink 1 cup daily to reduce inflammation and support metabolic health.

Benefits: Turmeric reduces systemic inflammation, and Black Pepper enhances nutrient absorption.

1051. Peppermint and Lemon Balm Craving Control Tea

Ingredients: 1 tablespoon Peppermint, 1 tablespoon Lemon Balm, 2 cups hot water.

Preparation: Steep Peppermint and Lemon Balm in hot water for 15 minutes. Strain and serve warm.

Suggested Usage: Drink as needed to reduce cravings and support digestion.

Benefits: Peppermint and Lemon Balm calm the nervous system, reducing emotional eating and cravings.

1052. Triphala Digestive Tonic Capsules

Ingredients: 1 tablespoon Triphala powder, empty gel capsules.

Preparation: Fill empty capsules with Triphala powder and seal.

Suggested Usage: Take 1 capsule daily to support digestion and detoxification.

Benefits: Triphala promotes bowel regularity, reduces bloating, and supports weight management.

1053. Fenugreek and Cinnamon Blood Sugar Balance Tea

Ingredients: 1 tablespoon Fenugreek seeds, 1 tablespoon Cinnamon, 2 cups hot water.
Preparation: Steep Fenugreek and Cinnamon in hot water for 15 minutes. Strain and serve warm.
Suggested Usage: Drink 1 cup before meals to balance blood sugar and reduce cravings.
Benefits: Fenugreek and Cinnamon stabilize blood sugar levels, preventing energy crashes and overeating.

1054. Ginger and Peppermint Appetite-Suppressing Capsules

Ingredients: 1 tablespoon Ginger powder, 1 tablespoon Peppermint powder, empty gel capsules.
Preparation: Mix Ginger and Peppermint powders thoroughly. Fill empty capsules and seal.
Suggested Usage: Take 1 capsule before meals to suppress appetite and reduce bloating.
Benefits: Ginger and Peppermint reduce hunger and improve digestion, supporting weight management.

1055. Lemon Balm and Skullcap Stress-Balancing Tea

Ingredients: 1 tablespoon Lemon Balm, 1 tablespoon Skullcap, 2 cups hot water.
Preparation: Steep Lemon Balm and Skullcap in hot water for 15 minutes. Strain and serve warm.
Suggested Usage: Drink 1 cup in the evening to reduce stress and prevent emotional eating.
Benefits: Lemon Balm and Skullcap calm

the nervous system, helping to reduce stress-related food cravings.

1056. Garcinia Cambogia and Cinnamon Metabolism Capsules

Ingredients: 1 tablespoon Garcinia Cambogia powder, 1 tablespoon Cinnamon, empty gel capsules.
Preparation: Mix Garcinia and Cinnamon powders thoroughly. Fill empty capsules and seal.
Suggested Usage: Take 1 capsule twice daily to enhance metabolism and reduce fat storage.
Benefits: Garcinia inhibits fat production, and Cinnamon helps balance blood sugar.

1057. Fennel and Lemon Detox Tea

Ingredients: 1 tablespoon Fennel seeds, 1 tablespoon fresh Lemon juice, 2 cups hot water.
Preparation: Steep Fennel seeds in hot water for 15 minutes. Strain, add Lemon juice, and serve warm.
Suggested Usage: Drink once daily to promote detoxification and reduce bloating.
Benefits: Fennel supports digestion and reduces water retention, while Lemon aids in detoxification.

1058. Green Tea and Cinnamon Weight-Loss Capsules

Ingredients: 1 tablespoon Green Tea powder, 1 tablespoon Cinnamon powder, empty gel capsules.
Preparation: Mix Green Tea and

Cinnamon powders thoroughly. Fill empty capsules and seal.

Suggested Usage: Take 1 capsule twice daily to boost metabolism and balance blood sugar.

Benefits: Green Tea promotes fat burning, while Cinnamon stabilizes blood sugar and curbs cravings.

Book 45: Enhancing Energy and Stamina with Herbs

Herbs to Boost Physical Energy

Maintaining high energy levels is crucial for productivity, physical performance, and overall vitality. Fatigue and low stamina can often be linked to nutritional deficiencies, stress, and lifestyle factors. While proper diet and regular exercise are essential for sustained energy, certain herbs can provide additional support to enhance physical stamina and combat fatigue naturally. These herbs work by improving adrenal function, supporting healthy energy production, and reducing the impact of stress on the body. Integrating these herbs into daily routines can help individuals achieve higher energy levels, improved endurance, and greater resilience to daily stressors.

One of the most powerful energy-boosting herbs is **Ginseng**, particularly **Panax Ginseng**, which has been used traditionally for centuries to combat fatigue, increase physical performance, and promote vitality. Ginseng works by enhancing the body's resistance to physical and mental stress, making it an excellent herb for individuals who experience low energy due to high stress levels. It improves oxygen utilization and stimulates adrenal function, thereby enhancing overall stamina and endurance.

Rhodiola Rosea is another adaptogenic herb known for its ability to combat fatigue and improve endurance. By balancing cortisol levels and supporting adrenal function, Rhodiola helps the body adapt to stress, resulting in increased energy and mental clarity. It has been shown to reduce feelings of exhaustion and enhance athletic performance, making it ideal for both mental and physical endurance.

Maca Root is a traditional Peruvian herb that is renowned for boosting energy, stamina, and endurance. It is rich in essential minerals and amino acids, which help support adrenal health and hormonal balance. Maca is often used by athletes to enhance physical performance and endurance, as it provides a steady source of energy without causing jitteriness.

Eleuthero, also known as **Siberian Ginseng**, is a powerful adaptogen that improves the body's response to stress and enhances physical endurance. It has been used traditionally to increase stamina, reduce fatigue, and improve mental performance. Eleuthero supports healthy adrenal function and can help combat the effects of chronic stress, making it a great choice for individuals who need sustained energy throughout the day.

Cordyceps Mushroom is another remarkable herb for energy and stamina. It enhances the body's production of ATP (adenosine triphosphate), the primary energy source for cellular function. By increasing ATP levels, Cordyceps improves energy, endurance, and athletic performance. It also supports lung function and oxygen utilization, making it beneficial for individuals who engage in intense physical activities.

Recipes for Energizing Elixirs

Herbal elixirs are an excellent way to boost energy levels naturally. These formulations can be prepared in various forms, such as teas, tinctures, and smoothies, and are easy to incorporate into daily routines. For example, a **Ginseng and Rhodiola Energy Tonic** can be prepared by combining 1 tablespoon of Ginseng Root and 1 tablespoon of Rhodiola Root in 2 cups of hot water. Steep for 15-20 minutes, strain, and drink 1 cup in the morning to enhance energy levels and reduce fatigue throughout the day.

A **Maca and Ashwagandha Stamina-Boosting Smoothie** is another excellent option. Blend 1 tablespoon of Maca Root powder, 1 teaspoon of Ashwagandha powder, 1 banana, and 1 cup of almond milk. This smoothie provides sustained energy and helps combat stress, making it perfect for starting the day with a burst of vitality.

For individuals looking for a more soothing formulation, a **Cordyceps and Eleuthero Endurance Tea** can be prepared by simmering 1 tablespoon of Cordyceps and 1 tablespoon of Eleuthero Root in 2 cups of water for 20 minutes. Strain and drink 1 cup before exercise or physical activity to enhance stamina and reduce fatigue.

Another powerful energy-enhancing formula is a **Schisandra and Holy Basil Adaptogen Elixir**, which can be prepared by combining 1 tablespoon of Schisandra berries and 1 tablespoon of dried Holy Basil in 2 cups of hot water. Steep for 15 minutes, strain, and drink 1 cup in the afternoon to combat afternoon slumps and boost mental clarity.

By incorporating these herbs and elixirs into daily routines, individuals can naturally enhance their energy, improve physical performance, and build greater resilience to physical and mental stress. These herbs not only provide immediate energy boosts but also support overall vitality and endurance in the long term. Regular use of these herbs, combined with a healthy lifestyle, can help individuals maintain high energy levels and stamina throughout the day.

Remedies for Energy and Stamina

1059. Ginseng and Rhodiola Energy Tonic

Ingredients: 1 tablespoon Ginseng Root, 1 tablespoon Rhodiola Root, 2 cups hot water.
Preparation: Steep Ginseng and Rhodiola in hot water for 15-20 minutes. Strain and serve warm.

Suggested Usage: Drink 1 cup in the morning to boost energy levels and reduce fatigue.
Benefits: Ginseng enhances stamina and vitality, while Rhodiola supports adrenal health and reduces stress-induced fatigue.

1060. Maca and Ashwagandha Stamina-Boosting Smoothie

Ingredients: 1 tablespoon Maca Root powder, 1 teaspoon Ashwagandha powder, 1 banana, 1 cup almond milk, 1 teaspoon honey (optional).
Preparation: Blend all ingredients together until smooth. Serve immediately.
Suggested Usage: Drink in the morning or before a workout to enhance physical performance and stamina.
Benefits: Maca boosts energy and endurance, while Ashwagandha reduces stress and promotes balanced energy levels.

1061. Cordyceps and Eleuthero Endurance Tea

Ingredients: 1 tablespoon Cordyceps powder, 1 tablespoon Eleuthero Root, 2 cups water.
Preparation: Simmer Cordyceps and Eleuthero in water for 20 minutes. Strain and serve warm.
Suggested Usage: Drink 1 cup before physical activity to support endurance and reduce fatigue.
Benefits: Cordyceps enhances oxygen utilization, and Eleuthero improves stamina and resilience.

1062. Schisandra and Holy Basil Adaptogen Elixir

Ingredients: 1 tablespoon Schisandra berries, 1 tablespoon dried Holy Basil leaves, 2 cups hot water.
Preparation: Steep Schisandra and Holy Basil in hot water for 15 minutes. Strain and serve warm.
Suggested Usage: Drink 1 cup in the afternoon to boost energy and mental clarity.

Benefits: Schisandra enhances focus and vitality, while Holy Basil reduces stress and improves energy balance.

1063. Siberian Ginseng and Licorice Adrenal Support Tea

Ingredients: 1 tablespoon Siberian Ginseng Root, 1 teaspoon Licorice Root, 2 cups hot water.
Preparation: Steep Siberian Ginseng and Licorice in hot water for 15 minutes. Strain and serve warm.
Suggested Usage: Drink 1 cup in the morning to support adrenal function and reduce fatigue.
Benefits: Siberian Ginseng enhances stamina, while Licorice supports adrenal health and combats stress.

1064. Maca Root and Cinnamon Energy Capsules

Ingredients: 1 tablespoon Maca Root powder, 1 teaspoon Cinnamon powder, empty gel capsules.
Preparation: Mix Maca and Cinnamon powders thoroughly. Fill empty capsules and seal.
Suggested Usage: Take 1 capsule twice daily to boost energy and support metabolic function.
Benefits: Maca enhances energy and endurance, while Cinnamon supports healthy blood sugar levels.

1065. Green Tea and Ginseng Metabolic Boost Tea

Ingredients: 1 tablespoon Green Tea leaves, 1 tablespoon Ginseng Root, 2 cups hot water.

Preparation: Steep Green Tea and Ginseng in hot water for 10 minutes. Strain and serve warm.

Suggested Usage: Drink 1 cup mid-morning to increase metabolic rate and enhance energy.

Benefits: Green Tea boosts metabolism, and Ginseng provides sustained energy.

1066. Holy Basil and Reishi Stress-Resilience Capsules

Ingredients: 1 tablespoon Holy Basil powder, 1 tablespoon Reishi Mushroom powder, empty gel capsules.

Preparation: Mix Holy Basil and Reishi powders thoroughly. Fill empty capsules and seal.

Suggested Usage: Take 1 capsule twice daily to reduce stress and support energy levels.

Benefits: Holy Basil and Reishi enhance stress resilience and promote balanced energy.

1067. Ginger and Turmeric Anti-Fatigue Elixir

Ingredients: 1 tablespoon grated Ginger, 1 teaspoon Turmeric powder, 1 cup hot water, 1 teaspoon honey (optional).

Preparation: Steep Ginger and Turmeric in hot water for 10 minutes. Strain, add honey if desired, and serve warm.

Suggested Usage: Drink once daily to reduce fatigue and inflammation.

Benefits: Ginger stimulates circulation, and Turmeric reduces inflammation, supporting overall vitality.

1068. Eleuthero and Astragalus Immune-Boosting Tonic

Ingredients: 1 tablespoon Eleuthero Root, 1 tablespoon Astragalus Root, 2 cups hot water.

Preparation: Simmer Eleuthero and Astragalus in hot water for 20 minutes. Strain and serve warm.

Suggested Usage: Drink 1 cup in the morning to boost energy and immunity.

Benefits: Eleuthero enhances endurance, and Astragalus strengthens immune function.

1069. Gotu Kola and Rosemary Cognitive Clarity Tea

Ingredients: 1 tablespoon Gotu Kola, 1 tablespoon dried Rosemary, 2 cups hot water.

Preparation: Steep Gotu Kola and Rosemary in hot water for 15 minutes. Strain and serve warm.

Suggested Usage: Drink 1 cup mid-morning to enhance focus and mental clarity.

Benefits: Gotu Kola supports brain health, and Rosemary enhances memory and cognitive function.

1070. Lemon Balm and Peppermint Refreshing Tea

Ingredients: 1 tablespoon Lemon Balm, 1 tablespoon Peppermint, 2 cups hot water.

Preparation: Steep Lemon Balm and Peppermint in hot water for 10-15 minutes. Strain and serve warm or chilled.

Suggested Usage: Drink 1 cup in the afternoon to refresh the mind and body.

Benefits: Lemon Balm reduces stress, and Peppermint invigorates the senses, enhancing energy.

1071. Ginkgo Biloba and Gotu Kola Focus Capsules

Ingredients: 1 tablespoon Ginkgo Biloba powder, 1 tablespoon Gotu Kola powder, empty gel capsules.
Preparation: Mix Ginkgo and Gotu Kola powders thoroughly. Fill empty capsules and seal.
Suggested Usage: Take 1 capsule in the morning to enhance concentration and cognitive function.
Benefits: Ginkgo improves circulation to the brain, and Gotu Kola supports memory and focus.

1072. Cordyceps and Reishi Adaptogen Latte

Ingredients: 1 tablespoon Cordyceps powder, 1 tablespoon Reishi Mushroom powder, 1 cup warm almond milk, 1 teaspoon honey.
Preparation: Mix Cordyceps and Reishi powders in warm almond milk. Stir well, add honey, and serve warm.
Suggested Usage: Drink mid-afternoon to support stamina and reduce stress.
Benefits: Cordyceps enhances energy production, and Reishi promotes stress resilience.

1073. Ginger and Cayenne Metabolism-Boosting Tonic

Ingredients: 1 tablespoon grated Ginger, 1/4 teaspoon Cayenne pepper, 1 cup hot water.
Preparation: Steep Ginger and Cayenne in hot water for 10 minutes. Strain and serve warm.
Suggested Usage: Drink before meals to boost metabolism and enhance energy.
Benefits: Ginger and Cayenne stimulate circulation and metabolism, supporting weight management and energy.

1074. Schisandra and Rhodiola Vitality Capsules

Ingredients: 1 tablespoon Schisandra berry powder, 1 tablespoon Rhodiola powder, empty gel capsules.
Preparation: Mix Schisandra and Rhodiola powders thoroughly. Fill empty capsules and seal.
Suggested Usage: Take 1 capsule in the morning to enhance vitality and reduce stress.
Benefits: Schisandra supports endurance and vitality, while Rhodiola improves stamina and mental resilience.

1075. Peppermint and Lemon Verbena Energizing Tea

Ingredients: 1 tablespoon Peppermint leaves, 1 tablespoon Lemon Verbena, 2 cups hot water.
Preparation: Steep Peppermint and Lemon Verbena in hot water for 10-15 minutes. Strain and serve warm.
Suggested Usage: Drink 1 cup in the morning to invigorate and refresh the body and mind.
Benefits: Peppermint enhances alertness, and Lemon Verbena calms and invigorates the senses.

1076. Ginseng and Matcha Green Energy Smoothie

Ingredients: 1 teaspoon Matcha powder, 1 teaspoon Ginseng powder, 1 cup almond milk, 1/2 banana, 1 teaspoon honey (optional).
Preparation: Blend all ingredients until smooth. Serve immediately.
Suggested Usage: Drink in the morning to boost energy and mental focus.
Benefits: Matcha and Ginseng work synergistically to increase energy, enhance focus, and reduce fatigue.

1077. Maca and Cacao Energy-Boosting Drink

Ingredients: 1 tablespoon Maca powder, 1 tablespoon Cacao powder, 1 cup warm almond milk, 1 teaspoon honey.
Preparation: Mix Maca and Cacao powders into warm almond milk. Stir well, add honey, and serve warm.
Suggested Usage: Drink mid-morning to promote sustained energy and endurance.
Benefits: Maca and Cacao enhance energy, stamina, and mood, making it an ideal natural pick-me-up.

1078. Holy Basil and Lemon Balm Calming Energy Tea

Ingredients: 1 tablespoon dried Holy Basil, 1 tablespoon Lemon Balm, 2 cups hot water.
Preparation: Steep Holy Basil and Lemon Balm in hot water for 15 minutes. Strain and serve warm.
Suggested Usage: Drink 1 cup in the afternoon to support calm energy and reduce stress.
Benefits: Holy Basil balances energy, and Lemon Balm reduces stress, promoting balanced vitality.

1079. Ashwagandha and Rhodiola Adrenal Support Capsules

Ingredients: 1 tablespoon Ashwagandha powder, 1 tablespoon Rhodiola powder, empty gel capsules.
Preparation: Mix Ashwagandha and Rhodiola powders thoroughly. Fill empty capsules and seal.
Suggested Usage: Take 1 capsule twice daily to support adrenal function and reduce fatigue.
Benefits: Ashwagandha and Rhodiola work together to promote adrenal health, enhancing resilience and energy levels.

1080. Reishi and Schisandra Endurance Tea

Ingredients: 1 tablespoon Reishi Mushroom powder, 1 tablespoon Schisandra berries, 2 cups hot water.
Preparation: Simmer Reishi and Schisandra in water for 20 minutes. Strain and serve warm.
Suggested Usage: Drink 1 cup before physical activities to boost endurance and reduce fatigue.
Benefits: Reishi enhances stamina, and Schisandra supports physical and mental endurance.

1081. Yerba Mate and Ginseng Vitality Brew

Ingredients: 1 tablespoon Yerba Mate, 1 tablespoon Ginseng Root, 2 cups hot water.
Preparation: Steep Yerba Mate and Ginseng in hot water for 10 minutes. Strain and serve warm or iced.
Suggested Usage: Drink 1 cup in the morning to increase energy and support mental alertness.
Benefits: Yerba Mate stimulates metabolism, and Ginseng provides a steady source of energy.

1082. Ginkgo and Holy Basil Focus-Enhancing Tea

Ingredients: 1 tablespoon Ginkgo Biloba, 1 tablespoon Holy Basil, 2 cups hot water.
Preparation: Steep Ginkgo and Holy Basil in hot water for 15 minutes. Strain and serve warm.
Suggested Usage: Drink 1 cup in the afternoon to enhance mental clarity and reduce brain fog.
Benefits: Ginkgo improves circulation to the brain, and Holy Basil enhances focus and cognitive function.

1083. Maca and Ginseng Physical Endurance Capsules

Ingredients: 1 tablespoon Maca powder, 1 tablespoon Ginseng powder, empty gel capsules.
Preparation: Mix Maca and Ginseng powders thoroughly. Fill empty capsules and seal.
Suggested Usage: Take 1 capsule before exercise to improve physical endurance and energy.
Benefits: Maca enhances stamina and endurance, while Ginseng provides steady energy for physical performance.

1084. Cordyceps and Rhodiola Athletic Performance Tea

Ingredients: 1 tablespoon Cordyceps powder, 1 tablespoon Rhodiola Root, 2 cups hot water.
Preparation: Simmer Cordyceps and Rhodiola in water for 20 minutes. Strain and serve warm.
Suggested Usage: Drink 1 cup before workouts to enhance physical performance and endurance.
Benefits: Cordyceps improves oxygen utilization, and Rhodiola supports physical and mental endurance.

1085. Astragalus and Reishi Immune Support Capsules

Ingredients: 1 tablespoon Astragalus powder, 1 tablespoon Reishi Mushroom powder, empty gel capsules.
Preparation: Mix Astragalus and Reishi powders thoroughly. Fill empty capsules and seal.
Suggested Usage: Take 1 capsule twice daily to support immune function and enhance vitality.
Benefits: Astragalus strengthens immunity, and Reishi supports energy and resilience.

1086. Tulsi and Peppermint Invigorating Tea

Ingredients: 1 tablespoon dried Tulsi, 1 tablespoon Peppermint, 2 cups hot water.
Preparation: Steep Tulsi and Peppermint

in hot water for 15 minutes. Strain and serve warm or chilled.
Suggested Usage: Drink 1 cup mid-afternoon to refresh and energize the mind and body.
Benefits: Tulsi enhances resilience, and Peppermint invigorates the senses, promoting alertness.

1087. Eleuthero and Licorice Root Anti-Stress Capsules

Ingredients: 1 tablespoon Eleuthero Root powder, 1 tablespoon Licorice Root powder, empty gel capsules.
Preparation: Mix Eleuthero and Licorice powders thoroughly. Fill empty capsules and seal.
Suggested Usage: Take 1 capsule in the morning to support adrenal health and reduce stress.
Benefits: Eleuthero improves endurance and stamina, while Licorice supports adrenal function.

1088. Schisandra and Lemon Peel Adaptogen Tea

Ingredients: 1 tablespoon Schisandra berries, 1 tablespoon dried Lemon Peel, 2 cups hot water.
Preparation: Steep Schisandra and Lemon Peel in hot water for 15 minutes. Strain and serve warm.
Suggested Usage: Drink 1 cup daily to reduce stress and enhance vitality.
Benefits: Schisandra supports energy and endurance, while Lemon Peel promotes digestion and vitality.

1089. Ginseng and Nettle Energy-Boosting Capsules

Ingredients: 1 tablespoon Ginseng powder, 1 tablespoon Nettle powder, empty gel capsules.
Preparation: Mix Ginseng and Nettle powders thoroughly. Fill empty capsules and seal.
Suggested Usage: Take 1 capsule twice daily to enhance energy and reduce fatigue.
Benefits: Ginseng promotes physical energy, and Nettle provides essential minerals for vitality and stamina.

1090. Gotu Kola and Ginseng Mental Clarity Tonic

Ingredients: 1 tablespoon Gotu Kola, 1 tablespoon Ginseng Root, 2 cups hot water.
Preparation: Steep Gotu Kola and Ginseng in hot water for 15 minutes. Strain and serve warm.
Suggested Usage: Drink 1 cup mid-morning to improve focus and mental clarity.
Benefits: Gotu Kola enhances cognitive function, while Ginseng boosts energy and focus.

1091. Rhodiola and Schisandra Adaptogen Capsules

Ingredients: 1 tablespoon Rhodiola powder, 1 tablespoon Schisandra berry powder, empty gel capsules.
Preparation: Mix Rhodiola and Schisandra powders thoroughly. Fill empty capsules and seal.

Suggested Usage: Take 1 capsule in the afternoon to reduce stress and boost resilience.
Benefits: Rhodiola supports adrenal health, and Schisandra enhances stamina and endurance.

1092. Lemon Balm, Holy Basil, and Ashwagandha Relaxation Tea

Ingredients: 1 tablespoon Lemon Balm, 1 tablespoon Holy Basil, 1 teaspoon Ashwagandha Root, 2 cups hot water.
Preparation: Steep all herbs in hot water for 15 minutes. Strain and serve warm.
Suggested Usage: Drink 1 cup in the evening to promote relaxation and stress reduction.
Benefits: Lemon Balm and Holy Basil calm the nervous system, while Ashwagandha supports balanced energy.

1093. Ginger and Ginseng Digestion and Energy Tea

Ingredients: 1 tablespoon grated Ginger, 1 tablespoon Ginseng Root, 2 cups hot water.
Preparation: Simmer Ginger and Ginseng in water for 15 minutes. Strain and serve warm.
Suggested Usage: Drink 1 cup before meals to stimulate digestion and increase energy.
Benefits: Ginger stimulates digestion, while Ginseng enhances energy and vitality.

1094. Holy Basil and Peppermint Revitalizing Capsules

Ingredients: 1 tablespoon Holy Basil powder, 1 tablespoon Peppermint powder, empty gel capsules.
Preparation: Mix Holy Basil and Peppermint powders thoroughly. Fill empty capsules and seal.
Suggested Usage: Take 1 capsule in the afternoon to refresh and revitalize the body and mind.
Benefits: Holy Basil promotes balanced energy, while Peppermint invigorates the senses.

1095. Maca and Ginseng Energizing Elixir

Ingredients: 1 tablespoon Maca powder, 1 teaspoon Ginseng powder, 1 cup warm water, 1 teaspoon honey (optional).
Preparation: Mix Maca and Ginseng powders in warm water. Stir well, add honey if desired, and serve warm.
Suggested Usage: Drink in the morning for a natural energy boost and improved stamina.
Benefits: Maca and Ginseng enhance physical and mental energy, making it a perfect start-of-the-day elixir.

1096. Cordyceps and Licorice Adrenal Support Tea

Ingredients: 1 tablespoon Cordyceps powder, 1 teaspoon Licorice Root, 2 cups hot water.
Preparation: Simmer Cordyceps and Licorice in water for 15-20 minutes. Strain and serve warm.
Suggested Usage: Drink 1 cup daily to support adrenal function and reduce stress.
Benefits: Cordyceps supports energy

production, and Licorice helps restore adrenal health.

1097. Rhodiola and Schisandra Focus-Boosting Capsules

Ingredients: 1 tablespoon Rhodiola powder, 1 tablespoon Schisandra berry powder, empty gel capsules.
Preparation: Mix Rhodiola and Schisandra powders thoroughly. Fill empty capsules and seal.
Suggested Usage: Take 1 capsule twice daily to enhance mental focus and reduce fatigue.
Benefits: Rhodiola and Schisandra work synergistically to enhance concentration and mental clarity.

1098. Lemon Balm and Holy Basil Stress-Relief Capsules

Ingredients: 1 tablespoon Lemon Balm powder, 1 tablespoon Holy Basil powder, empty gel capsules.
Preparation: Mix Lemon Balm and Holy Basil powders thoroughly. Fill empty capsules and seal.
Suggested Usage: Take 1 capsule in the evening to reduce stress and promote relaxation.
Benefits: Lemon Balm and Holy Basil calm the nervous system and support emotional balance.

1099. Green Tea and Gotu Kola Brain Boost Tea

Ingredients: 1 tablespoon Green Tea leaves, 1 tablespoon Gotu Kola, 2 cups hot water.
Preparation: Steep Green Tea and Gotu Kola in hot water for 10-15 minutes. Strain and serve warm.
Suggested Usage: Drink 1 cup in the morning to support cognitive function and increase energy.
Benefits: Green Tea enhances focus and alertness, while Gotu Kola improves memory and brain health.

1100. Ginseng and Reishi Vitality Capsules

Ingredients: 1 tablespoon Ginseng powder, 1 tablespoon Reishi Mushroom powder, empty gel capsules.
Preparation: Mix Ginseng and Reishi powders thoroughly. Fill empty capsules and seal.
Suggested Usage: Take 1 capsule daily to increase energy and resilience to stress.
Benefits: Ginseng supports physical and mental energy, while Reishi promotes vitality and stress reduction.

1101. Peppermint and Ginger Refreshing Energy Tea

Ingredients: 1 tablespoon Peppermint, 1 tablespoon grated Ginger, 2 cups hot water.
Preparation: Steep Peppermint and Ginger in hot water for 10-15 minutes. Strain and serve warm or iced.
Suggested Usage: Drink 1 cup mid-morning to refresh and energize the mind and body.
Benefits: Peppermint and Ginger invigorate the senses, enhance circulation, and promote alertness.

1102. Cordyceps and Maca Athletic Performance Capsules

Ingredients: 1 tablespoon Cordyceps powder, 1 tablespoon Maca powder, empty gel capsules.
Preparation: Mix Cordyceps and Maca powders thoroughly. Fill empty capsules and seal.
Suggested Usage: Take 1 capsule before physical activity to boost endurance and stamina.
Benefits: Cordyceps and Maca enhance physical performance, energy, and endurance.

1103. Schisandra and Holy Basil Adaptogenic Tea

Ingredients: 1 tablespoon Schisandra berries, 1 tablespoon Holy Basil, 2 cups hot water.
Preparation: Steep Schisandra and Holy Basil in hot water for 15 minutes. Strain and serve warm.
Suggested Usage: Drink 1 cup in the afternoon to reduce stress and support balanced energy levels.
Benefits: Schisandra enhances focus and resilience, while Holy Basil calms the mind and promotes mental clarity.

Book 46: Natural Remedies for Skin Health

Herbs for Clear and Radiant Skin

Maintaining healthy, glowing skin is not just about external care—it requires nourishing the skin from the inside out. Herbs have long been used to support skin health by addressing internal imbalances and offering natural topical benefits. Many herbs contain high levels of antioxidants, vitamins, and anti-inflammatory compounds that can protect against free radical damage, reduce inflammation, and promote a clear complexion. Incorporating these herbs into your diet or skincare routine can help address common skin issues like acne, eczema, dryness, and premature aging.

One of the most popular herbs for skin health is **Calendula**, known for its powerful anti-inflammatory, antimicrobial, and wound-healing properties. Calendula is often used in creams and ointments to soothe irritated skin, reduce redness, and promote faster healing of minor cuts and abrasions. Internally, it can help detoxify the liver, which is key for maintaining clear skin.

Chamomile is another excellent herb for calming inflamed skin and reducing redness. It is packed with antioxidants and has gentle skin-soothing properties, making it suitable for sensitive skin types. Chamomile can be applied topically as a compress or used in facial steams to soothe irritation and promote a healthy glow.

Burdock Root is traditionally used to cleanse the blood and detoxify the body, which can help clear up stubborn skin conditions like acne, eczema, and psoriasis. Burdock also has anti-inflammatory and antibacterial properties that support skin healing and reduce the risk of infections.

Nettle Leaf is rich in vitamins A, C, and K, and it's known for its purifying and anti-inflammatory properties. Taken internally, nettle helps balance hormones and cleanse the blood, making it an effective herb for reducing acne and promoting clear skin.

Gotu Kola is widely used in traditional Ayurvedic and Chinese medicine for its ability to support collagen production, reduce scarring, and improve skin elasticity. It is a rejuvenating herb that can enhance skin firmness and texture, making it ideal for aging or mature skin.

Recipes for Skin-Enhancing Creams and Oils

Creating herbal formulations at home allows you to tailor products specifically for your skin type and needs. For example, a **Calendula and Chamomile Soothing Cream** can be made by infusing 1/4 cup of dried Calendula flowers and 1/4 cup of Chamomile flowers in 1 cup of jojoba oil. After 2 weeks of infusing in a warm, dark place, strain the oil and blend with 1/4 cup melted shea butter and 2 tablespoons beeswax until smooth. This cream is perfect for sensitive or irritated skin, providing hydration and reducing inflammation.

For a more targeted treatment, try a **Gotu Kola and Rosehip Facial Serum**. Combine 1 tablespoon Gotu Kola-infused oil, 1 tablespoon Rosehip Seed Oil, and 5 drops of Frankincense essential oil in a small dropper bottle. Apply a few drops to clean skin at night to promote healing, reduce fine lines, and even out skin tone.

Creating a daily skincare routine that incorporates these herbal ingredients can lead to a healthier complexion and a more radiant glow. Each formulation not only provides topical benefits but also supports overall skin health from within.

Remedies for Skin Health

1104. Calendula and Rosehip Skin-Repairing Serum

Ingredients: 1 tablespoon Calendula-infused oil, 1 tablespoon Rosehip Seed Oil, 5 drops Lavender essential oil.
Preparation: Combine all ingredients in a small dropper bottle and shake well.
Suggested Usage: Apply a few drops to the face at night to repair damaged skin and reduce the appearance of scars.
Benefits: Promotes skin cell regeneration, reduces scarring, and hydrates deeply.

1105. Nettle and Dandelion Clear Skin Detox Tea

Ingredients: 1 tablespoon Nettle Leaf, 1 tablespoon Dandelion Root, 2 cups water.
Preparation: Simmer Nettle and Dandelion in water for 15-20 minutes. Strain and serve warm.
Suggested Usage: Drink 1 cup daily to detoxify the body and support healthy skin.
Benefits: Detoxifies the liver, reduces acne, and improves skin clarity.

1106. Gotu Kola and Frankincense Anti-Aging Cream

Ingredients: 1/4 cup Gotu Kola-infused oil, 1/4 cup shea butter, 1 tablespoon coconut oil, 5 drops Frankincense essential oil.
Preparation: Blend Gotu Kola oil, shea butter, and coconut oil until smooth. Add Frankincense oil and mix well.
Suggested Usage: Apply to the face and neck at night to reduce wrinkles and improve elasticity.
Benefits: Stimulates collagen production, tightens skin, and reduces the appearance of fine lines.

1107. Lavender and Chamomile Calming Facial Mist

Ingredients: 1 tablespoon dried Lavender, 1 tablespoon dried Chamomile, 1 cup distilled water.
Preparation: Steep Lavender and Chamomile in hot water for 15 minutes. Strain and pour into a spray bottle.
Suggested Usage: Mist onto the face throughout the day to refresh and soothe

the skin.
Benefits: Calms redness, reduces inflammation, and hydrates the skin.

1108. Turmeric and Honey Brightening Face Mask

Ingredients: 1 tablespoon Turmeric powder, 1 tablespoon raw honey, 1 tablespoon yogurt.
Preparation: Mix all ingredients into a smooth paste.
Suggested Usage: Apply to the face, leave on for 15 minutes, then rinse with warm water.
Benefits: Brightens the complexion, evens out skin tone, and reduces dark spots.

1109. Rose Petal and Aloe Vera Hydrating Gel

Ingredients: 1/4 cup fresh Rose petals, 1/2 cup Aloe Vera gel, 1 tablespoon jojoba oil.
Preparation: Blend Rose petals and Aloe Vera gel until smooth. Stir in jojoba oil.
Suggested Usage: Apply to the face and body after sun exposure or when the skin needs extra hydration.
Benefits: Soothes irritated skin, hydrates deeply, and promotes a glowing complexion.

1110. Chamomile and Oatmeal Exfoliating Scrub

Ingredients: 1/4 cup ground oatmeal, 1 tablespoon dried Chamomile flowers, 2 tablespoons honey.
Preparation: Mix all ingredients to form a thick paste.

Suggested Usage: Gently massage onto damp skin in circular motions, then rinse.
Benefits: Gently exfoliates dead skin cells, soothes inflammation, and softens the skin.

1111. Burdock Root and Red Clover Acne Tonic

Ingredients: 1 tablespoon Burdock Root, 1 tablespoon Red Clover, 2 cups water.
Preparation: Simmer Burdock and Red Clover in water for 20 minutes. Strain and serve warm.
Suggested Usage: Drink 1 cup daily to clear acne and detoxify the body.
Benefits: Purifies the blood, reduces inflammation, and prevents breakouts.

1112. Calendula and Plantain Healing Salve

Ingredients: 1/4 cup Calendula flowers, 1/4 cup Plantain leaves, 1 cup olive oil, 2 tablespoons beeswax.
Preparation: Infuse the herbs in olive oil for 2 weeks. Strain, then blend with melted beeswax.
Suggested Usage: Apply to minor skin irritations, cuts, or rashes as needed.
Benefits: Promotes wound healing, reduces inflammation, and soothes itching.

1113. Milk Thistle and Dandelion Liver Support Tea

Ingredients: 1 tablespoon Milk Thistle seeds, 1 tablespoon Dandelion Root, 2 cups hot water.
Preparation: Steep the herbs in hot water for 15 minutes. Strain and serve warm.

Suggested Usage: Drink 1 cup daily to support liver function and promote clear skin.

Benefits: Enhances liver detoxification, reduces acne, and improves overall skin health.

1114. Gotu Kola and Licorice Root Anti-Aging Capsules

Ingredients: 1 tablespoon Gotu Kola powder, 1 tablespoon Licorice Root powder, empty gel capsules.

Preparation: Mix the powders thoroughly and fill empty capsules.

Suggested Usage: Take 1 capsule daily to promote youthful skin and reduce inflammation.

Benefits: Reduces signs of aging, evens skin tone, and promotes skin regeneration.

1115. Calendula and Green Tea Facial Toner

Ingredients: 1 tablespoon dried Calendula flowers, 1 tablespoon Green Tea leaves, 1 cup distilled water.

Preparation: Steep the herbs in hot water for 15 minutes. Strain and cool. Pour into a spray bottle.

Suggested Usage: Use as a facial toner morning and night after cleansing.

Benefits: Reduces redness, balances skin tone, and provides antioxidant protection.

1116. Nettle and Lemon Balm Pore-Refining Steam

Ingredients: 1 tablespoon dried Nettle leaves, 1 tablespoon Lemon Balm leaves, 4 cups boiling water.

Preparation: Place herbs in a large bowl, pour boiling water over them, and cover your head with a towel to capture the steam.

Suggested Usage: Steam for 10 minutes to open pores and deeply cleanse the skin.

Benefits: Purifies the skin, tightens pores, and promotes a clear complexion.

1117. Gotu Kola and Tulsi Face Serum

Ingredients: 1 tablespoon Gotu Kola-infused oil, 1 tablespoon Tulsi-infused oil, 5 drops Vitamin E oil.

Preparation: Combine all ingredients in a dropper bottle and shake well.

Suggested Usage: Apply a few drops to the face nightly to promote collagen production and reduce signs of aging.

Benefits: Enhances skin elasticity, smoothens fine lines, and improves skin tone.

1118. Lavender and Peppermint Refreshing Body Oil

Ingredients: 1/4 cup dried Lavender, 1/4 cup dried Peppermint, 1 cup sweet almond oil.

Preparation: Infuse Lavender and Peppermint in almond oil for 2 weeks. Strain and store in a dark bottle.

Suggested Usage: Massage onto the body after a shower to refresh and moisturize the skin.

Benefits: Soothes sore muscles, hydrates the skin, and leaves a refreshing scent.

1119. Turmeric and Honey Anti-Acne Spot Treatment

Ingredients: 1 teaspoon Turmeric powder, 1 teaspoon raw honey.
Preparation: Mix Turmeric and honey into a smooth paste.
Suggested Usage: Apply directly to acne spots. Leave on for 15 minutes, then rinse with warm water.
Benefits: Reduces redness, fights acne-causing bacteria, and speeds up healing.

1120. Calendula and Chamomile Skin-Soothing Bath Soak

Ingredients: 1/2 cup dried Calendula flowers, 1/2 cup dried Chamomile flowers, 1 cup Epsom salts.
Preparation: Combine all ingredients and place in a muslin bag. Add the bag to warm bathwater and soak for 20 minutes.
Suggested Usage: Use during a bath to soothe irritated skin and relax the body.
Benefits: Reduces skin inflammation, calms the nervous system, and promotes relaxation.

1121. Dandelion and Burdock Root Clear Skin Elixir

Ingredients: 1 tablespoon Dandelion Root, 1 tablespoon Burdock Root, 2 cups water, 1 tablespoon raw honey.
Preparation: Simmer Dandelion and Burdock roots in water for 20 minutes. Strain, cool, and add honey.
Suggested Usage: Drink 1 cup daily to support detoxification and clear up the skin.
Benefits: Cleanses the blood, promotes liver health, and reduces acne.

1122. Rose and Aloe Vera Anti-Aging Eye Gel

Ingredients: 1/4 cup Aloe Vera gel, 1 tablespoon Rose water, 5 drops Rosehip Seed Oil.
Preparation: Mix all ingredients thoroughly and store in a small glass jar.
Suggested Usage: Gently dab under the eyes at night to reduce puffiness and fine lines.
Benefits: Reduces dark circles, hydrates, and tightens the delicate skin around the eyes.

1123. Nettle and Mint Cooling Facial Toner

Ingredients: 1 tablespoon dried Nettle leaves, 1 tablespoon dried Mint leaves, 1 cup distilled water.
Preparation: Steep Nettle and Mint in hot water for 15 minutes. Strain and cool. Pour into a spray bottle.
Suggested Usage: Use as a facial toner morning and night to refresh and balance the skin.
Benefits: Tightens pores, reduces oiliness, and calms inflammation.

1124. Licorice Root and Chamomile Skin-Brightening Cream

Ingredients: 1 tablespoon Licorice Root extract, 1/4 cup Chamomile-infused oil, 1/4 cup shea butter, 1 tablespoon beeswax.
Preparation: Melt the shea butter and beeswax together, then add Chamomile oil and Licorice extract. Blend until smooth.
Suggested Usage: Apply to dark spots or

uneven skin tone areas nightly.

Benefits: Fades dark spots, evens skin tone, and soothes irritated skin.

1125. Marshmallow Root and Plantain Skin-Healing Gel

Ingredients: 1/4 cup Marshmallow Root, 1/4 cup Plantain leaves, 1 cup Aloe Vera gel.

Preparation: Infuse Marshmallow Root and Plantain leaves in Aloe Vera gel for 1 week. Strain and store in a glass jar.

Suggested Usage: Apply to cuts, scrapes, or burns as needed.

Benefits: Speeds up healing, reduces inflammation, and hydrates the skin.

1126. Lavender and Sage Antiseptic Skin Spray

Ingredients: 1/4 cup dried Lavender flowers, 1/4 cup dried Sage, 1 cup distilled water, 1 tablespoon witch hazel.

Preparation: Steep Lavender and Sage in hot water for 20 minutes. Strain, add witch hazel, and pour into a spray bottle.

Suggested Usage: Spray onto the skin to cleanse and prevent infection in minor cuts or scrapes.

Benefits: Kills bacteria, prevents infection, and promotes healing.

1127. Gotu Kola and Turmeric Scar-Reducing Balm

Ingredients: 1 tablespoon Gotu Kola-infused oil, 1 teaspoon Turmeric powder, 1/4 cup shea butter, 2 tablespoons beeswax.

Preparation: Melt shea butter and beeswax together. Add Gotu Kola oil and Turmeric, stirring until well combined.

Suggested Usage: Apply to scars twice daily to reduce their appearance.

Benefits: Promotes collagen production, reduces scar tissue, and evens skin tone.

1128. Rosehip and Pomegranate Anti-Aging Facial Oil

Ingredients: 1 tablespoon Rosehip Seed Oil, 1 tablespoon Pomegranate Seed Oil, 5 drops Frankincense essential oil.

Preparation: Combine all ingredients in a small dropper bottle and shake well.

Suggested Usage: Apply 2-3 drops to the face at night to reduce wrinkles and promote a youthful glow.

Benefits: Rich in antioxidants, reduces fine lines, and improves skin elasticity.

1129. Yarrow and Calendula Itch-Relief Salve

Ingredients: 1/4 cup dried Yarrow, 1/4 cup Calendula flowers, 1 cup olive oil, 2 tablespoons beeswax.

Preparation: Infuse Yarrow and Calendula in olive oil for 2 weeks. Strain and blend with melted beeswax.

Suggested Usage: Apply to itchy or irritated skin as needed.

Benefits: Reduces itching, soothes irritation, and promotes skin healing.

1130. Holy Basil and Nettle Hormone-Balancing Tea

Ingredients: 1 tablespoon dried Holy Basil, 1 tablespoon dried Nettle leaves, 2 cups hot water.

Preparation: Steep Holy Basil and Nettle in hot water for 15 minutes. Strain and serve warm.

Suggested Usage: Drink 1 cup daily to balance hormones and improve skin clarity.

Benefits: Reduces hormonal acne, purifies the blood, and supports overall skin health.

1131. Green Tea and Aloe Vera Anti-Redness Toner

Ingredients: 1 tablespoon Green Tea leaves, 1/2 cup Aloe Vera gel, 1 cup distilled water.

Preparation: Steep Green Tea leaves in hot water for 10 minutes. Cool and mix with Aloe Vera gel.

Suggested Usage: Use as a facial toner morning and night to reduce redness and inflammation.

Benefits: Calms irritated skin, reduces redness, and provides antioxidant protection.

Pour into a spray bottle.

Suggested Usage: Apply to acne-prone skin daily to reduce oiliness and breakouts.

Benefits: Tightens pores, reduces acne, and balances oil production.

1132. Chamomile and Plantain Eczema Relief Cream

Ingredients: 1/4 cup dried Chamomile flowers, 1/4 cup dried Plantain leaves, 1 cup coconut oil, 2 tablespoons beeswax.

Preparation: Infuse Chamomile and Plantain in coconut oil for 2 weeks. Strain and blend with melted beeswax.

Suggested Usage: Apply to eczema-prone areas as needed.

Benefits: Soothes itchy, inflamed skin and reduces redness and irritation.

1133. Peppermint and Witch Hazel Blemish-Fighting Toner

Ingredients: 1 tablespoon dried Peppermint, 1/2 cup Witch Hazel, 1/2 cup distilled water.

Preparation: Steep Peppermint in hot water for 15 minutes. Cool, then add Witch Hazel.

Book 47: Herbal Supports for Eye Health

Promoting Vision and Eye Health with Herbs

Healthy vision and strong eye function are crucial components of overall well-being, and several herbs have been traditionally used to support and protect eye health. These herbs can help prevent common issues such as dryness, strain, inflammation, and age-related vision loss. Herbal remedies can also provide essential nutrients like antioxidants, vitamins, and minerals that strengthen eye tissues and improve overall visual acuity.

Bilberry is one of the most popular herbs for eye health, known for its high content of anthocyanins, which are powerful antioxidants that support the strength and flexibility of blood vessels in the eyes. Bilberry helps improve night vision and may reduce the risk of cataracts and macular degeneration.

Eyebright is another well-known herb for eye support. Traditionally used as a natural remedy for eye infections and inflammation, it helps reduce redness, swelling, and irritation. Eyebright can be taken internally as a tea or used externally in compresses to soothe tired or infected eyes.

Ginkgo Biloba is an excellent herb for enhancing circulation to the eyes. By increasing blood flow, Ginkgo can help protect against oxidative damage and support visual function, making it ideal for age-related eye conditions.

Turmeric is a potent anti-inflammatory herb that can reduce the inflammation often associated with dry eyes and other eye conditions. Curcumin, the active compound in Turmeric, may also help protect the retina from damage due to excessive light exposure.

Fennel is traditionally used to treat eye strain and improve vision. It contains a variety of nutrients, including Vitamin C and antioxidants, that support eye health and reduce inflammation.

Goji Berry has been used in Chinese medicine for centuries to support healthy vision. Rich in carotenoids and zeaxanthin, Goji Berry helps protect the retina and prevent age-related eye diseases.

Recipes for Eye-Boosting Remedies

When creating eye-supporting remedies, it's essential to focus on formulations that incorporate these herbs either as teas, tinctures, or compresses. For instance, a **Bilberry and Eyebright Eye-Strengthening Tea** can be made by combining 1 tablespoon of dried Bilberry with 1 tablespoon of dried Eyebright in 2 cups of hot water. Steep for 10-15 minutes, strain, and enjoy 1 cup daily to promote healthy vision and reduce eye strain.

For an external application, a **Chamomile and Fennel Eye Compress** can be used to soothe tired, dry, or irritated eyes. Combine 1 tablespoon of dried Chamomile flowers with 1 tablespoon of dried Fennel seeds in 1 cup of hot water. Steep for 10 minutes, cool, and then soak two clean cotton pads in the infusion. Place the pads over closed eyes for 10-15 minutes to reduce redness and inflammation.

Incorporating these herbs into your daily routine can provide essential nutrients to maintain optimal eye health and prevent vision-related issues. Creating a comprehensive eye-support plan that includes both internal and external herbal formulations can lead to clearer, brighter, and healthier eyes for years to come.

Remedies for Eye Health

1134. Bilberry and Eyebright Eye-Strengthening Tea

Ingredients: 1 tablespoon dried Bilberry, 1 tablespoon dried Eyebright, 2 cups hot water.
Preparation: Steep Bilberry and Eyebright in hot water for 15 minutes. Strain and serve warm.
Suggested Usage: Drink 1 cup daily to enhance vision and support overall eye health.
Benefits: Improves night vision, supports healthy blood flow to the eyes, and reduces eye strain.

1135. Ginkgo and Turmeric Vision Support Capsules

Ingredients: 1 tablespoon Ginkgo powder, 1 tablespoon Turmeric powder, empty gel capsules.
Preparation: Mix Ginkgo and Turmeric powders thoroughly. Fill empty capsules and seal.
Suggested Usage: Take 1 capsule daily to reduce inflammation and improve circulation to the eyes.
Benefits: Protects the retina, reduces inflammation, and enhances overall visual acuity.

1136. Chamomile and Fennel Eye-Soothing Compress

Ingredients: 1 tablespoon dried Chamomile, 1 tablespoon dried Fennel seeds, 1 cup hot water.
Preparation: Steep Chamomile and Fennel in hot water for 10 minutes. Cool, soak cotton pads in the mixture, and place over closed eyes.
Suggested Usage: Use the compress for 10-15 minutes to relieve tired or irritated eyes.
Benefits: Reduces redness, soothes inflammation, and relieves eye strain.

1137. Goji Berry and Licorice Vision Tonic

Ingredients: 1 tablespoon dried Goji Berries, 1 teaspoon Licorice Root, 2 cups hot water.
Preparation: Steep Goji Berries and Licorice Root in hot water for 15 minutes. Strain and serve warm.
Suggested Usage: Drink 1 cup daily to nourish and protect the eyes.

Benefits: Supports healthy vision, protects the retina, and prevents age-related eye disorders.

1138. Turmeric and Black Pepper Eye Health Capsules

Ingredients: 1 tablespoon Turmeric powder, 1/2 teaspoon Black Pepper powder, empty gel capsules.
Preparation: Mix Turmeric and Black Pepper thoroughly. Fill empty capsules and seal.
Suggested Usage: Take 1 capsule daily to reduce inflammation and support retinal health.
Benefits: Anti-inflammatory properties protect the eyes from oxidative damage and reduce inflammation.

1139. Blueberry and Hibiscus Antioxidant Tea

Ingredients: 1 tablespoon dried Blueberries, 1 tablespoon dried Hibiscus, 2 cups hot water.
Preparation: Steep Blueberries and Hibiscus in hot water for 15 minutes. Strain and serve warm.
Suggested Usage: Drink 1 cup daily to provide antioxidant support to the eyes.
Benefits: Reduces free radical damage, promotes clear vision, and enhances eye health.

1140. Calendula and Goldenseal Eye Rinse

Ingredients: 1 tablespoon dried Calendula flowers, 1 teaspoon Goldenseal Root, 2 cups boiling water.
Preparation: Steep Calendula and Goldenseal in hot water for 15 minutes. Strain and cool. Use as an eye rinse twice daily.
Suggested Usage: Use 2-3 drops of the solution in each eye for relief from dryness and irritation.
Benefits: Reduces redness, soothes dry eyes, and prevents infections.

1141. Fennel and Rosemary Vision-Boosting Tea

Ingredients: 1 tablespoon dried Fennel, 1 tablespoon Rosemary, 2 cups hot water.
Preparation: Steep Fennel and Rosemary in hot water for 10-15 minutes. Strain and serve warm.
Suggested Usage: Drink 1 cup daily to enhance visual clarity and reduce eye strain.
Benefits: Improves blood circulation to the eyes, supports clear vision, and reduces inflammation.

1142. Gotu Kola and Lavender Eye-Calming Capsules

Ingredients: 1 tablespoon Gotu Kola powder, 1 tablespoon Lavender powder, empty gel capsules.
Preparation: Mix Gotu Kola and Lavender powders thoroughly. Fill empty capsules and seal.
Suggested Usage: Take 1 capsule before bedtime to relieve eye strain and promote restful sleep.
Benefits: Calms the nervous system, relieves stress-related eye tension, and supports clear vision.

1143. Eyebright and Goldenseal Anti-Inflammatory Eye Drops

Ingredients: 1 teaspoon dried Eyebright, 1 teaspoon Goldenseal Root, 1 cup distilled water.
Preparation: Simmer Eyebright and Goldenseal in water for 15 minutes. Cool, strain, and pour into a sterilized dropper bottle.
Suggested Usage: Use 1-2 drops in each eye twice daily to reduce inflammation and irritation.
Benefits: Soothes irritated eyes, reduces redness, and helps fight infections.

1144. Bilberry and Nettle Eye Health Tea

Ingredients: 1 tablespoon dried Bilberry, 1 tablespoon Nettle leaves, 2 cups hot water.
Preparation: Steep Bilberry and Nettle in hot water for 15 minutes. Strain and serve warm.
Suggested Usage: Drink 1 cup daily to support overall eye health and reduce the risk of vision loss.
Benefits: Rich in antioxidants, supports clear vision, and nourishes the eyes.

1145. Turmeric and Ginkgo Vision Support Capsules

Ingredients: 1 tablespoon Turmeric powder, 1 tablespoon Ginkgo powder, empty gel capsules.
Preparation: Mix Turmeric and Ginkgo powders thoroughly. Fill empty capsules and seal.
Suggested Usage: Take 1 capsule daily to improve circulation and reduce inflammation.
Benefits: Enhances blood flow to the eyes, protects against oxidative stress, and supports healthy vision.

1146. Elderflower and Chamomile Eye Compress

Ingredients: 1 tablespoon dried Elderflower, 1 tablespoon dried Chamomile, 1 cup hot water.
Preparation: Steep Elderflower and Chamomile in hot water for 15 minutes. Cool, soak cotton pads in the mixture, and place over closed eyes.
Suggested Usage: Use the compress for 10-15 minutes to relieve puffiness and soothe irritation.
Benefits: Soothes puffy eyes, reduces inflammation, and refreshes tired eyes.

1147. Goji Berry and Ginger Eye Health Tonic

Ingredients: 1 tablespoon dried Goji Berries, 1 tablespoon grated Ginger, 2 cups hot water.
Preparation: Steep Goji Berries and Ginger in hot water for 15 minutes. Strain and serve warm.
Suggested Usage: Drink 1 cup daily to protect against age-related vision loss.
Benefits: Supports eye health, improves circulation, and enhances overall vision.

1148. Gotu Kola and Ashwagandha Vision Tonic

Ingredients: 1 tablespoon Gotu Kola, 1 tablespoon Ashwagandha Root, 2 cups hot water.

Preparation: Simmer Gotu Kola and Ashwagandha in water for 15 minutes. Strain and serve warm.

Suggested Usage: Drink 1 cup daily to strengthen eye function and improve visual clarity.

Benefits: Reduces eye strain, promotes clear vision, and supports cognitive health.

1149. Saffron and Chamomile Vision-Enhancing Tea

Ingredients: 1 teaspoon Saffron threads, 1 tablespoon dried Chamomile, 2 cups hot water.

Preparation: Steep Saffron and Chamomile in hot water for 10 minutes. Strain and serve warm.

Suggested Usage: Drink 1 cup daily to improve visual acuity and reduce eye fatigue.

Benefits: Enhances vision clarity, reduces eye strain, and supports retinal health.

1150. Blueberry and Rosehip Antioxidant Eye Tea

Ingredients: 1 tablespoon dried Blueberries, 1 tablespoon dried Rosehip, 2 cups hot water.

Preparation: Steep Blueberries and Rosehip in hot water for 15 minutes. Strain and serve warm.

Suggested Usage: Drink 1 cup daily to support eye health and protect against oxidative damage.

Benefits: High in antioxidants, reduces free radical damage, and promotes clear vision.

1151. Carrot and Ginger Vision-Boosting Juice

Ingredients: 3 large carrots, 1-inch piece of fresh Ginger, 1 apple.

Preparation: Juice the carrots, ginger, and apple together. Stir and serve immediately.

Suggested Usage: Drink 1 cup daily to support overall eye health and provide essential nutrients.

Benefits: Rich in beta-carotene and Vitamin A, improves night vision, and reduces inflammation.

1152. Eyebright and Licorice Soothing Eye Drops

Ingredients: 1 teaspoon Eyebright herb, 1 teaspoon Licorice Root, 1 cup distilled water.

Preparation: Simmer Eyebright and Licorice Root in water for 15 minutes. Cool, strain, and pour into a sterilized dropper bottle.

Suggested Usage: Use 1-2 drops in each eye twice daily to reduce redness and soothe irritation.

Benefits: Relieves eye irritation, reduces inflammation, and promotes healing.

1153. Goldenrod and Sage Eye Health Capsules

Ingredients: 1 tablespoon dried Goldenrod powder, 1 tablespoon Sage powder, empty gel capsules.

Preparation: Mix the powders thoroughly and fill the capsules.

Suggested Usage: Take 1 capsule daily to support healthy vision and reduce

inflammation.
Benefits: Reduces oxidative stress, enhances blood flow to the eyes, and supports overall eye health.

1154. Chamomile and Aloe Vera Eye Gel

Ingredients: 1/4 cup Aloe Vera gel, 1 tablespoon Chamomile-infused oil, 5 drops Lavender essential oil.
Preparation: Mix all ingredients thoroughly and store in a small glass jar.
Suggested Usage: Apply gently around the eyes at night to reduce puffiness and soothe tired eyes.
Benefits: Reduces puffiness, hydrates delicate skin, and soothes irritation.

1155. Ginkgo and Gotu Kola Cognitive Vision Tea

Ingredients: 1 tablespoon dried Ginkgo, 1 tablespoon Gotu Kola, 2 cups hot water.
Preparation: Steep Ginkgo and Gotu Kola in hot water for 15 minutes. Strain and serve warm.
Suggested Usage: Drink 1 cup daily to improve circulation to the eyes and support cognitive function.
Benefits: Enhances blood flow to the eyes, improves memory and focus, and reduces visual fatigue.

1156. Calendula and Peppermint Eye-Restoring Compress

Ingredients: 1 tablespoon dried Calendula flowers, 1 tablespoon dried Peppermint leaves, 1 cup hot water.
Preparation: Steep Calendula and Peppermint in hot water for 15 minutes. Cool, soak cotton pads in the mixture, and place over closed eyes.
Suggested Usage: Use the compress for 10-15 minutes to refresh and soothe tired eyes.
Benefits: Reduces puffiness, cools and refreshes the eyes, and alleviates redness.

1157. Elderberry and Chamomile Vision Tea

Ingredients: 1 tablespoon dried Elderberries, 1 tablespoon Chamomile, 2 cups hot water.
Preparation: Steep Elderberries and Chamomile in hot water for 15 minutes. Strain and serve warm.
Suggested Usage: Drink 1 cup daily to support healthy vision and reduce inflammation.
Benefits: Rich in antioxidants, promotes eye health, and reduces eye inflammation.

1158. Turmeric and Ginger Eye Health Elixir

Ingredients: 1 tablespoon Turmeric powder, 1 tablespoon grated Ginger, 1 cup warm water, 1 tablespoon honey.
Preparation: Mix Turmeric and Ginger in warm water, add honey, and stir well.
Suggested Usage: Drink 1 cup daily to reduce inflammation and protect the eyes.
Benefits: Anti-inflammatory properties reduce oxidative damage and support retinal health.

1159. Rosemary and Lavender Vision-Boosting Tea

Ingredients: 1 tablespoon dried Rosemary, 1 tablespoon dried Lavender, 2 cups hot water.
Preparation: Steep Rosemary and Lavender in hot water for 15 minutes. Strain and serve warm.
Suggested Usage: Drink 1 cup daily to improve circulation and reduce eye strain.
Benefits: Enhances blood flow, reduces tension in the eyes, and promotes visual clarity.

1160. Sage and Eyebright Eye-Soothing Capsules

Ingredients: 1 tablespoon dried Sage powder, 1 tablespoon Eyebright powder, empty gel capsules.
Preparation: Mix Sage and Eyebright powders thoroughly and fill capsules.
Suggested Usage: Take 1 capsule daily to reduce inflammation and support healthy vision.
Benefits: Soothes inflammation, reduces redness, and protects against eye infections.

1161. Calendula and Licorice Anti-Inflammatory Tea

Ingredients: 1 tablespoon dried Calendula, 1 teaspoon Licorice Root, 2 cups hot water.
Preparation: Steep Calendula and Licorice Root in hot water for 15 minutes. Strain and serve warm.
Suggested Usage: Drink 1 cup daily to reduce inflammation and support eye health.
Benefits: Reduces inflammation, soothes irritated eyes, and promotes clear vision.

1162. Eyebright and Chamomile Anti-Irritation Eye Drops

Ingredients: 1 teaspoon Eyebright, 1 tablespoon dried Chamomile, 1 cup distilled water.
Preparation: Simmer Eyebright and Chamomile in water for 15 minutes. Cool, strain, and pour into a sterilized dropper bottle.
Suggested Usage: Use 1-2 drops in each eye twice daily to soothe irritation and redness.
Benefits: Reduces redness, soothes irritated eyes, and helps prevent infections.

1163. Blueberry and Goji Berry Eye Health Smoothie

Ingredients: 1/2 cup fresh Blueberries, 1/4 cup dried Goji Berries, 1 banana, 1 cup almond milk.
Preparation: Blend all ingredients until smooth.
Suggested Usage: Drink daily to provide essential nutrients for optimal eye health.
Benefits: Rich in antioxidants and vitamins, reduces eye strain, and supports healthy vision.

1164. Bilberry and Turmeric Night Vision Tea

Ingredients: 1 tablespoon dried Bilberry, 1/2 teaspoon Turmeric, 2 cups hot water.
Preparation: Steep Bilberry and Turmeric in hot water for 15 minutes. Strain and serve warm.
Suggested Usage: Drink 1 cup daily to support night vision and reduce eye

fatigue.

Benefits: Improves night vision, reduces eye strain, and supports healthy blood flow to the eyes.

Book 48: Natural Hair Growth Remedies

Herbs to Stimulate Hair Growth

Healthy hair growth begins with a nourished scalp and strong hair follicles. Several herbs are renowned for their ability to promote hair growth, prevent hair loss, and enhance the overall health of the scalp. By incorporating these herbs into daily routines, you can create a holistic approach to hair care that not only promotes growth but also adds shine, strength, and resilience to your hair.

Horsetail is a powerful herb rich in silica, a mineral that strengthens hair strands and improves elasticity. Silica also enhances collagen production, which supports the health of hair and skin. Consuming Horsetail tea or applying it topically can lead to stronger, shinier hair.

Rosemary is known for its ability to improve circulation in the scalp, which helps deliver nutrients and oxygen to hair follicles. Rosemary is effective in promoting new hair growth and slowing down hair loss. Regular use of Rosemary oil or rinses can also darken gray hairs and add a healthy shine.

Nettle is a nutrient-rich herb containing vitamins A, C, D, and B, as well as calcium, iron, magnesium, and zinc. These nutrients support hair follicle health and help reduce hair shedding. Nettle can be consumed as a tea or applied topically in oil infusions or hair rinses.

Burdock Root is an herb known for its high levels of phytosterols and essential fatty acids, both of which support healthy scalp conditions and strengthen hair. Burdock Root promotes hair regrowth and soothes inflammation on the scalp.

Saw Palmetto is a popular herb for both men and women dealing with hair loss due to its ability to block DHT, a hormone associated with hair thinning and loss. Taking Saw Palmetto supplements or using it in scalp massages can help maintain hair density and prevent further loss.

Fenugreek is a powerful herb for combating hair thinning and promoting new growth. It is rich in protein, nicotinic acid, and lecithin, which strengthen hair from the roots. Fenugreek paste applied to the scalp helps prevent hair fall and boosts the strength and shine of hair strands.

Recipes for Hair-Strengthening Elixirs

Creating effective hair growth elixirs and treatments involves combining these herbs with other nourishing ingredients like oils and essential oils. A **Rosemary and Nettle Hair Growth Tonic** can be made by steeping 1 tablespoon each of dried Rosemary and Nettle leaves in 2 cups of hot water. Strain and store in a spray bottle, using it as a daily scalp spray to promote circulation and nourish the follicles.

For a **Fenugreek and Burdock Root Hair Mask**, soak 2 tablespoons of Fenugreek seeds in water overnight, then blend with 1 tablespoon of Burdock Root powder and 2 tablespoons of coconut oil to form a paste. Apply to the scalp and hair, leave on for 30 minutes, then rinse thoroughly. This mask strengthens the roots and boosts hair growth.

Remedies for Hair Growth

1165. Rosemary and Nettle Hair Growth Tonic

Ingredients: 1 tablespoon dried Rosemary, 1 tablespoon dried Nettle, 2 cups hot water.
Preparation: Steep Rosemary and Nettle in hot water for 15 minutes. Strain and store in a spray bottle.
Suggested Usage: Spray onto the scalp daily and massage gently to promote circulation and nourish hair follicles.
Benefits: Stimulates hair growth, strengthens roots, and improves scalp health.

1166. Horsetail and Lavender Strengthening Hair Rinse

Ingredients: 1 tablespoon dried Horsetail, 1 tablespoon dried Lavender, 3 cups water.
Preparation: Simmer Horsetail and Lavender in water for 20 minutes. Strain and use as a final rinse after shampooing.
Suggested Usage: Rinse hair with this herbal infusion 2-3 times a week to strengthen and add shine.
Benefits: Provides silica to strengthen hair strands, reduces breakage, and adds luster.

1167. Fenugreek and Aloe Vera Hair Regrowth Mask

Ingredients: 2 tablespoons Fenugreek seeds, 1/4 cup Aloe Vera gel.
Preparation: Soak Fenugreek seeds overnight, then blend with Aloe Vera gel to form a smooth paste.
Suggested Usage: Apply to the scalp and hair, leave on for 30 minutes, and rinse thoroughly.
Benefits: Nourishes the scalp, promotes hair regrowth, and reduces hair thinning.

1168. Brahmi and Bhringraj Scalp Oil

Ingredients: 1/4 cup Brahmi powder, 1/4 cup Bhringraj powder, 1/2 cup coconut oil.
Preparation: Heat the coconut oil and add Brahmi and Bhringraj powders. Simmer on low heat for 15 minutes, strain, and store in a glass jar.
Suggested Usage: Massage into the scalp 2-3 times a week and leave overnight for maximum benefit.
Benefits: Strengthens hair roots, reduces hair fall, and enhances hair thickness.

1169. Saw Palmetto and Peppermint Scalp Massage Oil

Ingredients: 1 tablespoon Saw Palmetto extract, 5 drops Peppermint essential oil, 1/4 cup jojoba oil.
Preparation: Mix all ingredients thoroughly and store in a glass bottle.
Suggested Usage: Massage into the scalp for 5-10 minutes, leave for an hour, and wash as usual.
Benefits: Blocks DHT to prevent hair loss, stimulates the scalp, and promotes healthy hair growth.

1170. Hibiscus and Amla Hair Strengthening Mask

Ingredients: 1/4 cup Hibiscus powder, 1/4 cup Amla powder, 1/2 cup yogurt.
Preparation: Mix all ingredients to form a thick paste.
Suggested Usage: Apply to the scalp and hair, leave on for 30 minutes, and rinse thoroughly.
Benefits: Promotes stronger hair, prevents premature graying, and adds shine.

1171. Burdock Root and Nettle Hair Health Tea

Ingredients: 1 tablespoon dried Burdock Root, 1 tablespoon Nettle leaves, 2 cups hot water.
Preparation: Steep Burdock Root and Nettle in hot water for 15 minutes. Strain and serve.
Suggested Usage: Drink 1 cup daily to nourish hair from within.
Benefits: Supports healthy hair growth, reduces hair fall, and improves scalp condition.

1172. Horsetail and Chamomile Silica-Boosting Hair Rinse

Ingredients: 1 tablespoon dried Horsetail, 1 tablespoon dried Chamomile, 2 cups water.
Preparation: Steep Horsetail and Chamomile in hot water for 20 minutes. Strain and use as a hair rinse after washing.
Suggested Usage: Use 2-3 times weekly for shiny, strong hair.
Benefits: Boosts silica content in hair, strengthens hair fibers, and reduces breakage.

1173. Ginger and Castor Oil Hair Regrowth Serum

Ingredients: 2 tablespoons Ginger juice, 1/4 cup castor oil.
Preparation: Mix Ginger juice and castor oil thoroughly.
Suggested Usage: Massage into the scalp for 5 minutes, leave for 1 hour, and wash out.
Benefits: Increases blood circulation, stimulates hair follicles, and promotes new hair growth.

1174. Nettle and Rosemary Hair Strength Capsules

Ingredients: 1 tablespoon dried Nettle powder, 1 tablespoon dried Rosemary powder, empty gel capsules.
Preparation: Mix Nettle and Rosemary powders and fill the capsules.
Suggested Usage: Take 1 capsule daily to strengthen hair from within.
Benefits: Provides essential nutrients,

reduces hair fall, and promotes thicker hair.

1175. Sage and Horsetail Hair Growth Tea

Ingredients: 1 tablespoon dried Sage, 1 tablespoon Horsetail, 2 cups hot water.
Preparation: Steep Sage and Horsetail in hot water for 15 minutes. Strain and serve.
Suggested Usage: Drink 1 cup daily to support hair growth and reduce thinning.
Benefits: Supports healthy hair, strengthens hair strands, and improves scalp health.

1176. Brahmi and Neem Hair Nourishing Oil

Ingredients: 1/4 cup Brahmi powder, 1/4 cup Neem powder, 1/2 cup sesame oil.
Preparation: Heat sesame oil, add Brahmi and Neem powders, and simmer for 15 minutes. Strain and store.
Suggested Usage: Massage into the scalp 2-3 times a week to nourish and strengthen hair.
Benefits: Prevents hair loss, improves scalp health, and reduces dandruff.

1177. Lavender and Cedarwood Scalp Stimulating Oil

Ingredients: 10 drops Lavender essential oil, 10 drops Cedarwood essential oil, 1/4 cup almond oil.
Preparation: Mix all ingredients and store in a glass bottle.
Suggested Usage: Massage into the scalp 2-3 times weekly to stimulate hair growth.
Benefits: Increases circulation,

strengthens hair roots, and promotes relaxation.

1178. Amla and Fenugreek Hair Thickening Mask

Ingredients: 2 tablespoons Amla powder, 2 tablespoons Fenugreek seeds (soaked), 1/4 cup coconut milk.
Preparation: Blend all ingredients into a smooth paste.
Suggested Usage: Apply to scalp and hair, leave on for 30 minutes, and rinse thoroughly.
Benefits: Strengthens hair roots, promotes hair density, and reduces shedding.

1179. Nettle and Peppermint Scalp Spray

Ingredients: 1 tablespoon dried Nettle, 1 tablespoon dried Peppermint, 2 cups hot water.
Preparation: Steep Nettle and Peppermint in hot water for 15 minutes. Strain and store in a spray bottle.
Suggested Usage: Spray onto the scalp daily to stimulate hair growth.
Benefits: Improves circulation, nourishes hair follicles, and reduces hair thinning.

1180. Chamomile and Lemon Hair Brightening Rinse

Ingredients: 1/4 cup Chamomile flowers, 1 tablespoon lemon juice, 2 cups hot water.
Preparation: Steep Chamomile in hot water for 15 minutes. Cool, add lemon juice, and use as a hair rinse.
Suggested Usage: Use once a week for

bright, shiny hair.

Benefits: Adds natural highlights, enhances shine, and soothes the scalp.

Book 49: Herbal Solutions for Bone Health

Supporting Bone Density and Strength

Bone health is essential for maintaining a strong and resilient skeletal system, especially as we age. The process of bone formation and resorption is continuous throughout life, but factors like diet, physical activity, and hormonal balance significantly impact bone density. Several herbs are known for their high mineral content, which supports bone strength and reduces the risk of osteoporosis.

Nettle is one of the most mineral-rich herbs, containing high levels of calcium, magnesium, iron, and silica. These minerals are crucial for maintaining bone density and preventing bone loss. Consuming Nettle tea or capsules regularly can help strengthen bones and reduce the risk of fractures.

Horsetail is another excellent herb for bone health due to its high silica content. Silica is a critical component of collagen, which is a major structural protein in bones. Regular intake of Horsetail tea or tincture helps maintain bone elasticity and strength.

Red Clover is known for its phytoestrogenic properties, which can help balance hormones and support bone health, particularly in postmenopausal women. Red Clover tea or supplements provide gentle hormonal support, promoting calcium retention in bones.

Alfalfa is a calcium-rich herb that helps build bone density. It also contains Vitamin K, which is essential for the proper utilization of calcium in the bones.

Oatstraw is another herb with high silica content, which promotes bone resilience. Its gentle, nutritive properties make it ideal for long-term use to support bone health and prevent bone-related conditions.

Recipes for Bone-Boosting Remedies

Incorporating these herbs into daily routines through teas, tinctures, and supplements can significantly enhance bone health. A **Nettle and Oatstraw Bone Strengthening Tea** can be made by combining 1 tablespoon of Nettle and 1 tablespoon of Oatstraw in 2 cups of hot water. Steep for 15-20 minutes, strain, and enjoy daily to support bone density.

For a more concentrated remedy, a **Horsetail and Red Clover Tincture** can be prepared by mixing equal parts of dried Horsetail and Red Clover in a jar and covering with high-proof alcohol. Let it steep for 4-6 weeks, strain, and take 1-2 teaspoons daily.

Remedies for Bone Health

1181. Nettle and Oatstraw Bone Strength Tea

Ingredients: 1 tablespoon dried Nettle, 1 tablespoon dried Oatstraw, 2 cups hot water.
Preparation: Steep Nettle and Oatstraw in hot water for 15-20 minutes. Strain and serve warm.
Suggested Usage: Drink 1 cup daily to support bone density and overall skeletal health.
Benefits: Rich in calcium, magnesium, and silica, promoting strong bones and reducing the risk of osteoporosis.

1182. Horsetail and Red Clover Mineral-Rich Capsules

Ingredients: 1 tablespoon dried Horsetail powder, 1 tablespoon dried Red Clover powder, empty gel capsules.
Preparation: Mix the powders thoroughly and fill empty capsules.
Suggested Usage: Take 1 capsule daily to boost mineral intake and support bone strength.
Benefits: Provides silica, calcium, and phytoestrogens that enhance bone density and resilience.

1183. Alfalfa and Nettle Bone Strength Tonic

Ingredients: 2 tablespoons Alfalfa powder, 2 tablespoons Nettle powder, 1 cup warm water, 1 tablespoon honey.
Preparation: Mix Alfalfa and Nettle powders in warm water, add honey, and stir well.
Suggested Usage: Drink daily to promote strong bones and overall mineral balance.
Benefits: High in calcium and magnesium, supports bone formation and reduces bone loss.

1184. Red Clover and Sage Hormone-Balancing Tea

Ingredients: 1 tablespoon dried Red Clover, 1 teaspoon dried Sage, 2 cups hot water.
Preparation: Steep Red Clover and Sage in hot water for 15 minutes. Strain and serve warm.
Suggested Usage: Drink 1 cup daily, especially beneficial for postmenopausal women.
Benefits: Contains phytoestrogens that balance hormones and support calcium retention in bones.

1185. Horsetail and Chamomile Silica Boost Tea

Ingredients: 1 tablespoon dried Horsetail, 1 tablespoon dried Chamomile, 2 cups hot water.
Preparation: Steep Horsetail and Chamomile in hot water for 15-20 minutes. Strain and serve.
Suggested Usage: Drink 1 cup daily to boost silica levels and support bone health.
Benefits: Silica strengthens bone matrix and improves bone flexibility, reducing the risk of fractures.

1186. Dandelion and Burdock Root Bone Health Tea

Ingredients: 1 tablespoon dried Dandelion Root, 1 tablespoon dried Burdock Root, 2 cups hot water.
Preparation: Simmer Dandelion and Burdock Root in water for 15 minutes. Strain and serve.
Suggested Usage: Drink 1 cup daily to support bone health and detoxification.
Benefits: Rich in minerals and detoxifying compounds that promote bone density and health.

1187. Comfrey and Oatstraw Bone Strengthening Oil

Ingredients: 1/4 cup dried Comfrey, 1/4 cup dried Oatstraw, 1/2 cup olive oil.
Preparation: Simmer Comfrey and Oatstraw in olive oil on low heat for 30 minutes. Strain and store.
Suggested Usage: Massage into joints and bones 2-3 times a week to support bone strength.
Benefits: Soothes inflammation, promotes bone healing, and enhances joint health.

1188. Alfalfa and Horsetail Bone-Strengthening Capsules

Ingredients: 1 tablespoon dried Alfalfa powder, 1 tablespoon dried Horsetail powder, empty gel capsules.
Preparation: Mix Alfalfa and Horsetail powders thoroughly and fill capsules.
Suggested Usage: Take 1 capsule daily for bone strengthening and mineral balance.
Benefits: Rich in silica and calcium, promotes bone resilience and reduces the risk of fractures.

1189. Nettle and Dandelion Leaf Calcium Tea

Ingredients: 1 tablespoon dried Nettle, 1 tablespoon dried Dandelion leaf, 2 cups hot water.
Preparation: Steep Nettle and Dandelion leaf in hot water for 15 minutes. Strain and serve warm.
Suggested Usage: Drink 1 cup daily to maintain bone density and overall mineral balance.
Benefits: High in calcium, magnesium, and other essential minerals for bone health.

1190. Sage and Red Clover Bone-Support Tincture

Ingredients: 1 tablespoon dried Sage, 1 tablespoon dried Red Clover, 1/2 cup vodka or glycerin.
Preparation: Place herbs in a jar and cover with alcohol or glycerin. Let steep for 4-6 weeks, strain, and store.
Suggested Usage: Take 1-2 teaspoons daily to support bone health and hormone balance.
Benefits: Balances hormones, promotes calcium absorption, and supports bone density.

1191. Basil and Thyme Bone Health Capsules

Ingredients: 1 tablespoon dried Basil powder, 1 tablespoon dried Thyme powder, empty gel capsules.

Preparation: Mix Basil and Thyme powders thoroughly and fill capsules.

Suggested Usage: Take 1 capsule daily to boost bone strength and density.

Benefits: Contains bone-supporting nutrients like calcium, magnesium, and Vitamin K.

1192. Shatavari and Ashwagandha Bone-Building Tea

Ingredients: 1 tablespoon dried Shatavari, 1 tablespoon dried Ashwagandha, 2 cups hot water.

Preparation: Steep Shatavari and Ashwagandha in hot water for 15 minutes. Strain and serve.

Suggested Usage: Drink 1 cup daily to support bone strength and reduce inflammation.

Benefits: Balances hormones, promotes bone density, and reduces bone loss.

1193. Gotu Kola and Ginger Bone-Strengthening Tea

Ingredients: 1 tablespoon Gotu Kola, 1 tablespoon grated Ginger, 2 cups hot water.

Preparation: Steep Gotu Kola and Ginger in hot water for 15 minutes. Strain and serve.

Suggested Usage: Drink 1 cup daily to support collagen production and strengthen bones.

Benefits: Enhances collagen synthesis, supports bone elasticity, and improves joint health.

1194. Ashwagandha and Nettle Adaptogen Capsules

Ingredients: 1 tablespoon Ashwagandha powder, 1 tablespoon Nettle powder, empty gel capsules.

Preparation: Mix Ashwagandha and Nettle powders thoroughly and fill capsules.

Suggested Usage: Take 1 capsule daily to support bone health and reduce stress-related bone loss.

Benefits: Supports bone health, reduces cortisol levels, and enhances calcium absorption.

1195. Red Clover and Alfalfa Bone Support Elixir

Ingredients: 1 tablespoon Red Clover, 1 tablespoon Alfalfa, 1 cup apple cider vinegar.

Preparation: Place herbs in a jar and cover with apple cider vinegar. Let steep for 4 weeks, strain, and store.

Suggested Usage: Take 1 tablespoon daily to enhance bone strength and balance hormones.

Benefits: Promotes bone density, balances hormones, and supports calcium absorption.

1196. Horsetail and Nettle Calcium-Boosting Capsules

Ingredients: 1 tablespoon dried Horsetail powder, 1 tablespoon dried Nettle powder, empty gel capsules.

Preparation: Mix Horsetail and Nettle powders thoroughly and fill empty gel capsules.

Suggested Usage: Take 1 capsule daily to enhance bone density and mineral content.

Benefits: High in calcium, silica, and

other essential minerals that strengthen bones and reduce bone loss.

1197. Comfrey and Arnica Bone-Healing Balm

Ingredients: 1/4 cup dried Comfrey, 1/4 cup dried Arnica, 1/2 cup coconut oil, 2 tablespoons beeswax.
Preparation: Infuse Comfrey and Arnica in coconut oil over low heat for 30 minutes. Strain, add beeswax, and pour into a small jar to solidify.
Suggested Usage: Apply topically to bones and joints 2-3 times a day to support healing and relieve pain.
Benefits: Promotes bone healing, reduces inflammation, and soothes aches and pains.

1198. Oatstraw and Licorice Root Bone Tonic Tea

Ingredients: 1 tablespoon Oatstraw, 1 teaspoon Licorice Root, 2 cups hot water.
Preparation: Steep Oatstraw and Licorice Root in hot water for 15 minutes. Strain and serve.
Suggested Usage: Drink 1 cup daily to nourish bones and balance hormones.
Benefits: Provides essential nutrients for bones, balances cortisol, and supports bone strength.

1199. Black Cohosh and Sage Bone Support Capsules

Ingredients: 1 tablespoon dried Black Cohosh powder, 1 tablespoon dried Sage powder, empty gel capsules.
Preparation: Mix Black Cohosh and Sage powders thoroughly and fill capsules.
Suggested Usage: Take 1 capsule daily to support bone health and maintain hormonal balance.
Benefits: Contains phytoestrogens that support bone density and prevent osteoporosis, especially in postmenopausal women.

1200. Dandelion Root and Alfalfa Bone Health Tea

Ingredients: 1 tablespoon Dandelion Root, 1 tablespoon Alfalfa, 2 cups hot water.
Preparation: Steep Dandelion Root and Alfalfa in hot water for 15 minutes. Strain and serve warm.
Suggested Usage: Drink 1 cup daily to promote bone strength and detoxification.
Benefits: High in calcium, magnesium, and other minerals that strengthen bones and support liver health.

1201. Licorice Root and Shatavari Bone-Balancing Tea

Ingredients: 1 tablespoon dried Licorice Root, 1 tablespoon Shatavari, 2 cups hot water.
Preparation: Steep Licorice Root and Shatavari in hot water for 15 minutes. Strain and serve.
Suggested Usage: Drink 1 cup daily to balance hormones and enhance bone strength.
Benefits: Supports bone density, balances cortisol, and reduces bone loss.

1202. Gotu Kola and Horsetail Bone Health Capsules

Ingredients: 1 tablespoon dried Gotu Kola powder, 1 tablespoon dried Horsetail powder, empty gel capsules.
Preparation: Mix Gotu Kola and Horsetail powders thoroughly and fill capsules.
Suggested Usage: Take 1 capsule daily to support bone strength and elasticity.
Benefits: Promotes collagen production, strengthens bone matrix, and supports joint health.

1203. White Willow Bark and Arnica Joint-Soothing Cream

Ingredients: 1/4 cup dried White Willow Bark, 1/4 cup dried Arnica, 1/2 cup shea butter, 2 tablespoons beeswax.
Preparation: Infuse White Willow Bark and Arnica in shea butter on low heat for 30 minutes. Strain, add beeswax, and let solidify.
Suggested Usage: Apply to joints and bones as needed to soothe pain and promote healing.
Benefits: Relieves joint pain, reduces inflammation, and supports bone healing.

1204. Sage and Licorice Bone Density Tea

Ingredients: 1 tablespoon dried Sage, 1 teaspoon dried Licorice Root, 2 cups hot water.
Preparation: Steep Sage and Licorice Root in hot water for 15 minutes. Strain and serve.
Suggested Usage: Drink 1 cup daily to

enhance bone density and hormonal health.
Benefits: Supports bone strength, balances hormones, and prevents bone loss.

1205. Ashwagandha and Nettle Hormone-Balancing Capsules

Ingredients: 1 tablespoon dried Ashwagandha powder, 1 tablespoon dried Nettle powder, empty gel capsules.
Preparation: Mix Ashwagandha and Nettle powders thoroughly and fill capsules.
Suggested Usage: Take 1 capsule daily to support bone health and reduce stress-related bone loss.
Benefits: Enhances calcium absorption, promotes bone resilience, and reduces the impact of stress on bone density.

1206. Alfalfa and Nettle Bone Restoring Tea

Ingredients: 1 tablespoon dried Alfalfa, 1 tablespoon dried Nettle, 2 cups hot water.
Preparation: Steep Alfalfa and Nettle in hot water for 15 minutes. Strain and serve warm.
Suggested Usage: Drink 1 cup daily to restore bone strength and mineral density.
Benefits: High in calcium, iron, and magnesium, which support bone formation and prevent osteoporosis.

1207. Comfrey and Calendula Bone-Healing Balm

Ingredients: 1/4 cup dried Comfrey, 1/4 cup dried Calendula, 1/2 cup olive oil, 2 tablespoons beeswax.

Preparation: Infuse Comfrey and Calendula in olive oil over low heat for 30 minutes. Strain, add beeswax, and let solidify in a jar.

Suggested Usage: Apply to bones and joints as needed to promote bone healing and reduce pain.

Benefits: Supports bone healing, reduces inflammation, and soothes muscle aches.

1208. Nettle and Chamomile Bone Support Capsules

Ingredients: 1 tablespoon dried Nettle powder, 1 tablespoon dried Chamomile powder, empty gel capsules.

Preparation: Mix Nettle and Chamomile powders thoroughly and fill capsules.

Suggested Usage: Take 1 capsule daily to support bone density and reduce bone loss.

Benefits: High in minerals that strengthen bones and prevent osteoporosis.

1209. Oatstraw and Licorice Root Bone-Balancing Tea

Ingredients: 1 tablespoon dried Oatstraw, 1 tablespoon Licorice Root, 2 cups hot water.

Preparation: Steep Oatstraw and Licorice Root in hot water for 15 minutes. Strain and serve warm.

Suggested Usage: Drink 1 cup daily to enhance bone health and balance hormones.

Benefits: Contains essential minerals that promote bone strength and reduce the risk of fractures.

Book 50: Enhancing Physical Performance Naturally

Herbs to Improve Athletic Performance

Optimizing physical performance requires a balance of strength, stamina, energy, and recovery. While regular exercise and a nutritious diet are foundational, certain herbs can provide an extra boost to enhance athletic capabilities. Herbs like **Ginseng**, **Rhodiola**, **Cordyceps**, and **Maca** have been used for centuries to increase endurance, reduce fatigue, and support muscle recovery.

Ginseng is a powerful adaptogen known for its ability to increase energy, enhance focus, and improve stamina. It reduces oxidative stress, allowing athletes to push through physical limitations and recover more efficiently.

Rhodiola is another adaptogen that reduces fatigue and enhances mental clarity, making it ideal for high-intensity training. It supports mitochondrial energy production, boosting both physical and cognitive performance.

Cordyceps, a medicinal mushroom, is revered for its ability to increase oxygen uptake and enhance stamina. By improving the efficiency of oxygen utilization, Cordyceps can enhance athletic performance and speed up recovery times.

Maca, a root vegetable from the Andes, is known for its ability to boost energy, increase libido, and improve overall endurance. It is rich in essential amino acids, vitamins, and minerals, making it a powerhouse for physical performance.

Recipes for Performance-Enhancing Elixirs

Creating herbal elixirs and tonics that incorporate these herbs can provide an extra edge for those looking to enhance their physical capabilities. A **Ginseng and Rhodiola Endurance Elixir** can be made by simmering 1 tablespoon of dried Ginseng root and 1 tablespoon of Rhodiola in 2 cups of water for 20 minutes. Strain and drink 1 cup before workouts to boost stamina and focus.

For a quick energy boost, a **Cordyceps and Maca Power Smoothie** can be blended using 1 teaspoon of Cordyceps powder, 1 teaspoon of Maca powder, 1 banana, and 1 cup of almond milk. This smoothie provides a rich source of energy and nutrients to support endurance and strength.

Remedies for Physical Performance

1210. Ginseng and Rhodiola Endurance Elixir

Ingredients: 1 tablespoon dried Ginseng root, 1 tablespoon Rhodiola root, 2 cups water.
Preparation: Simmer Ginseng and Rhodiola in water for 20 minutes. Strain and serve warm.
Suggested Usage: Drink 1 cup 30 minutes before exercise for enhanced stamina and endurance.
Benefits: Boosts energy, reduces fatigue, and improves physical and mental performance.

1211. Cordyceps and Maca Energy Smoothie

Ingredients: 1 teaspoon Cordyceps powder, 1 teaspoon Maca powder, 1 banana, 1 cup almond milk.
Preparation: Blend all ingredients until smooth.
Suggested Usage: Drink before or after workouts for sustained energy and recovery support.
Benefits: Increases energy, enhances endurance, and supports muscle recovery.

1212. Ashwagandha and Holy Basil Stress-Relief Capsules

Ingredients: 1 tablespoon dried Ashwagandha powder, 1 tablespoon dried Holy Basil powder, empty gel capsules.
Preparation: Mix Ashwagandha and Holy Basil powders thoroughly and fill capsules.
Suggested Usage: Take 1 capsule daily to reduce exercise-induced stress and promote recovery.
Benefits: Reduces cortisol levels, enhances endurance, and supports muscle recovery.

1213. Beetroot and Ginger Pre-Workout Tonic

Ingredients: 1/4 cup Beetroot juice, 1 teaspoon grated Ginger, 1 cup water.
Preparation: Mix all ingredients thoroughly.
Suggested Usage: Drink 30 minutes before exercise to boost nitric oxide levels and enhance performance.
Benefits: Improves blood flow, enhances stamina, and reduces muscle soreness.

1214. Eleuthero and Schisandra Endurance Tea

Ingredients: 1 tablespoon dried Eleuthero root, 1 tablespoon dried Schisandra berries, 2 cups water.
Preparation: Simmer Eleuthero and Schisandra in water for 15 minutes. Strain and serve.
Suggested Usage: Drink 1 cup before physical activity to enhance stamina and reduce fatigue.
Benefits: Increases energy, reduces oxidative stress, and improves physical performance.

1215. Reishi and Cordyceps Recovery Tea

Ingredients: 1 tablespoon dried Reishi mushroom, 1 tablespoon dried Cordyceps, 2 cups water.
Preparation: Simmer Reishi and Cordyceps in water for 20 minutes. Strain and serve.
Suggested Usage: Drink 1 cup post-exercise to speed up recovery and reduce inflammation.
Benefits: Enhances oxygen utilization, reduces inflammation, and supports immune health.

1216. Rhodiola and Ginseng Power Tonic

Ingredients: 1 teaspoon dried Rhodiola root, 1 teaspoon Ginseng root, 1 cup hot water.
Preparation: Steep Rhodiola and Ginseng in hot water for 15 minutes. Strain and serve.
Suggested Usage: Drink 1 cup daily to boost energy and focus during training.
Benefits: Improves energy, enhances focus, and supports endurance.

1217. Holy Basil and Lemon Balm Post-Workout Relaxation Tea

Ingredients: 1 tablespoon dried Holy Basil, 1 tablespoon dried Lemon Balm, 2 cups hot water.
Preparation: Steep Holy Basil and Lemon Balm in hot water for 15 minutes. Strain and serve.
Suggested Usage: Drink 1 cup after exercise to reduce stress and support muscle recovery.

Benefits: Reduces cortisol levels, promotes relaxation, and enhances recovery.

1218. Maca and Ginseng Energy Capsules

Ingredients: 1 tablespoon dried Maca powder, 1 tablespoon dried Ginseng powder, empty gel capsules.
Preparation: Mix Maca and Ginseng powders and fill capsules.
Suggested Usage: Take 1 capsule daily for a natural energy boost.
Benefits: Increases stamina, reduces fatigue, and enhances physical strength.

1219. Cordyceps and Reishi Mushroom Adaptogen Capsules

Ingredients: 1 tablespoon dried Cordyceps powder, 1 tablespoon dried Reishi powder, empty gel capsules.
Preparation: Mix powders thoroughly and fill capsules.
Suggested Usage: Take 1 capsule daily to enhance endurance and promote overall vitality.
Benefits: Supports energy, boosts immunity, and improves physical endurance.

1220. Eleuthero and Maca Pre-Workout Smoothie

Ingredients: 1 teaspoon Eleuthero powder, 1 teaspoon Maca powder, 1 cup oat milk, 1 banana.
Preparation: Blend all ingredients until

smooth.

Suggested Usage: Drink 30 minutes before exercise for sustained energy and stamina.

Benefits: Increases stamina, enhances strength, and supports mental clarity.

1221. Schisandra and Rhodiola Performance Tonic

Ingredients: 1 tablespoon dried Schisandra berries, 1 teaspoon Rhodiola root, 2 cups water.

Preparation: Simmer Schisandra and Rhodiola in water for 20 minutes. Strain and serve.

Suggested Usage: Drink 1 cup daily to boost endurance and reduce fatigue.

Benefits: Enhances physical performance, reduces fatigue, and improves mental focus.

1222. Ginseng and Turmeric Anti-Inflammatory Capsules

Ingredients: 1 tablespoon dried Ginseng powder, 1 tablespoon dried Turmeric powder, empty gel capsules.

Preparation: Mix powders and fill capsules.

Suggested Usage: Take 1 capsule daily to reduce exercise-induced inflammation.

Benefits: Reduces inflammation, supports joint health, and enhances recovery.

1223. Ashwagandha and Gotu Kola Resilience Tea

Ingredients: 1 tablespoon dried Ashwagandha root, 1 tablespoon dried Gotu Kola, 2 cups water.

Preparation: Simmer Ashwagandha and Gotu Kola in water for 20 minutes. Strain and serve.

Suggested Usage: Drink 1 cup before exercise to reduce fatigue and increase resilience.

Benefits: Enhances endurance, reduces fatigue, and supports mental focus.

1224. Ginseng and Peppermint Energizing Tea

Ingredients: 1 tablespoon dried Ginseng root, 1 tablespoon dried Peppermint, 2 cups hot water.

Preparation: Steep Ginseng and Peppermint in hot water for 15 minutes. Strain and serve.

Suggested Usage: Drink 1 cup before exercise to enhance focus and boost energy.

Benefits: Enhances mental clarity, boosts physical energy, and supports stamina.

1225. Maca and Schisandra Vitality-Enhancing Smoothie

Ingredients: 1 teaspoon Maca powder, 1 teaspoon Schisandra powder, 1 cup almond milk, 1 teaspoon honey.

Preparation: Blend all ingredients until smooth.

Suggested Usage: Drink in the morning or pre-workout for increased vitality and stamina.

Benefits: Enhances endurance, boosts energy, and supports hormone balance.

1226. Rhodiola and Holy Basil Adaptogen Tea

Ingredients: 1 teaspoon dried Rhodiola root, 1 teaspoon dried Holy Basil, 2 cups hot water.
Preparation: Steep Rhodiola and Holy Basil in hot water for 15 minutes. Strain and serve.
Suggested Usage: Drink 1 cup daily to reduce stress and improve physical resilience.
Benefits: Reduces fatigue, enhances endurance, and supports mental and physical balance.

1227. Cordyceps and Turmeric Recovery Capsules

Ingredients: 1 tablespoon dried Cordyceps powder, 1 tablespoon dried Turmeric powder, empty gel capsules.
Preparation: Mix Cordyceps and Turmeric powders thoroughly and fill capsules.
Suggested Usage: Take 1 capsule daily post-exercise for faster recovery.
Benefits: Reduces inflammation, supports muscle repair, and enhances recovery.

1228. Eleuthero and Ashwagandha Endurance Tonic

Ingredients: 1 teaspoon Eleuthero root powder, 1 teaspoon Ashwagandha powder, 1 cup hot water, 1 teaspoon honey.
Preparation: Steep powders in hot water for 15 minutes. Add honey and stir.
Suggested Usage: Drink before physical activity to increase stamina and reduce fatigue.
Benefits: Boosts endurance, enhances strength, and supports mental clarity.

1229. Ginseng and Ginger Performance Tea

Ingredients: 1 tablespoon Ginseng root, 1 tablespoon grated Ginger, 2 cups water.
Preparation: Simmer Ginseng and Ginger in water for 20 minutes. Strain and serve.
Suggested Usage: Drink 1 cup before workouts to boost energy and reduce fatigue.
Benefits: Increases physical endurance, enhances mental clarity, and supports immune health.

1230. Maca and Cordyceps Energy Boost Capsules

Ingredients: 1 tablespoon Maca powder, 1 tablespoon Cordyceps powder, empty gel capsules.
Preparation: Mix powders and fill capsules.
Suggested Usage: Take 1 capsule daily to support energy and vitality.
Benefits: Boosts stamina, enhances endurance, and supports overall energy levels.

1231. Schisandra and Reishi Mushroom Stress-Relief Tea

Ingredients: 1 tablespoon dried Schisandra berries, 1 tablespoon Reishi mushroom, 2 cups water.
Preparation: Simmer Schisandra and Reishi in water for 20 minutes. Strain and

serve.

Suggested Usage: Drink 1 cup after workouts to reduce stress and support recovery.

Benefits: Reduces cortisol, enhances recovery, and supports immune function.

1232. Rhodiola and Eleuthero Focus Capsules

Ingredients: 1 tablespoon dried Rhodiola powder, 1 tablespoon dried Eleuthero powder, empty gel capsules.

Preparation: Mix powders thoroughly and fill capsules.

Suggested Usage: Take 1 capsule before intense physical or mental activities to enhance focus and stamina.

Benefits: Boosts energy, improves mental focus, and supports physical performance.

1233. Turmeric and Black Pepper Anti-Inflammatory Tea

Ingredients: 1 teaspoon dried Turmeric, 1/2 teaspoon Black Pepper, 2 cups hot water, 1 teaspoon honey.

Preparation: Steep Turmeric and Black Pepper in hot water for 15 minutes. Add honey and stir.

Suggested Usage: Drink post-exercise to reduce inflammation and promote recovery.

Benefits: Reduces inflammation, supports joint health, and enhances muscle recovery.

1234. Lion's Mane and Rhodiola Cognitive-Boosting Capsules

Ingredients: 1 tablespoon dried Lion's Mane powder, 1 tablespoon dried Rhodiola powder, empty gel capsules.

Preparation: Mix powders and fill capsules.

Suggested Usage: Take 1 capsule daily for enhanced mental clarity and physical performance.

Benefits: Supports cognitive function, enhances focus, and reduces physical and mental fatigue.

1235. Holy Basil and Lemon Balm Calm Focus Tea

Ingredients: 1 tablespoon Holy Basil, 1 tablespoon Lemon Balm, 2 cups hot water.

Preparation: Steep Holy Basil and Lemon Balm in hot water for 15 minutes. Strain and serve.

Suggested Usage: Drink 1 cup before or after workouts for calm energy and mental focus.

Benefits: Enhances mental clarity, reduces stress, and supports balanced energy levels.

1236. Reishi and Schisandra Vitality Elixir

Ingredients: 1 tablespoon Reishi powder, 1 tablespoon Schisandra powder, 2 cups water, 1 teaspoon honey.

Preparation: Simmer Reishi and Schisandra in water for 20 minutes. Strain, add honey, and serve.

Suggested Usage: Drink 1 cup daily to support endurance and overall vitality.

Benefits: Enhances stamina, reduces fatigue, and supports immune health.

1237. Ginseng and Rhodiola Adaptogen Tonic

Ingredients: 1 teaspoon dried Ginseng, 1 teaspoon dried Rhodiola, 2 cups hot water.
Preparation: Steep Ginseng and Rhodiola in hot water for 15 minutes. Strain and serve.
Suggested Usage: Drink 1 cup daily to increase resilience to physical stress.
Benefits: Enhances endurance, boosts energy, and reduces exercise-induced stress.

1238. Eleuthero and Reishi Stress-Relief Capsules

Ingredients: 1 tablespoon Eleuthero powder, 1 tablespoon Reishi powder, empty gel capsules.
Preparation: Mix powders and fill capsules.
Suggested Usage: Take 1 capsule post-exercise to support stress reduction and recovery.
Benefits: Reduces cortisol, enhances mental clarity, and supports immune function.

Conclusion

Herbal medicine offers an abundant variety of remedies that can be seamlessly woven into our lives, enriching our health and well-being. This guide has explored numerous ways herbs can be used to address specific ailments, boost vitality, enhance mental clarity, and support overall wellness. Now, as we reach the conclusion, it's time to focus on how to effectively and sustainably integrate these herbal remedies into daily life. Establishing a sustainable routine, embracing continuous learning, and adopting a holistic lifestyle will help you get the most out of herbal medicine for the long term.

Integrating herbal remedies into everyday routines is a deeply personal journey, shaped by individual health needs, lifestyle preferences, and goals. The key to a successful herbal regimen is creating one that feels manageable and meaningful, encouraging consistent use without feeling overwhelming. Herbs work best when used regularly over time, allowing their beneficial properties to gently harmonize with your body. As you begin to build your routine, it's essential to understand your health priorities and choose herbs that align with those goals.

Start by reflecting on your primary health objectives. Consider whether your focus is on managing stress, enhancing digestion, boosting immunity, or maintaining cognitive function. Defining these goals will help narrow down the selection of herbs and guide your approach. For example, if stress relief is a priority, you might begin with adaptogens like Ashwagandha or Holy Basil. For digestive support, consider incorporating herbs such as Dandelion Root or Peppermint into your routine. By focusing on one or two health concerns initially, you can avoid overwhelming yourself and allow time to observe how your body responds to the remedies.

Choosing the right herbal formulations is equally important. Teas, tinctures, capsules, and topical applications each offer distinct benefits depending on your needs and lifestyle. If you prefer a comforting evening ritual, herbal teas might be your preferred option, while capsules are convenient for those with a busy schedule. Tinctures are potent and easily absorbed, making them ideal for quick results, while salves and oils are beneficial for topical issues like sore muscles or skin conditions. The form you choose should align with how you wish to experience the herbs and integrate them into your day.

Start with a small selection of herbs and a simple regimen that you can follow consistently. As you become more comfortable, you can gradually expand your repertoire to include additional herbs or try new formulations. Perhaps you begin with a morning tea to support energy and a calming tincture before bed. Over time, you might add a midday digestive bitters before meals or a nourishing herbal infusion in the evening. The key is to build slowly, paying attention to how your body feels and adapting as needed.

Creating a sustainable herbal routine also means considering your practical constraints. If your mornings are hectic, opt for pre-made capsules or a ready-to-use tincture. If you enjoy a slow, mindful start to your day, a morning tea ritual might be more suitable. Tailoring your regimen to fit your lifestyle ensures that it becomes a lasting habit rather than a passing phase. Making herbs an enjoyable part of your daily routine—whether through delicious teas, soothing baths, or aromatic diffusions—will cultivate a positive association and encourage long-term adherence.

Once your routine is in place, consistency is crucial. Herbs work gradually, and their full benefits often become apparent only after weeks or even months of regular use. Think of your herbal routine as an ongoing commitment to yourself and your well-being, similar to regular exercise or healthy eating. Stay patient and mindful, noting any changes in your health and adjusting as needed. The more consistently you use herbs, the more deeply they can support your body's natural healing processes.

Herbal medicine is a field of endless depth and variety, inviting continual learning and exploration. As you begin integrating herbs into your life, consider this the starting point of a lifelong journey. Deepening your understanding of herbs not only enriches your experience but also empowers you to make informed choices that are best suited to your unique needs.

One of the most rewarding aspects of herbal medicine is the opportunity to cultivate a deeper relationship with plants. Learning to identify herbs in the wild, understanding their growing cycles, and experimenting with making your own preparations can significantly deepen your appreciation for the healing power of nature. Consider starting with a few key herbs that resonate with you. Study their history, learn about their traditional uses, and experiment with different ways to prepare and use them. If possible, grow a few herbs yourself, even if it's just a small pot of Basil or Mint on a windowsill. Connecting with the plants in this way makes their use feel more personal and meaningful.

There are numerous resources available for those wishing to continue their education in herbal medicine. Books, online courses, local workshops, and herbal apprenticeships provide various levels of learning, from basic knowledge to advanced clinical training. Look for trusted herbalists and educators who offer programs that align with your interests, whether that's herbal crafting, medicinal plant identification, or holistic health practices. The more you learn, the more empowered you'll become in choosing, preparing, and using herbs to support your health.

Additionally, engaging with the herbal community can be both inspiring and supportive. Connecting with others who share your passion for herbal medicine—whether through online forums, local herb groups, or social media—allows for the exchange of ideas, recipes, and personal experiences. Sharing your own journey and learning from others can help solidify your understanding and keep you motivated. The herbal community is vast and diverse, filled with people who are eager to share their knowledge and support your growth.

Continued learning isn't just about acquiring knowledge; it's about fostering a deep sense of respect and reverence for the plants that provide us with healing. Every new herb you learn about, every new preparation you master, brings you closer to understanding the intricate relationships between plants, people, and health. This process of discovery can be profoundly fulfilling, transforming herbal medicine from a mere health practice into a way of life.

While herbal remedies can have a significant positive impact on health, they are most effective when integrated into a holistic lifestyle that encompasses not only physical health but also mental, emotional, and spiritual well-being. A holistic approach recognizes that true health is multifaceted, requiring attention to diet, exercise, stress management, sleep, relationships, and the environment. Herbs are one piece of a larger puzzle, complementing other practices that together promote sustained wellness.

Adopting a holistic lifestyle means approaching health proactively rather than reactively. Instead of using herbs solely to address symptoms, consider using them to build resilience, prevent illness, and support overall vitality. Adaptogens like Rhodiola or Ashwagandha, for example, can be taken daily to help the body manage stress and maintain balance, while nutritive herbs like Nettle or Oatstraw can nourish the body over time. Viewing herbs as daily allies rather than occasional remedies fosters a deeper, more sustainable relationship with natural medicine.

This holistic approach also invites mindfulness into everyday practices. When preparing a cup of tea or applying a herbal salve, take a moment to connect with the herbs, appreciating their unique qualities and the nourishment they provide. These small rituals can bring a sense of peace and groundedness, transforming routine actions into moments of mindfulness. Similarly, incorporating practices like yoga, meditation, deep breathing, and nature walks can enhance the effects of herbal remedies, creating a synergistic approach to health.

Nutrition is another cornerstone of holistic health. A diet rich in whole foods—fruits, vegetables, whole grains, healthy fats, and lean proteins—forms the foundation of physical well-being. Herbs can play a complementary role, providing concentrated nutrients and phytochemicals that enhance overall health. Infusing daily meals with herbs like Turmeric, Rosemary, or Ginger not only adds flavor but also boosts the medicinal value of food. Experiment with adding herbs to smoothies, soups, salads, and even desserts to make your diet both delicious and health-supportive.

Physical activity is equally vital. Exercise not only strengthens the body but also promotes mental clarity, emotional resilience, and energy flow. Herbs can support these benefits by enhancing stamina, aiding muscle recovery, and reducing inflammation. Combining regular movement with herbal tonics that support physical performance, such as a Cordyceps and Maca blend, can optimize your fitness regimen.

Stress management is perhaps the most crucial aspect of a holistic lifestyle. Chronic stress has a profound impact on health, contributing to a range of physical and mental conditions. Herbs like Holy Basil, Lemon Balm, and Passionflower are invaluable in calming the nervous system and promoting relaxation. Incorporating these herbs into your daily routine—whether through teas, tinctures, or aromatherapy—can help mitigate the effects of stress and maintain emotional balance.

Sleep is another pillar of health that is often overlooked. Herbs such as Valerian, Hops, and Chamomile have long been used to promote restful sleep, supporting the body's natural rhythms and enhancing recovery. Establishing a calming evening routine that includes herbal teas or a warm bath infused with Lavender and Chamomile can set the stage for deep, restorative sleep.

Finally, cultivating a sense of purpose, joy, and connection is essential for holistic well-being. Whether through relationships, creative pursuits, or spiritual practices, finding what nourishes your spirit is as important as caring for your body. Herbal medicine, with its roots in nature and tradition, can be a beautiful way to connect with something greater than oneself. Growing herbs, foraging, or simply enjoying a cup of tea can foster a deep appreciation for the natural world and our place within it.

In conclusion, embracing a holistic lifestyle supported by herbal medicine is a journey of self-discovery and empowerment. By creating a sustainable herbal routine, continuing your education, and adopting practices that nurture the body, mind, and spirit, you can cultivate lifelong health and vitality. Herbs offer a path to wellness that is both ancient and accessible, inviting you to explore their healing power and weave them into the fabric of your everyday life. As you continue to deepen your understanding and relationship with these plants, may you find joy, peace, and vibrant health on your herbal journey.

Made in United States
Orlando, FL
20 November 2024